CLINICAL GASTROENTEROLOGY

Series Editor
George Y. Wu
University of Connecticut Health Center, Farmington, CT, USA

For further volumes:
http://www.springer.com/series/7672

Elizabeth J. Carey • Keith D. Lindor
Editors

Cholestatic Liver Disease

Second Edition

Humana Press

Editors
Elizabeth J. Carey
Division of Gastroenterology
and Hepatology
Mayo Clinic
Phoenix, AZ, USA

Keith D. Lindor
Mayo Clinic
Phoenix, AZ, USA

ISSN 2197-7399 ISSN 2197-7704 (electronic)
ISBN 978-1-4939-1012-0 ISBN 978-1-4939-1013-7 (eBook)
DOI 10.1007/978-1-4939-1013-7
Springer New York Heidelberg Dordrecht London

Library of Congress Control Number: 2014943498

Printed on acid-free paper

Humana Press is a brand of Springer
Springer is part of Springer Science+Business Media (www.springer.com)

Preface

Despite advances in the understanding and management of the cholestatic liver diseases, these disorders continue to pose clinical challenges to patients and their medical practitioners. This second edition of *Cholestatic Liver Disease* aims to update the reader on the classic entities of primary biliary cirrhosis and primary sclerosing cholangitis while also providing insights on more recently described problems: IgG4-associated cholangitis, cholestasis after hematologic transplantation, advances in biliary endoscopy, and new treatment options such as the farnesoid X receptor agonists.

We hope that *Cholestatic Liver Disease* will be a valuable resource for those interested in learning about these diseases and for those who treat patients affected by the cholestatic liver disorders. The goal of this textbook is to provide scientific updates from leading experts while reviewing thc clinical evaluation, management, and recent advances in the cholestatic liver diseases. It is our hope that *Cholestatic Liver Disease* will be a useful reference for learners and practitioners alike.

Phoenix, AZ, USA

Elizabeth J. Carey, M.D.
Keith D. Lindor, M.D., B.S.

Contents

Contributors

Abrar Ahmed, M.D. Division of Digestive & Liver Diseases, University of Texas Southwestern Medical Center, Dallas, TX, USA

Bashar Aqel, M.D. Division of Gastroenterology & Hepatology, Mayo Clinic Arizona, Scottsdale, AZ, USA

Mary A. Atia, M.D. Division of Gastroenterology & Hepatology, Mayo Clinic Arizona, Scottsdale, AZ, USA

Todd H. Baron, M.D. Division of Gastroenterology & Hepatology, Advanced Therapeutic Endoscopy, Department of Medicine, University of North Carolina, Chapel Hill, NC, USA

Einar S. Björnsson, M.D., Ph.D. Gastroenterology and Hepatology, Landspitali University Hospital, Reykjavik, Iceland

Meredith Borman, M.D., Ph.D., F.R.C.P.C. Snyder Institute for Chronic Diseases, University of Calgary, Calgary, AB, Canada

Division of Hepatology and Gastroenterology, University of Calgary, Calgary, AB, Canada

Ozlem Pinar Bulut, M.D. Pediatric Gastroenterology, Hepatology & Nutrition, Phoenix Children's Hospital, Phoenix, AZ, USA

Elizabeth J. Carey, M.D. Division of Gastroenterology and Hepatology, Mayo Clinic, Phoenix, AZ, USA

Roger W. Chapman, M.D., F.R.C.P. Translational Gastroenterology, Oxford University Hospital Trust, Oxford, UK

Emma L. Culver, B.Sc. (Hons), M.B.Ch.B., M.R.C.P. Translational Gastroenterology Unit, John Radcliffe Hospital, Oxford, UK

Bertus Eksteen, M.B.Ch.B., Ph.D., F.R.C.P. Medicine, Division of Hepatology and Gastroenterology, Foothills Hospital, University of Calgary, Calgary, AB, Canada

Andrea A. Gossard, M.S., C.N.P. Division of Gastroenterology and Hepatology, Mayo Clinic, Rochester, MN, USA

Denise M. Harnois, D.O. Department of Transplant, Mayo Clinic, Jacksonville, FL, USA

Anne M. Larson, M.D. Swedish Liver Center, Swedish Health Systems, Seattle, WA, USA

Said Al Mamari, M.D., M.R.C.P. (UK) Liver Unit, Sultan Qaboos Hospital, Salalah, Dhofar, Oman

Marlyn J. Mayo, M.D. Division of Digestive & Liver Diseases, University of Texas Southwestern Medical Center, Dallas, TX, USA

Tamir Miloh, M.D. Pediatrics Department, Phoenix Children's Hospital, Phoenix, AZ, USA

Marina G. Silveira, M.D. Gastroenterology and Hepatology, Cleveland, OH, USA

James H. Tabibian, M.D. Division of Gastroenterology & Hepatology, Department of Medicine, Mayo Clinic, Rochester, MN, USA

Kymberly D.S. Watt, M.D. Gastroenterology and Hepatology, Mayo Clinic, Rochester, MN, USA

Anitha Yadav, M.D. Transplant Hepatology, Mayo Clinic Arizona, Phoenix, AZ, USA

Chapter 1
Diagnosis of Cholestasis

Andrea A. Gossard

Key Points

- Cholestasis may be identified through blood work or may be clinically evident.
- Causes of cholestasis require a thorough review of the patient's medical and surgical history, medication list, and symptomatology.
- Initial evaluation of the cholestatic patient should include imaging of the liver and biliary tree in addition to laboratory work.
- Management of reversible conditions may require endoscopic intervention.

Introduction

Bile is formulated in the bile canaliculi, the smallest bile duct branches. It is then secreted by the liver and deposited into the duodenum at the ampulla of Vater. The primary role of bile is to aid in the digestion of fats. Cholestasis may be defined as a condition in which bile cannot flow from the liver to the small intestine.

Cholestatic liver disease may be broadly attributed to either hepatocellular dysfunction, leading to impaired bile formation by hepatocytes, or to obstructive processes within the extrahepatic ducts and/or intrahepatic bile ducts. Obstructive cholestasis is usually the result of physical obstruction of the biliary system at the level of the extrahepatic bile ducts, often by stone, stricture, or tumor. However, obstruction or paucity of small bile ducts can result in functional obstruction of the entire biliary system. Early identification of cholestasis typically involves elevations of serum alkaline phosphatase and conjugated bilirubin levels.

A.A. Gossard, M.S., C.N.P. (✉)
Division of Gastroenterology and Hepatology, Mayo Clinic,
200 First Street SW, Rochester, MN 55901, USA
e-mail: Gossard.Andrea@mayo.edu

E.J. Carey and K.D. Lindor (eds.), *Cholestatic Liver Disease*, Clinical Gastroenterology,
DOI 10.1007/978-1-4939-1013-7_1, © Springer Science+Business Media New York 2014

Approach to the Diagnosis

Cholestasis may be identified in the symptomatic patient, or may be an incidental finding at the time of routine blood work. When present, symptoms may include pruritus, fever, and fatigue. Symptoms such as jaundice, dark urine, and acholic stools are not common in the setting of intrahepatic bile duct disease but may be evident with large duct obstruction. Many patients, however, are entirely asymptomatic and are diagnosed with cholestatic liver disease only after the discovery of liver test abnormalities.

Alkaline phosphatase levels are the most commonly elevated in patients with cholestasis. The increased serum levels of alkaline phosphatase are thought to be caused by the damaging effect of high concentrations of bile acids on intracellular and biliary membranes causing "leakage" of this enzyme into the blood [1].

In the setting of an isolated alkaline phosphatase elevation, care should be given to ensure the source is indeed hepatic in origin. This may be accomplished by either obtaining alkaline phosphatase isoenzymes, or serum 5'-nucleotidase levels. One may also corroborate hepatic origin by testing the gamma glutamyltranspeptidase (GGT). If normal, this would direct the clinician to pursue non-hepatic etiologies [2]. If elevated, this would suggest the alkaline phosphatase elevation is indeed of hepatic origin. Limitations of GGT, however, include marked sensitivity and lack of specificity. Alkaline phosphatase isoenzymes also allow the clinician to determine whether the source of the elevation is hepatic, or from bone or gastrointestinal sources. Serum bile acids are considered the most sensitive and however are not readily available in most clinical settings.

Many cholestatic patients present with conjugated hyperbilirubinemia. Normal serum bilirubin is largely unconjugated [3]. Bilirubin is bound to serum proteins for transport to the liver where conjugation occurs. Conjugated bilirubin may be secreted into bile as it is water soluble. Elevated bilirubin levels may develop due to overproduction, decreased uptake, decreased conjugation, decreased excretion, or regurgitation of bilirubin from damaged hepatocytes or bile ducts [4]. In the setting of extrahepatic biliary obstruction, conjugated hyperbilirubinemia will be evident in up to 80 % of patients. The degree of bilirubin elevation is helpful when evaluating the status of chronic cholestatic liver diseases such as primary biliary cirrhosis (PBC) and primary sclerosing cholangitis (PSC) [5, 6].

Clinically, a cholestatic disorder may be initially differentiated from a primarily hepatocellular disorder by the enzyme pattern. A proportionally greater elevation in the alkaline phosphatase compared to the aminotransferases is consistent with cholestasis and should direct the clinician toward the biliary tree. Once cholestasis is identified, it is helpful to characterize the probable site of bile flow obstruction with imaging studies.

Assessment of the biliary tree may be accomplished with many different diagnostic studies. Noninvasive methods of assessment include abdominal ultrasound (US), computed tomography (CT), or magnetic resonance imaging (MRI). Endoscopically, assessment of the biliary tree is accomplished by endoscopic ultrasound (EUS) and endoscopic retrograde cholangiopancreatogram (ERCP). In addition to ERCP, direct assessment of the biliary tree may also be accomplished by percutaneous transhepatic cholangiography (PTC). Magnetic resonance cholangiopancreatography (MRCP) and computed tomography cholangiography (CT cholangiogram) allow for noninvasive assessment of the biliary tree in addition to imaging of the hepatic parenchyma. Histologic assessment via liver biopsy may be helpful in some cases but oftentimes is unnecessary. These will be discussed in greater detail later in this chapter.

Cholestasis is considered chronic when present for greater than 6 months. It may be further defined as primarily intrahepatic or extrahepatic, and many cases are acute on chronic. Most cases of chronic cholestasis are intrahepatic and approximately 50 % of these patients will demonstrate conjugated hyperbilirubinemia.

Evaluating Cholestasis

The evaluation of cholestasis begins with the identification of an elevated alkaline phosphatase and confirmation that it is hepatic in origin. The most sensitive test to evaluate for impaired bile flow involves obtaining serum bile acids. This test is not widely available, however; so use of serum alkaline phosphatase is more common. Bilirubin levels may or may not be elevated so may not be helpful. Aminotransferase levels are useful when suspecting overlap syndromes.

The next step involves review of possible causes. First, a patient's medication list should be reviewed for potentially offending agents. The list of possible medicines to consider is extensive and may include estrogens, oral contraceptives, anabolic steroids, phenytoin, cyclosporin, dapsone, and erythromycin among others (Table 1.1). Use of herbal medicines or teas, vitamins, and other supplements should be reviewed and discontinued, when possible. Total parenteral nutrition may also cause cholestasis. Oftentimes the specific offending medicine or supplement is not identified.

A history of fever, especially when accompanied by rigors or right upper quadrant abdominal pain, may be suggestive of cholangitis. Cholangitis may develop in patients with obstructive processes such as choledocholithiasis or biliary tract strictures. These symptoms may be seen in alcoholic disease and rarely in the setting of viral hepatitis as well [1]. Recent surgery in the region of the biliary system may have resulted in an inadvertent injury to a bile duct and should also be considered as a possible cause. This type of trauma may lead to the development of secondary sclerosing cholangitis.

The differential diagnosis beyond medicines includes the most common cause of extrahepatic cholestasis which is choledocholithiasis [7, 8]. In the setting of cholelithiasis, it is estimated that up to 20 % of patients will develop choledocholithiasis [9]. Other causes to consider include extra-biliary tumors, cysts, parasites, and lymphoma (Table 1.2). Once cholestasis is confirmed, imaging is useful at defining the source of obstruction.

Table 1.1 Common drugs that may cause cholestasis

Anabolic steroids, estrogens
Amoxicillin–clavulanic acid
Azathioprine
Cetirizine
Chlorpromazine
Cyclosporin
Dapsone
Diltiazem
Erythromycin
Fenofibrate
Floxuridine
Gold salts
Infliximab
Itraconazole
Metolazone
Nitrofurantoin
Oral contraceptives
Phenytoin
Rifampicin
Trimethoprim–sulfamethoxazole
5-Fluorouracil or floxuridine

Table 1.2 Causes of extrahepatic biliary obstruction

Intraductal obstruction
Choledocholithiasis
Benign bile duct tumors (rare)
Bile duct strictures including those from IgG4 related disease cholangiocarcinoma
Cysts
AIDS cholangiopathy
Parasites
Extrinsic compression
Extra-biliary tumors
Lymphoma
Acute and chronic pancreatitis

Imaging

Ultrasound

Abdominal ultrasound (US) is often the initial imaging performed when evaluating cholestasis. Advantages of US include relatively low cost, wide availability, noninvasive nature, and the absence of radiation. Ultrasound can effectively evaluate for intrahepatic and extrahepatic bile duct dilation and the presence of mass lesions; however, operator variability can be an issue. Ultrasound is highly dependent on the skill of the sonographer and the experience of the interpreter. In addition, technical limitations include the inability to penetrate bone, as well as the risk of excess abdominal adipose tissue or bowel gas obstructing the view. Ultrasound can differentiate between intrahepatic and extrahepatic causes of biliary tract disease, however, and can readily identify gallbladder pathology particularly when the patient is fasting [10, 11]. In cases of obstructive jaundice, the sensitivity and specificity of US may exceed 80 % [12]. US may not be reliable, however, at detecting choledocholithiasis [13]. Use of US as an initial evaluation is reasonable although additional diagnostics may be necessary.

Computed Tomography

Computed tomography (CT) is less operator dependent than US, more effective when imaging obese patients, and is less susceptible to bowel gas when evaluating the distal bile ducts. Computed tomography is more accurate than US at identifying the level (88–97 % vs. 23–95 %) as well as the cause (70–94 % vs. 38–94 %) of biliary obstruction if present [14]. It is not as able to identify choledocholithiasis, however, and exposes the patient to radiation [15]. Computed tomography is therefore reserved for equivocal US findings rather than for first-line imaging.

Magnetic Resonance Imaging/Cholangiopancreatography

MRI is useful in the diagnosis of chronic versus acute etiologies of cholestasis. Use of magnetic resonance cholangiopancreatogram (MRCP) is considered a safe, noninvasive tool for evaluating the biliary tree and hepatic parenchyma. Advantages include the lack of ionizing radiation and sharp contrast resolution between normal and abnormal tissues. The accuracy of MRCP in evaluating the bile ducts is comparable to endoscopic cholangiography. In fact, a review of 67 studies found MRCP sensitivity and specificity to diagnose biliary obstruction to be 95 % and 97 % respectively [16, 17]. As the bile ducts are visualized in their normal physiologic state, MRCP may be a better indicator than endoscopic cholangiogram when assessing true caliber of the bile ducts. The sensitivity for biliary strictures is, however, lower [17]. In addition, MRCP has limited specificity for the diagnosis of malignant strictures [18]. Although stenosis may be identified, direct visualization of the bile duct narrowing is not possible by MRCP. Further disadvantages include the relatively high cost, inability to perform on patients with implanted metallic devices, and the potential for suboptimal images due to motion-related artifacts.

CT Cholangiography

For patients who are unable to undergo MRI, CT cholangiography may be an option. Multidetector helical CT imaging allows for evaluation of the biliary tree more rapidly than MRCP. The study requires use of oral or intravenous contrast. Early studies suggest the accuracy is similar to MRCP [8].

Endoscopic and Percutaneous Assessment

Extrahepatic causes of chronic cholestatic liver disease should be excluded early as they are potentially reversible and failure to do so may result in complications such as recurrent cholangitis or secondary biliary cirrhosis. When suspicion is high or signs on cross-sectional imaging point to mechanical obstruction, direct cholangiography either endoscopically or percutaneously may be necessary. The primary advantage of direct cholangiography, as with endoscopic retrograde cholangiography (ERC) or PTC, is the ability to diagnose and intervene therapeutically when indicated.

Endoscopic Retrograde Cholangiography

ERC is the "gold standard" for diagnosing PSC. The procedure involves cannulation of the ampulla of Vater (the opening where the common bile duct and pancreatic duct meet the duodenum) followed by the injection of contrast to opacify the biliary tree. The combination of endoscopy and fluoroscopy allows the clinician to evaluate for the presence of stones or blockage of the bile duct. Many patients will undergo sphincterotomy by cutting the Sphincter of Oddi, the muscular ring at the ampulla, during the first ERC. When indicated, this may allow for improved access for stone extraction in the setting of choledocholithiasis or treatment of a biliary stricture with balloon dilation or an expandable stent. In patients with obstructive jaundice, ERC can effectively identify the location in 92–99 % and may identify the cause in 75–87 % of cases [19].

Unfortunately, 3–5 % of all patients who undergo ERC will experience complications the most common of which is pancreatitis [20]. Other procedure related complications may include perforation, hemorrhage, and cholangitis [21].

Percutaneous Transhepatic Cholangiography

PTC allows for radiographic assessment of the biliary tree and for interventions such as bile duct dilation, intraductal biopsy, and stone removal. The procedure involves transhepatic insertion of a needle into a bile duct after which X-rays are obtained. The test should be reserved for patients in whom ERC is precluded for anatomic reasons and when need for therapeutic intervention is evident. When the intrahepatic bile ducts are dilated, this technique tends to work well. The complication rate increases in patients with small, non-dilated ducts due to the frequent need for multiple attempts at cannulation of the bile ducts [22]. Bacteremia is also a concern, although the risk is low [23].

Endoscopic Ultrasound

EUS is a highly reliable method of detecting extrahepatic sources of bile duct obstruction. The procedure is performed by passing the endoscope with the transducer into the first or second part of the duodenum. From this position, evaluation of the biliary tree, pancreas, and surrounding structures can be performed. If concerning, fine needle aspiration may be performed at the time of the procedure. The ultrasound probe can be used to assess for stones within the common bile duct.

Use of EUS in one study demonstrated 98 % sensitivity and 99 % specificity in the setting of choledocholithiasis. In this study, 46 % of the patients were able to avoid more invasive testing as a result of undergoing EUS [24]. In another study of patients with suspected choledocholithiasis, 67.1 % of patients were able to avoid ERC after EUS revealed no evidence of stones [25]. A benefit of EUS is avoidance of sphincterotomy and more invasive procedures if indeed choledocholithiasis is suspected but ultimately not identified [26]. Limitations include the inability to intervene therapeutically if indicated.

Many of the conditions in the differential diagnosis may be excluded by history, laboratory tests, and imaging studies. A liver biopsy may be useful when suspecting unusual conditions such as autoimmune cholangitis, overlap syndromes, or in patients with suspected sarcoidosis.

Intrahepatic Causes of Cholestasis

The most common diseases that cause intrahepatic cholestasis include immune-mediated diseases such as PBC, PSC, and sarcoidosis (Table 1.3). Hepatocellular diseases which may cause intrahepatic cholestatic liver disease include viral hepatitis B and C. Hepatitis C has been associated with chronic cholestasis although the usual biochemical abnormalities reflect hepatocellular damage. Alcoholic hepatitis may present with clinical and biochemical features of cholestatic liver disease. This type of hepatocellular disease may also coexist with other liver diseases, so a detailed history is imperative.

The most common cause of chronic intrahepatic cholestatic liver disease in adults is PBC [27]. PBC is a chronic, inflammatory autoimmune liver disease that affects the cholangiocytes of the interlobular bile ducts. It is estimated that in the USA the prevalence of PBC is about 150–400 cases per million individuals. PBC may have a very long natural history. The presence of antimitochondrial antibodies

Table 1.3 Causes of intrahepatic cholestasis

Immune mediated disease
Primary biliary cirrhosis
Primary sclerosing cholangitis
Sarcoidosis
Hepatocellular disease
Alcoholic hepatitis
Autoimmune hepatitis
Hepatitis B
Hepatitis C
Other causes
Drug induced cholestasis
Idiopathic adult ductopenia
Benign recurrent intrahepatic cholestasis
Cystic fibrosis
Sepsis
Sickle cell disease
Total parenteral nutrition

is noted in over 95 % of PBC patients and is helpful in making the diagnosis. Presence of a positive antimitochondrial antibody (AMA) in a woman with cholestasis is essentially diagnostic of PBC. The specificity of AMA for PBC is 95 % [28]. Over 80 % of patients with PBC are female. The terms autoimmune cholangitis and "AMA negative PBC" have been used for patients who have clinical and histologic features of PBC but are AMA negative. These patients are generally positive for antinuclear or anti-smooth muscle antibodies. Autoimmune cholangitis and PBC appear to be part of a disease spectrum with very similar clinical and histologic features and a similar response to therapy. Liver biopsy is helpful in confirmation of this disease, but in patients who have prominent cholestatic liver biochemistries and a strongly positive AMA, the diagnosis of PBC is highly likely and liver biopsy is usually unnecessary.

PSC is the second most common cause of intrahepatic cholestatic liver disease. PSC is characterized by an inflammatory and fibrotic process that damages both the intrahepatic and extrahepatic ducts and causes chronic cholestasis [29]. The etiology is not well understood. The prevalence of PSC is estimated to range from 50 to 70 cases per million individuals. The natural history of PSC is more variable than that of PBC with varying rates of disease progression. The disease is more common in men with a 2:1 male to female ratio and strongly associated with inflammatory bowel disease. More than 80 % of patients have concurrent inflammatory bowel disease. Approximately 80 % of these patients will have chronic ulcerative colitis (CUC), 10 % have Crohn's colitis, and another 10 % may have mixed features or indeterminate colitis [30]. Patients with both PSC and CUC are at an increased risk of developing colorectal cancer as well as cholangiocarcinoma. Antimitochondrial antibodies are typically absent in patients who have PSC. Other antibodies such as antinuclear antibodies and antineutrophil cytoplasmic antibodies, however, are frequently found.

Bile duct imaging with magnetic resonance cholangiography is very helpful in confirming the diagnosis of PSC. Classic cholangiographic features of PSC include multifocal stricturing and saccular segmental dilatation causing a beaded appearance [31]. Usually both the intrahepatic and extrahepatic ducts are involved, but up to 20 % of patients have only intrahepatic duct disease. Involvement of only the extrahepatic ducts is rare and should prompt evaluation for IgG4 associated cholangiopathy. Liver biopsy is useful for histologic confirmation and in staging the disease, but it is not typically necessary.

Dominant bile duct strictures can contribute to intrahepatic and extrahepatic cholestasis in the setting of PSC. Dominant strictures are defined as stenosis of ≤1.5 mm in the common bile duct of ≤1 mm in the hepatic duct [32]. The prevalence of dominant strictures in PSC is unknown but is estimated at 50 % [33].

Occasionally, patients present with histologic features of PSC in the setting of chronic colitis but have normal cholangiograms. These patients are considered to have small duct PSC and comprise approximately 5 % of all PSC patients [34]. Small duct PSC may develop into cholangiographically evident disease in up to 20 % of patients over a 7–10-year period of time [34, 35].

Overlap syndromes are not uncommon in the setting of PSC and this has been reported in up to 6 % of cases [36, 37]. Autoimmune hepatitis (AIH)—PSC overlap syndrome should be suspected when there is cholangiographic evidence of PSC and biochemical features of AIH. These patients typically have marked elevations of aminotransferase levels with an autoantibody profile, positive antinuclear antibody or positive smooth-muscle antibody that is consistent with AIH. Histologic findings would reveal lymphoplasmacytic portal-based infiltrates and significant interface hepatitis.

AIH may present quite similarly to PBC and some degree of overlap is not uncommon [38]. The precise prevalence is unknown but perhaps 10 % of patients could be classified in this overlap category [39–41]. The majority of patients with AIH have antinuclear antibodies and anti-smooth muscle antibodies in the serum, however, and histologically there is rarely destruction of the bile ducts. Pruritus is less common in AIH than it is in PBC, and the serum alkaline phosphatase level is typically only minimally elevated. In some cases differentiating between AIH and PBC is difficult, but under these circumstances patients with AIH will experience a dramatic response to immunosuppressive therapy whereas PBC patients will not.

Chronic cholestatic sarcoidosis, a disease most common in young African-American men, can present with features that are histologically similar to PBC and in some cases PSC. Granulomatous destruction of small ducts is the hallmark of this condition. The granulomas are typically large and well defined, in contrast to the small and poorly defined granulomas seen in PBC. Most of these patients have hilar adenopathy on chest roentgenograms and other features of sarcoidosis, and do not have AMA.

Benign familial recurrent cholestasis is a rare syndrome characterized by recurrent attacks of pruritus and jaundice. During the attack, serum alkaline phosphatase levels are elevated and cholestasis is noted histologically. The cholangiogram is normal, however, and all cases eventually will go into remission. Cirrhosis does not develop and the prognosis is excellent [42].

Patients with cystic fibrosis may have neonatal jaundice that resolves yet recurs later in life [43]. Histologic examination of the liver reveals mucus-plugged cholangioles without significant parenchymal damage; consequently portal hypertension is a prominent manifestation. Approximately one-third of patients have abnormalities of the gallbladder or cystic duct. Prognosis is largely determined by the status of the pulmonary disease.

Summary

Elevations of serum alkaline phosphatase levels are the hallmark of cholestasis. Evaluation hinges on identifying the probable etiology with laboratory work and imaging studies. Treatment of reversible causes with cholangiography may be indicated. Liver biopsy may be helpful in characterizing overlap syndromes. PBC and PSC are important causes of chronic cholestasis and are the most common causes of cholestatic liver disease.

References

1. Carleton BC, Smith MA, Gelin MN, Heathcote SC. Paediatric adverse drug reaction reporting: understanding and future directions. Can J Clin Pharmacol. 2007;14(1):e45–57 [Research Support, Non-U.S. Gov't].
2. Whitfield JB, Pounder RE, Neale G, Moss DW. Serum-glytamyl transpeptidase activity in liver disease. Gut. 1972;13(9):702–8.
3. Billing BH. Twenty-five years of progress in bilirubin metabolism (1952-77). Gut. 1978;19(6):481–91 [Review].
4. Luketic VA, Shiffman ML. Benign recurrent intrahepatic cholestasis. Clinics in liver disease. 2004;8(1):133–49, vii [Review].
5. Wiesner RH, Porayko MK, Dickson ER, Gores GJ, LaRusso NF, Hay JE, et al. Selection and timing of liver transplantation in primary biliary cirrhosis and primary sclerosing cholangitis. Hepatology. 1992;16(5):1290–9 [Review].
6. Levy C, Lindor KD. Primary sclerosing cholangitis: epidemiology, natural history, and prognosis. Semin Liver Dis. 2006;26(1):22–30 [Review].
7. Mark DH, Flamm CR, Aronson N. Evidence-based assessment of diagnostic modalities for common bile duct stones. Gastrointest Endosc. 2002;56(6 Suppl):S190–4 [Comparative Study Research Support, U.S. Gov't, P.H.S. Review].
8. Baillie J, Paulson EK, Vitellas KM. Biliary imaging: a review. Gastroenterology. 2003;124(6):1686–99 [Review].
9. Mitchell SE, Clark RA. A comparison of computed tomography and sonography in choledocholithiasis. AJR Am J Roentgenol. 1984;142(4):729–33 [Comparative Study].
10. Bennett WF, Bova JG. Review of hepatic imaging and a problem-oriented approach to liver masses. Hepatology. 1990;12(4 Pt 1):761–75 [Comparative Study Review].
11. Pedersen OM, Nordgard K, Kvinnsland S. Value of sonography in obstructive jaundice. Limitations of bile duct caliber as an index of obstruction. Scand J Gastroenterol. 1987;22(8):975–81.
12. Reddy SI, Grace ND. Liver imaging. A hepatologist's perspective Clinics in liver disease. 2002;6(1):297–310, ix [Review].

13. Varghese JC, Liddell RP, Farrell MA, Murray FE, Osborne DH, Lee MJ. Diagnostic accuracy of magnetic resonance cholangiopancreatography and ultrasound compared with direct cholangiography in the detection of choledocholithiasis. Clin Radiol. 2000;55(1):25–35 [Comparative Study Research Support, Non-U.S. Gov't].
14. Reddy SI, Grace ND. Liver imaging. A hepatologist's perspective Clin Liver Dis. 2002;6(1): 297–310, ix [Review].
15. Saini S. Imaging of the hepatobiliary tract. N Engl J Med. 1997;336(26):1889–94 [Review].
16. Romagnuolo J, Bardou M, Rahme E, Joseph L, Reinhold C, Barkun AN. Magnetic resonance cholangiopancreatography: a meta-analysis of test performance in suspected biliary disease. Ann Intern Med. 2003;139(7):547–57 [Meta-Analysis Research Support, Non-U.S. Gov't].
17. Varghese JC, Liddell RP, Farrell MA, Murray FE, Osborne H, Lee MJ. The diagnostic accuracy of magnetic resonance cholangiopancreatography and ultrasound compared with direct cholangiography in the detection of choledocholithiasis. Clin Radiol. 1999;54(9):604–14 [Comparative Study Research Support, Non-U.S. Gov't].
18. Rosch T, Meining A, Fruhmorgen S, Zillinger C, Schusdziarra V, Hellerhoff K, et al. A prospective comparison of the diagnostic accuracy of ERCP, MRCP, CT, and EUS in biliary strictures. Gastrointest Endosc. 2002;55(7):870–6 [Clinical Trial Comparative Study Randomized Controlled Trial].
19. Pasanen PA, Partanen KP, Pikkarainen PH, Alhava EM, Janatuinen EK, Pirinen AE. A comparison of ultrasound, computed tomography and endoscopic retrograde cholangiopancreatography in the differential diagnosis of benign and malignant jaundice and cholestasis. Eur J Surg. 1993;159(1):23–9 [Comparative Study].
20. Freeman ML, Nelson DB, Sherman S, Haber GB, Herman ME, Dorsher PJ, et al. Complications of endoscopic biliary sphincterotomy. N Engl J Med. 1996;335(13):909–18 [Multicenter Study Research Support, Non-U.S. Gov't].
21. Andriulli A, Loperfido S, Napolitano G, Niro G, Valvano MR, Spirito F, et al. Incidence rates of post-ERCP complications: a systematic survey of prospective studies. Am J Gastroenterol. 2007;102(8):1781–8 [Research Support, Non-U.S. Gov't Review].
22. Teplick SK, Flick P, Brandon JC. Transhepatic cholangiography in patients with suspected biliary disease and nondilated intrahepatic bile ducts. Gastrointest Radiol. 1991 Summer; 16(3):193–7.
23. Ginat D, Saad WE, Davies MG, Saad NE, Waldman DL, Kitanosono T. Incidence of cholangitis and sepsis associated with percutaneous transhepatic biliary drain cholangiography and exchange: a comparison between liver transplant and native liver patients. AJR Am J Roentgenol. 2011;196(1):W73–7 [Comparative Study].
24. Buscarini E, Tansini P, Vallisa D, Zambelli A, Buscarini L. EUS for suspected choledocholithiasis: do benefits outweigh costs? A prospective, controlled study. Gastrointest Endosc. 2003;57(4):510–8 [Clinical Trial Controlled Clinical Trial].
25. Petrov MS, Savides TJ. Systematic review of endoscopic ultrasonography versus endoscopic retrograde cholangiopancreatography for suspected choledocholithiasis. Br J Surg. 2009; 96(9):967–74 [Comparative Study Meta-Analysis Research Support, Non-U.S. Gov't Review].
26. Prat F, Amouyal G, Amouyal P, Pelletier G, Fritsch J, Choury AD, et al. Prospective controlled study of endoscopic ultrasonography and endoscopic retrograde cholangiography in patients with suspected common-bileduct lithiasis. Lancet. 1996;347(8994):75–9 [Clinical Trial Comparative Study Controlled Clinical Trial Research Support, Non-U.S. Gov't].
27. Ludwig J. Idiopathic adulthood ductopenia: an update. Mayo Clin Proc. 1998;73(3):285–91 [Review].
28. Invernizzi P, Lleo A, Podda M. Interpreting serological tests in diagnosing autoimmune liver diseases. Semin Liver Dis. 2007;27(2):161–72 [Review].
29. Maggs JR, Chapman RW. An update on primary sclerosing cholangitis. Curr Opin Gastroenterol. 2008;24(3):377–83 [Review].
30. Loftus Jr EV, Harewood GC, Loftus CG, Tremaine WJ, Harmsen WS, Zinsmeister AR, et al. PSC-IBD: a unique form of inflammatory bowel disease associated with primary sclerosing cholangitis. Gut. 2005;54(1):91–6.

31. MacCarty RL, LaRusso NF, Wiesner RH, Ludwig J. Primary sclerosing cholangitis: findings on cholangiography and pancreatography. Radiology. 1983;149(1):39–44.
32. Chapman R, Fevery J, Kalloo A, Nagorney DM, Boberg KM, Shneider B, et al. Diagnosis and management of primary sclerosing cholangitis. Hepatology. 2010;51(2):660–78 [Practice Guideline].
33. Stiehl A, Rudolph G, Kloters-Plachky P, Sauer P, Walker S. Development of dominant bile duct stenoses in patients with primary sclerosing cholangitis treated with ursodeoxycholic acid: outcome after endoscopic treatment. J Hepatol. 2002;36(2):151–6 [Clinical Trial].
34. Bjornsson E, Olsson R, Bergquist A, Lindgren S, Braden B, Chapman RW, et al. The natural history of small-duct primary sclerosing cholangitis. Gastroenterology. 2008;134(4):975–80.
35. Bjornsson E, Boberg KM, Cullen S, Fleming K, Clausen OP, Fausa O, et al. Patients with small duct primary sclerosing cholangitis have a favourable long term prognosis. Gut. 2002; 51(5):731–5.
36. Kaya M, Angulo P, Lindor KD. Overlap of autoimmune hepatitis and primary sclerosing cholangitis: an evaluation of a modified scoring system. J Hepatol. 2000;33(4):537–42.
37. Al-Chalabi T, Portmann BC, Bernal W, McFarlane IG, Heneghan MA. Autoimmune hepatitis overlap syndromes: an evaluation of treatment response, long-term outcome and survival. Aliment Pharmacol Ther. 2008;28(2):209–20 [Comparative Study].
38. Heathcote EJ. Overlap of autoimmune hepatitis and primary biliary cirrhosis: an evaluation of a modified scoring system. Am J Gastroenterol. 2002;97(5):1090–2.
39. Poupon R, Chazouilleres O, Corpechot C, Chretien Y. Development of autoimmune hepatitis in patients with typical primary biliary cirrhosis. Hepatology. 2006;44(1):85–90.
40. Rust C, Beuers U. Overlap syndromes among autoimmune liver diseases. World J Gastroenterol. 2008;14(21):3368–73 [Case Reports Review].
41. Czaja AJ. The variant forms of autoimmune hepatitis. Ann Intern Med. 1996;125(7):588–98.
42. Nakamuta M, Sakamoto S, Miyata Y, Sato M, Nawata H. Benign recurrent intrahepatic cholestasis: a long-term follow-up. Hepatogastroenterology. 1994;41(3):287–9 [Case Reports].
43. Colombo C, Battezzati PM, Crosignani A, Morabito A, Costantini D, Padoan R, et al. Liver disease in cystic fibrosis: a prospective study on incidence, risk factors, and outcome. Hepatology. 2002;36(6):1374–82.

Chapter 2
Drug-Induced Cholestasis

Einar S. Björnsson

Background

Cholestatic liver disease has a wide variety of causes which often requires radiological examination to rule out extrahepatic and intrahepatic causes. Drug-induced cholestasis is frequent among the differential diagnoses in patients with cholestasis and normal hepatobiliary imaging. Cholestasis is mostly defined by a biochemical pattern with predominant increase in alkaline phosphatase (AlkPhos) in comparison with aminotransferases, whereas the hepatocellular pattern is evident when elevation in aminotransferases is more prominent than the AlkPhos [1, 2]. The understanding of the pathophysiology of hepatocellular type of liver injury is scarce whereas advances in the understanding of the pathogenesis of cholestatic liver disease have increased in recent years. It has become clear that drugs or metabolites of drugs interfere in many cases with the hepatobiliary transport systems found at the basolateral and canalicular membranes of hepatocytes.

Patients who present with cholestatic liver test abnormalities can have many differential diagnoses. In some cases the diagnosis is straightforward, such as in a patient recently treated with an antibiotic with known hepatotoxicity. However, in other patients with systemic illness, who are often treated with multiple drugs, it can be very difficult to establish the diagnosis of DILI. It is not common that a diagnosis of DILI is proven. Thus, in most cases DILI is suspected and is labeled as highly probable, probable, or possible. However, if a rechallenge with the same drug results in identical liver test abnormalities as previously observed, the diagnosis of DILI can be established. Rechallenge nowadays usually occurs inadvertently and the diagnosis DILI is often based on circumstantial evidence and exclusion of competing etiologies. The extent of diagnostic workup such as serological tests and radiological

E.S. Björnsson, M.D., Ph.D. (✉)
Gastroenterology and Hepatology, Landspitali University Hospital, Hringbraut, 101, Reykjavik, Iceland
e-mail: einarsb@landspitali.is

E.J. Carey and K.D. Lindor (eds.), *Cholestatic Liver Disease*, Clinical Gastroenterology,
DOI 10.1007/978-1-4939-1013-7_2,

imaging relies heavily on the clinical context. Although symptomatic cholestatic DILI can cause considerable morbidity and lead to hospitalizations and investigational costs, the long-term prognosis is favorable in most cases. Although liver test abnormalities will reverse with the cessation of the suspected offending drug, this can lead in rare circumstances to vanishing bile duct syndrome (VBDS) [3, 4], a condition that may or may not be reversible. Furthermore, in the worst case scenario this may lead to biliary fibrosis and cirrhosis with decompensated liver disease [3].

Incidence and Outcome

Incidence

The true incidence of hepatic adverse drug reactions has previously been largely unknown. Except within clinical trials which give reliable information about development of abnormal liver tests, great uncertainty exists about the occurrence of DILI associated with the clinical use of drugs. Only two studies have been undertaken to investigate the incidence of DILI in the general population [5, 6]. These studies were prospective and based on careful search for DILI in a defined population and probably underestimate rather than overestimate the incidence of DILI.

A retrospective population based case–control study in the General Practice Research Database in the UK identified patients referred or hospitalized for a liver related diagnosis [7]. In this study cholestatic drug reactions were the most common manifestations of DILI. The strongest associated hepatotoxicity was observed for chlorpromazine, amoxicillin–clavulanic acid, flucloxacillin, and macrolides among other drugs [7]. The highest crude incidence rates were found for chlorpromazine, azathioprine (AZA), and sulfasalazine (approximately 1 per 1,000 users). A dose effect was observed for diclofenac, amoxicillin–clavulanic acid, and flucloxacillin and higher risk associated with longer duration of drug treatment observed for sulfasalazine, flucloxacillin, and diclofenac [7].

Hepatotoxicity due to drugs has been reported to occur in 2–10 % of patients hospitalized for jaundice [8–12]. Thus, DILI is not a common cause of jaundice. However, the majority of patients with jaundice have obvious etiology such as hepatobiliary malignancy, alcoholic liver disease, gallstone disease, and a much higher proportion of DILI is found among those without obvious etiology [11]. In several large retrospective DILI studies, cholestatic pattern has been found in 20–40 % of patients, mixed pattern in 12–20 %, and hepatocellular in 48–58 % [13–16] (Table 2.1). Limited data exists on the incidence of DILI with cholestatic reactions in the general population. The first population-based study on the incidence of DILI was undertaken in France in a defined population and revealed an incidence of 13.9 cases per 100,000 per year [5]. A total of 33 % of cases had a cholestatic or mixed pattern [5]. Another population-based study from Iceland, with an incidence of 19 cases per 100,000, showed that 32 % of the patients had a cholestatic and 26 %

Table 2.1 Type of liver injury in several large DILI studies

	Cholestatic (%)	Mixed (%)	Hepatocellular (%)
Bjornsson and Olsson [13]	26	22	52
De Valle et al. [16]	40	12	48
Andrade et al. [14]	20	22	58
Chalasani et al. [15]	23	20	56

Table 2.2 Types of liver injury and mortality rates in the largest studies on DILI

	Cholestatic pattern (%)	Mixed pattern (%)	Hepatocellular pattern (%)
Bjornsson and Olsson [13]	8	2	13
Andrade et al. [14]	5	2	7
Chalasani et al. [15]	14	2	8

mixed type of liver injury, whereas the rest had a hepatocellular type [6]. Patients with a cholestatic/mixed type of injury were older than those with a hepatocellular type, 60 years vs. 46 years of age ($P=0.004$), which is in line with the results from other studies [5, 13–16].

Outcome

Drug-induced jaundice has been associated with a poor prognosis and a severe drug liver reaction was found by Dr. Hy Zimmerman to lead to at least 10 % mortality [17]. This has been named Hy's law and was later validated in a large series of patients with DILI showing a mortality/liver transplantation rate of 9–12 % [13–15] (Table 2.2). Originally, this association was thought to be true only for hepatocellular jaundice, and the prognosis of those with cholestatic injury was mainly related to comorbidities and age [4].

In recent series, cholestatic DILI has also been associated with mortality of 5–14 % [13–15]. However, in general the prognosis in patients with hepatocellular liver injury due to drugs is worse than in those with cholestatic/mixed pattern [13–15]. In the Drug Induced Liver Injury Network (DILIN) study, not all these patients had a liver related mortality [15]. Mortality and liver transplantation among patients with different patterns of liver injury is shown in Table 2.2.

Vanishing Bile Duct Syndrome

DILI of cholestatic type has been associated with a chronic intrahepatic cholestatic pattern called the vanishing bile duct syndrome [4]. Although well documented, VBDS is a very rare syndrome and has been considered to be only 0.5 % of all cases of small duct biliary disease [18]. The liver histology can mimic that of PBC with granulomatous duct injury [4]. In a minority of patients progressive ductopenia occurs, which can lead to near complete absence of ducts with variable amounts of inflammation [19]. This is mainly observed in patients with prolonged cholestasis for months or years, often with jaundice. This can in rare cases lead to cirrhosis [3, 4, 19–23]. The prototype of drugs leading to this syndrome is chlorpromazine [3]. Many other drugs have been implicated and ductopenia has been associated with more than 40 drugs [21, 24]. Ductopenia can also be progressive, without resolution of jaundice and lead to fibrosis and biliary cirrhosis [3, 20, 25–28]. Inability of bile duct ductular proliferation is the likely explanation, leading to prolonged and occasionally irreversible changes resulting in death from cholestatic cirrhosis [28]. However, VBDS has been shown to be reversible in some cases with disappearance of jaundice during long-term follow-up [29, 30]. Animal experiments have demonstrated neoductular proliferation accompanied by improved biliary drainage [31]. Reversal of the vanishing bile duct syndrome due to drugs has been reported [30]. A sequence of changes documented with repeated liver biopsies demonstrating restoration of bile ducts has been nicely illustrated [30]. This is most likely due to regeneration of the terminal branches of the biliary tree from a progenitor cell compartment located at the interface of bile ducts with hepatic parenchyma [30].

Chronic Evolution During Long-Term Follow-Up

A prospective follow-up of patients from the Spanish Hepatotoxicity Registry revealed development of chronic liver injury in approximately 6 % of patients [32]. Chronic liver injury was defined differently in different types of DILI: hepatocellular pattern of damage was defined as chronic if liver tests showed persistent abnormality more than 3 months after stopping the drug therapy and in case of cholestatic/mixed type of injury, if abnormality was present for more than 6 months following drug discontinuation [32]. The most frequent drug associated with chronicity was amoxicillin–clavulanate. Patients with cholestatic liver injury were more likely to develop chronic liver injury [32]. Ductal lesions developed in three patients in the cholestatic/mixed group [32]. Similarly, a single center study from Sweden also found 6 % of patients previously diagnosed with DILI with persistently abnormal liver biochemistries at follow-up [33]. The rate of chronic liver injury at 6 months was 13.6 % in the first 300 cases enrolled in the DILIN study [15]. Features of the implicated agent, pattern of DILI or patient age were not associated with chronicity [15]. However, long-term outcome of these patients is unknown, as these patients were followed for 20 months [32], 48 months [33] and 6 months [15]. A follow-up study of DILI patients who originally all had DILI and concomitant jaundice with a mean follow-up of 10 years revealed that development of a clinically important liver disease after severe DILI was rare [34]. A total of 23/685 (3.4 %) DILI patients who had survived acute DILI were hospitalized for liver disease during the study period and five had liver-related mortality [34]. Among these patients five out of eight with cirrhosis did not have an identifiable cause of cirrhosis, in which DILI might have played a role for this development and two of these had cholestatic liver injury. A significantly longer duration of drug therapy prior to the detection of DILI was observed in those who developed liver-related morbidity and mortality during follow-up [34]. Interestingly, the most common cause of hospitalization for DILI during follow-up was a protracted course of the DILI. Most patients with protracted courses (86 %) were of cholestatic/mixed type and had a mean follow-up of 13 years. In this subgroup of patients, all patients except one (with 6 years follow-up) normalized their liver tests at last follow-up and remained free of liver morbidity thereafter [34].

Diagnostic Workup

Definitions

Cholestasis is defined biochemically as an increase in AlkPhos >2× the upper limit of normal (ULN) and/or with an ALT/AlkPhos ratio <2 [1, 2]. Mixed liver injury is the intermediate between cholestatic and hepatocellular injury with an ALT/AlkPhos ratio greater than 2 and less than 5. Mixed injury is considered to have more in common with cholestatic than hepatocellular injury and cholestatic and mixed patterns are sometimes taken together as one condition [13–15]. The traditional classification of cholestasis has been into acute and prolonged cholestasis. Furthermore, drug-induced cholestasis is often classified into: (1) acute pure ("bland") cholestasis, defined histologically as features of cholestasis such as hepatocyte cholestasis and canalicular dilatation often with bile plugs without occurrence of significant inflammation; (2) acute drug-induced cholestatic hepatitis characterized histologically by cholestasis with concomitant inflammatory reaction and sometimes hepatocyte necrosis; (3) drug-induced cholestasis with bile duct injury, ductular, cholangiolar, or cholangiolytic with minimal parenchymal liver cell injury; and (4) vanishing bile duct syndrome (see section "Outcomes").

Symptoms and Signs

The clinical presentation of cholestatic liver disease is very variable. Asymptomatic elevation of liver enzymes can be observed with dominating increase in AlkPhos but jaundice with or without pruritus is a common presentation. Some patients present with fever and abdominal pain that can simulate gallstone disease. As some patients can have stones in the gallbladder, this can lead to unnecessary cholecystectomies.

Clinical information about the patient is very important to establish the diagnosis of the cholestatic reaction. Abdominal pain can occur as part of a cholestatic hepatitis due to drugs but abdominal discomfort is probably more prevalent. Painless jaundice is also a frequent presentation of DILI. If abdominal pain dominates the picture it argues against a drug as the etiology. In these cases, even though a suspicion of a drug etiology has been raised it may be necessary to do an MRCP or ERCP despite a normal abdominal ultrasound. In all types of alcoholic liver disease, cholestasis can be a prominent feature both biochemically and histologically [35]. Thus, alcohol abuse needs to be ruled out in the workup of suspected cholestatic injury due to drugs.

Different medical conditions such as sepsis [36] and cardiac failure [37] can be associated with pure cholestasis and it is of great importance to distinguish these conditions from a suspected cholestatic DILI. Although infectious hepatitis presents most often with hepatocellular pattern, a biochemical cholestatic pattern can occur in infectious hepatitis such as hepatitis A [38] and Epstein-Barr virus [39]. Other infections such as acute Q fever due to *Coxiella burnetii* [40] and typhoid fever [41] can present with cholestasis. In the appropriate clinical setting, rare infectious diseases have to be ruled out before the diagnosis of DILI can be established. Jaundice and cholestatic hepatitis due to hyperthyroidism has been reported [42]. Thus, the number of serological tests and the extent of radiological imaging to exclude other competing etiologies rely entirely on the clinical context.

Causality Assessment

At the current time, no marker of hepatotoxicity exists that is completely reliable and specific for DILI. A reasonable suspicion of a drug etiology and thorough exclusion of other potential causes is necessary to make a diagnosis of DILI. In clinical research on DILI the most common causality assessment method that has been used is the Roussel Uclaf Assessment model (RUCAM) [1, 2]. RUCAM is based on factors that are important to consider when taking a history in a patient with suspected DILI. These factors include the time from initial drug intake until start of the reaction, course of the liver injury after termination of the suspected drug, risk factors for DILI, concomitant drugs, exclusion of other causes, documented hepatotoxicity of this particular drug and if available the results of rechallenge. In most DILI cases a rapid biochemical and clinical improvement is observed after discontinuation of the implicated drug, that is positive dechallenge. However, for some drugs causing hepatotoxicity liver injury may worsen initially for days or sometimes weeks between discontinuation of the drug and clinical presentation of liver injury. It has been well documented that the regression of cholestasis is slower than in those with hepatocellular injury and the RUCAM instrument takes that into the equation. Some drugs have a "signature pattern," that is, they tend to give similar type of liver injury and liver injury develops following a similar duration of drug intake.

A common cause of cholestatic hepatitis is associated with amoxicillin–clavulanate and liver injury can be difficult to recognize, as there can be a considerable delay, sometimes 3–4 weeks, between discontinuation of drug intake and symptoms of the liver injury such as itching and jaundice [43]. Thus, knowledge of the known hepatotoxicity of various drugs is important for establishing a correct diagnosis. Recently a comprehensive Web site on the documentation of liver injury for a wide range of drugs has been established, which can be of great help for physicians who wonder about the known hepatoxicity of a particular drug [44].

Risk Factors

To predict the susceptibility for DILI in an individual patient is almost impossible. If the patient has already experienced a liver injury from a particular drug, there is a great risk that this will happen again in the same subject. Also a past history of DILI from one drug has been shown to be a predictor of future DILI [2, 34]. Genetic variability in the hepatic metabolism of drugs has been considered to be the most important risk factor for DILI but clinical utility of genetic testing in this context is not available at the current time.

Genetic Studies

One of the most common drugs leading to DILI is amoxicillin–clavulanate [13–15], which is mostly associated with cholestatic or mixed injury. One of the first HLA haplotypes associated with DILI, HLA B1*1501-DRB5*0101-DQB1*0602,149 was found in 57 % of patients with amoxicillin/clavulanate-induced DILI, but in only 12 % of controls [45]. Another study confirmed the association between HLA DRB1*15 and liver injury from amoxicillin–clavulanate [46]. Patients with amoxicillin–clavulanate-associated DILI had a significantly higher prevalence of HLA-DQR1*06 than controls [46]. A study from the Spanish Hepatotoxicity Registry revealed that those with cholestatic/mixed DILI had a significantly higher frequency of HLA-DRB1*15 and HLADQB1*06 alleles and a lower frequency of DRB1*07 and DQB1*02 alleles [47].

Results of genome-wide association studies of flucloxacillin induced liver injury, a drug mostly associated with cholestasis, showed an association peak in the major histocompatibility complex region with the strongest association observed for rs2395029, a marker in complete linkage disequilibrium with HLA B*570.1 [48]. Direct genotyping for HLA-B*5701 in 51 cases and 63 drug-exposed controls revealed a very strong relationship between this allele and flucloxacillin-induced liver injury with an odds ratio of 80. Increased susceptibility of cholestatic injury due to contraceptives has been reported to be associated with BSEP 1331T to C polymorphism [49].

Underlying Condition

Rifampicin, a tuberculostatica later shown to be effective in the treatment of pruritus in primary biliary cirrhosis (PBC), has been shown to lead to cholestatic hepatitis [45]. Rifampicin seems to be associated with an increased risk for hepatotoxicity in patients with PBC. In two studies that tested rifampicin for treating pruritus in patients with primary biliary cirrhosis, a high frequency of hepatotoxicity was observed [50, 51] and much higher than previously reported.

Susceptibility to oral contraceptives or postmenopausal hormone replacement therapy appears to be increased in patients with intrahepatic cholestasis of pregnancy [52, 53]. These results support the concept of a genetically determined canalicular transporter deficiency as a common denominator. In general it is controversial whether preexisting liver disease is a risk factor the development of DILI.

Effect of Age

The cholestatic type of DILI is more common among the elderly, whereas hepatocellular DILI appears to be more common in younger individuals [6, 16, 54]. In one study older age was independently associated with cholestatic type of injury [54]. Advancing age has also been shown to be a risk factor for the development of amoxicillin–clavulanate cholestatic type of injury [54]. The reason for this age related susceptibility for cholestatic liver injury is unclear. It is conceivable that expression of hepatocellular transporters could be related to age. In a recent study, a significant inter-individual variability could be demonstrated in canalicular transporter proteins [55]. However, this variability in the susceptibility to develop drug-induced cholestasis was not related to age differences in baseline expression levels of these canalicular transporter proteins [55].

Drug Properties

Limited data exist on the risk of DILI associated with the chemical properties of drugs. Temafloxacin and Trovafloxacin known to be able to cause cholestasis have a unique difluorinated side chain that does not occur in other quinolones with much less hepatotoxicity [55]. Drugs given orally in a daily dose of more than 50 mg have recently been shown to be more likely to lead to DILI than those with a lower daily dose [56]. Among US prescription medicines, daily doses of oral medications were associated significantly with liver failure, liver transplantation, and death from DILI. In approximately one-third of cases the observed pattern was of cholestatic type [56]. These results were reproduced in a study of approximately 600 DILI cases from the Spanish Hepatotoxicity Registry, demonstrating that 77 % of patients with DILI received medications with daily doses greater than 50 mg [54], 50 % having cholestatic or mixed pattern [54].

The same group of investigators also demonstrated that drugs with 50 % or greater hepatic metabolism caused a significantly higher frequency (compared with drugs with less hepatic metabolism) of hepatic adverse events [56]. Interestingly, compared with medications without biliary excretion, compounds with biliary excretion significantly increased the incidence of jaundice (74 % vs. 40 %; $P<0.0001$) [56]. Cholestatic drug reactions per se were not further analyzed and need further study. Although some drugs are given in high doses and metabolized to a great extent in the liver they do not seem to be prone to lead to hepatotoxicity. Interestingly, a recent study demonstrated that apart from the high daily dose found to be important for the risk of DILI, the lipophilicity of drugs contributed significantly to the risk [57]. The dose and the lipophilicity of the drug, called by the authors as the "rule-of-two" seems to be able to better estimate the risk of DILI than the dose alone [57]. However, the hepatic metabolism of the drugs was not taken into this equation and needs further study.

Pathophysiology

Hepatic metabolism of drugs involves phase I reactions followed by phase II reactions or phase I alone or rarely only phase II [58]. Phase II reactions result in their anionic conjugates with sulfate, glucuronate or glutathione. These drug metabolites are transported across hepatocyte membranes by transporters (uptake or efflux transporters) on the apical or the canalicular membranes [59]. This hepatic drug transport has been shown to be involved in the pathophysiology of cholestatic adverse effects due to drugs [59, 60]. Transport at the apical membrane into hepatocytes involves the organic anion transporting polypeptide [59]. Little data exist on defects in these uptake transporters and risk for cholestatic liver injury [59]. Basolateral transport processes probably determine hepatic exposure to drugs and their metabolites, which reach the canalicular membrane [60, 61]. Inhibition of this basolateral transport does not seem to increase the risk of cholestasis due to drugs [62]. In contrast, inhibition of efflux proteins can lead to cholestatic liver injury caused by certain compounds or their metabolites [60, 61]. The efflux of drugs into bile involves canalicular transporters of the MRP family, includes certain glycoproteins of the MDR family and bile salt export pump (BSEP, ABCB11) [62]. The bile salt export pump (BSEP) has been shown to be a major transporter of bile salts and drug metabolites from hepatocytes into bile [62]. Drugs that inhibit export on the canalicular side through inhibition of BSEP can lead to cholestasis in susceptible subjects [62].

Many cholestatic drug reactions result from a drug- or metabolite-mediated inhibition of hepatobiliary transporter systems [60, 61]. Cholestatic liver disease associated with rifampicin, troglitazone, glibenclamide, and bosentan has in animal experiments been related to inhibition of bile salt export pump function in cholestatic liver disease [60, 61]. Cholestasis due to flucloxacillin, terbinafine, sulindac, and bosentan has been associated with inhibition of the canalicular BSEP [63–65]. Bosentan, a drug with well-known hepatotoxicity, has been shown to inhibit BSEP, leading to accumulation of toxic bile acids within the hepatocytes [66, 67]. Mutations that disturb BSEP function have been identified in patients with a history of cholestasis due to drugs [68]. Patients with mutations in genes that encode BSEP or MDR3 have a threefold increase in risk of cholestatic DILI from oral contraceptives, psychotropic drugs, proton pump inhibitors and certain antibiotics [68]. Other molecular mechanisms of cholestasis have been reported such as destruction of the cytoskeleton, impaired trafficking and disruption of the tight junction network, inhibition of ATP-dependent transporters and modulation of fluidity of the canalicular membrane [68].

Specific Agents

As the list of drugs associated with cholestatic injury is very long [44, 69] only the most important drugs and type of drugs will be covered.

Antibiotics are the most common type of drugs associated with DILI [13–16].

Penicillanase-Resistant Penicillins and Other Penicillins

Flucloxacillin-induced cholestasis is well documented [20, 22, 70, 71]. Flucloxacillin is on the market and commonly prescribed in Australia, Sweden, and UK, whereas this drug has never been marketed in the USA and many other countries. Flucloxacillin is the most common reason of *idiosyncratic* liver injury in Sweden, with 16 % of all DILI cases [13] and the second most common cause of drug-induced jaundice in the UK [72]. Female sex, age and high daily doses have been shown to be associated with higher risk of liver injury due to flucloxacillin [20, 71]. A total of 7/129 (5 %) who had reported flucloxacillin liver injury, in Sweden from 1970–2004, which is probably anunderestimation as not all cases were have been reported to the authorities [13]. Ductopenia [22] and cholestatic cirrhosis leading to liver transplantation has been reported [20, 70]. Also other semi-synthetic penicillanase resistant penicillins such as cloxacillin, dicloxacillins, and oxacillins have been shown to induce cholestatic hepatitis [15, 20, 70]. Treatment with penicillinase-sensitive penicillins very rarely causes liver damage [73], but a prolonged and severe cholestasis has been reported for benzylpenicillin [74].

Amoxicillin–Clavulanate

Amoxicillin–Clavulanate (A–C) is a commonly prescribed antibiotic in many countries and in most DILI studies it is among the most common antibiotics leading to DILI [14, 15]. One-third of drug-induced jaundice was associated with A–C in a study from the UK [72] and the most common cause of DILI in Spain [14]. In the USA A–C was the most common antibiotic associated with DILI [15]. Liver injury can develop early in the course of treatment but also late in the course of prolonged treatment and furthermore following discontinuation of therapy [75]. Most cases of A–C induced liver injury have a cholestatic or mixed pattern. Liver injury is mainly related to the clavulanic acid component, as the incidence of DILI with A–C combination is markedly higher than that of amoxicillin alone [76]. Risk factors for hepatotoxicity are age over 65 years, female sex and repeated course of the antibiotic [75–77]. Most cases are mild but a protracted course is also possible and can in rare cases lead to acute liver failure or require transplantation [75, 77].

Tetracyclines

Tetracycline hepatotoxicity was originally associated with large doses that were often given intravenously and in pregnancy [78]. Incidence of hepatotoxicity associated with normal and low dose tetracyclines such as doxycycline, seems to be lower than most reported antibiotics leading to DILI with a generally favorable prognosis [79, 80]. The liver injury was designated as cholestatic, hepatocellular, and mixed, with similar frequencies [79]. No cases of death due to tetracyclines have been reported to the Swedish authorities by spontaneous reporting [13, 79].

Trimethoprim–Sulfamethoxazole

In most studies on DILI, this drug is commonly associated with DILI [13–16]. After A–C, nitrofurantoin and isoniazid, Trimethoprim–Sulfamethoxazole (T–S) was the fourth most common antibiotic inducing DILI in the North American DILIN study [15]. The sulphonamide component is considered to be responsible and sulfonamides mostly lead to cholestatic patterns [81]. Almost 60 % of reactions are of cholestatic nature [82]. In one study approximately 10 % of patients with jaundice due to T–S either died or underwent liver transplantation [13].

Macrolides

Erythromycin is a well-documented cause of cholestatic liver injury [73]. Erythromycin was the second most commonly reported antibiotic leading to DILI in Sweden [13]. In a collection of case reports from the literature, cholestatic injury was observed in 69 % of cases [82]. Prognosis is generally favorable and it has extremely rarely been reported to lead to acute liver failure and death [13, 82]. Clarithromycin and azithromycin have both been associated with cholestatic liver injury [83, 84].

Other Antibiotics

The antifungal Terbinafine has been shown to induce cholestatic injury that can be very severe and lead to acute liver failure and/or require liver transplantation [85, 86]. Terbinafine induced hepatotoxicity has been reported in a number of patients from previous studies on DILI [13, 15]. Other antibiotics in common use and shown to lead to cholestatic hepatitis are ciprofloxacin [87, 88] and cephalosporins [89, 90]. DILI due to cephalosporins has previously been considered to be extremely rare. However, a recent study from the DILIN network in the USA, described 32 out of a total of 655 cases (5 %) enrolled between 2004 and 2010 [90]. The majority demonstrated a cholestatic pattern and in several cases the toxicity occurred after therapy had been stopped; at least one fatal outcome was attributed to the cephalosporin-induced hepatotoxicity [90].

Immunosuppressive Agents

A number of cases of severe cholestatic hepatitis due to AZA have been reported in the literature [91–93]. Nodular regenerative liver hyperplasia (NRH) is a rare but potentially serious complication of treatment with AZA [94].

Most patients develop liver injury during the first 3 months of therapy [94]. The frequency of DILI associated with AZA is unclear. According to a systematic review, the mean prevalence of AZA or 6-mercaptopurine (MP)-induced liver injury in IBD was approximately 3 %, and the mean annual drug-induced liver disorder rate was only 1.4 % [95]. This low figure was based on retrospective studies and contrasts with an approximately 10 % incidence reported by a prospective study [94]. In this prospective study hepatotoxicity occurred in 16/161 (10 %) after a median of 85 days, but only in approximately one-third of cases azathioprine therapy had to be discontinued [94]. In a recent prospective study, as much as 1 out of 133 users of azathioprine developed liver injury [6], which is the highest frequency of idiosyncratic liver injury associated with drugs, reported so far.

Psychotropic Drugs

Chlorpromazine has been the prototype of cholestatic type of injury and can lead to cholestatic hepatitis, ductopenia and in rare cases to cholestatic cirrhosis [3]. Other antipsychotic drugs such as risperidone have also been reported to cause cholestatic liver injury [96, 97]. Cholestatic hepatitis has also been observed after tricyclic antidepressants such as imipramine and amitryptyline [44]. Duloxetine, a commonly used antidepressant, nowadays has recently been associated with cholestatic hepatitis [98].

Drugs Against HIV

Liver injury has been attributed to highly active antiretroviral therapy (HAART) [99]. DILI was the most likely cause in one-third of patients with AIDS and jaundice [100]. Among cases of suspected DILI reported to the WHO monitoring center, HIV drugs such as stavudine, didanosine, and nevirapine were among the top ten most common causes of fatal liver injury due to drugs [101]. Non-cirrhotic portal hypertension (NCPH) in HIV infected persons has been associated with antiretroviral therapy, particularly the drug didanosine [102–105]. Most patients present with cholestatic liver disease for months or years before signs manifestations of portal hypertension such as variceal bleeding and ascites became apparent [102, 104]. The prognosis seems to be favorable until symptoms and signs of portal hypertension develop [105]. Approximately one-fourth of patients with NCPH and esophageal varices had liver related mortality [105]. In multivariate analysis, the only independent predictor of NCPH was didanosine exposure [105].

Other Types of Drugs Associated With Cholestatic Liver Injury

Although cholestatic liver disease has been associated with oral contraceptives (OC) for many decades, less than 1 % of cases in Sweden, Spain, and the USA were attributed to OC [13–15]. The long-term use of OC has been associated with an increased risk of certain types of liver disease such as acute intrahepatic canalicular cholestasis, hepatic adenoma, focal nodular hyperplasia, hepatic vein thrombosis, and portal vein thrombosis [52, 106]. In a Swedish study on adverse liver reactions attributed to OC over 25 years, there was a sharp decline in the number of reports during the studied period, suggesting changes in reporting habits [107]. There was also a significantly lower incidence of reports for medium-compared to high-estrogen dose OC, and a further decrease in incidence with low-estrogen dose OC [107]. Cholestatic and hepatocellular liver enzyme patterns were equally frequent in patients with adverse reactions from low-dose estrogen OC and both types had favorable prognosis [107]. The duration of therapy until the hepatic reaction was detected ranged from 3 to 360 days (median of 60 days) [107]. Lower doses of estrogens and gestagens seem to lead to a decreased incidence of adverse liver reactions [107]. Anabolic steroids have a well-documented hepatotoxicity, mainly in the form of intrahepatic cholestasis [108]. Hepatotoxicity associated with dietary supplements containing anabolic steroids has been increasingly recognized in the USA [108, 109]. Several other dietary supplements have been associated with cholestasis, although for some reason hepatocellular pattern is more frequently observed associated with dietary supplements [109].

Management

Once DILI is suspected in a patient with new onset liver disease prompt discontinuation of the drug implicated is usually the first step in the management of these patients. At the same time it is also of major importance to assess the severity of the liver disease. Symptomatic patients with jaundice should be hospitalized. Once coagulopathy and/or encephalopathy develops an immediate contact should be taken with a transplant center if the patient does not have an obvious contraindication for liver transplantation. Patients with suspected DILI and concomitant jaundice should be carefully looked after and liver transplantation considered before they develop severe encephalopathy. Patients with DILI-related acute liver failure should be considered for liver transplantation early in the course of the disease as acute liver failure due to drugs has a generally poor prognosis without transplantation [110]. Transplantation free survival in non-acetaminophen-induced liver failure was better in patients receiving *N*-acetylcysteine (NAC) than those who were randomized to placebo [110]. Approximately one-fourth of these patients had drugs other than acetaminophen induced acute liver failure [110]. Other than NAC specific treatment options of the liver injury associated with drugs are very limited. Although ursodeoxycholic acid has been used in long-standing cholestatic drug reactions, no data is available that has documented its efficacy. Rechallenge with the suspected drug leading to DILI for diagnostic of therapeutic purposes is generally not recommended as there is usually a more severe reactions associated with rechallenge [111].

Summary

Cholestasis due to drugs is a diagnosis that needs to be considered in most patients presenting with a biochemical cholestatic pattern. Detailed information on the drug use, results of dechallenge, the documented hepatotoxicity of the drug, and exclusion of competing etiologies are important to support a diagnosis of DILI. Most cases of cholestatic DILI are mild but in rare cases, ductopenia and cholestatic cirrhosis can develop. Patients with cholestatic jaundice due to drugs can develop liver failure in approximately 10 % of cases.

References

1. Benichou C, Danan G, Flahault A. Causality assessment of adverse reactions to drugs—II. An original model for validation of drug causality assessment methods: case reports with positive rechallenge. J Clin Epidemiol. 1993;46:1331–6.
2. Danan G, Benichou C. Causality assessment of adverse reactions to drugs–I. A novel method based on the conclusions of international consensus meetings: application to drug-induced liver injuries. J Clin Epidemiol. 1993;46:1323–30.

3. Moradpour D, Altorfer J, Flury R, Greminger P, Meyenberger C, Jost R, Schmid M. Chlorpromazine-induced vanishing bile duct syndrome leading to biliary cirrhosis. Hepatology. 1994;20:1437–41.
4. Kleiner DE. The pathology of drug-induced liver injury. Semin Liver Dis. 2009;29:364–72.
5. Sgro C, Clinard F, Ouazir K, Chanay H, Allard C, Guilleminet C, et al. Incidence of drug-induced hepatic injuries: a French population-based study. Hepatology. 2002;36:451–5.
6. Bjornsson ES, Bergmann OM, Bjornsson HK, Kvaran RB, Olafsson S. Incidence, presentation and outcomes in patients with drug-induced liver injury in the general population of Iceland. Gastroenterology. 2013;144(7):1419–25, 1425.e1–3; quiz e19–20 [Epub ahead of print]
7. de Abajo FJ, Montero D, Madurga M, Garcia Rodriguez LA. Acute and clinically relevant drug-induced liver injury: a population based case-control study. Br J Clin Pharmacol. 2004;58:71–80.
8. Bjørneboe M, Iversen O, Olsen S. Infective hepatitis and toxic jaundice in a municipal hospital during a five year period: Incidence and prognosis. Acta Med Scand. 1967;182:491–501.
9. Malchow-Møller A, Matzen P, Bjerregaard B, Hilden J, Holst-Christensen J, Staehr Johansen T, et al. Causes and characteristics of 500 consecutive causes of jaundice. Scand J Gastroenterol. 1981;16:1–6.
10. Whitehead MW, Hainsworth I, Kingham JGC. The causes of obvious jaundice in South West Wales: 2000. Gut. 2001;48:409–13.
11. Björnsson E, Ismael S, Nejdet S, Kilander A. Severe jaundice in Sweden in the new millennium: causes, investigations, treatment and prognosis. Scand J Gastroenterol. 2003;38:86–94.
12. Vuppalanchi R, Liangpunsakul S, Chalasani N. Etiology of new-onset jaundice: how often is it caused by idiosyncratic drug-induced liver injury in the United States. Am J Gastroenterol. 2006;101:1–5.
13. Bjornsson E, Olsson R. Outcome and prognostic markers in severe drug-induced liver disease. Hepatology. 2005;42:481–9.
14. Andrade RJ, Lucena MI, Fernandez MC, et al. Drug-induced liver injury: an analysis of 461 incidences submitted to the Spanish registry over a 10-year period. Gastroenterology. 2005;129:512–21.
15. Chalasani N, Fontana RJ, Bonkovsky HL, et al. Causes, clinical features, and outcomes from a prospective study of drug-induced liver injury in the United States. Gastroenterology 2008;135:1924–34, 34 e1–4.
16. De Valle MB, Av Klinteberg V, Alem N, et al. Drug-induced liver injury in a Swedish University hospital out-patient hepatology clinic. Aliment Pharmacol Ther. 2006;24:1187–95.
17. Zimmerman H. Hepatotoxicity: the adverse effects of drugs and other chemicals on the liver. Philadelphia: Lippincott, Williams & Wilkins; 1999.
18. Ludwig J. Idiopathic adulthood ductopenia: an update. Mayo Clin Proc. 1998;73:193–9.
19. Degott C, Feldmann G, Larrey D, Durand-Schneider AM, Grange D, Machayekhi JP, Moreau A, Potet F, Benhamou JP. Drug-induced prolonged cholestasis in adults: a histological semi-quantitative study demonstrating progressive ductopenia. Hepatology. 1992;15:244–51.
20. Olsson R, Wiholm BE, Sand C, Hultcrantz R, Myrhed M. Liver damage from flucloxacillin, cloxacillin and dicloxacillin. J Hepatol. 1992;15:154–61.
21. Desmet V. Vanishing bile duct syndrome in drug-induced liver disease. J Hepatol. 1997;26:31–5.
22. Davies MH, Harrison RF, Elias E, Hübscher SG. Antibiotic-associated acute vanishing bile duct syndrome: a pattern associated with severe, prolonged, intrahepatic cholestasis. J Hepatol. 1994;20:112–6.
23. Forbes GM, Jeffrey GP, Shilkin KB, Reed WD. Carbamazepine hepatotoxicity: another cause of the vanishing bile duct syndrome. Gastroenterology. 1992;102:1385–8.
24. Padda MS, Sanchez M, Akhtar AJ, Boyer JL. Drug-induced cholestasis. Hepatology. 2011;53:1377–87.
25. Gregory DH, Zaki GF, Sarcosi GA, Carey JB. Chronic cholestasis following prolonged tolbutamide administration. Arch Pathol. 1967;84:194–201.

26. Glober GA, Wilkenson JA. Biliary cirrhosis following administration of methyltestosterone. JAMA. 1968;204:170–3.
27. Ishii M, Miyazaki Y, Yamamoto T, Miura M, Ueno Y, Takahashi T, Toyota T. A case of drug-induced ductopenia resulting in fatal biliary cirrhosis. Liver. 1993;13:227–31.
28. Eckstein RP, Dowsett JF, Lunzer MR. Flucloxacillin induced liver disease: histopathological findings at biopsy and autopsy. Pathology. 1993;25:223–38.
29. Ramos AM, Gayotto LC, Clemente CM, Mello ES, Luz KG, Freitas ML. Reversible vanishing bile duct syndrome induced by carbamazepine. Eur J Gastroenterol Hepatol. 2002;14:1019–22.
30. Vuppalanchi R, Chalasani N, Saxena R. Restoration of bile ducts in drug-induced vanishing bile duct syndrome due to zonisamide. Am J Surg Pathol. 2006;30:1619–23.
31. Alpini G, Lenzi R, Sarkozi L, Tavoloni N. Biliary physiology in rats with bile ductular cell hyperplasia. Evidence for a secretory function of proliferated bile ductules. J Clin Invest. 1988;81:569–78.
32. Andrade RJ, Lucena MI, Kaplowitz N, García-Muņoz B, Borraz Y, Pachkoria K, et al. Outcome of acute idiosyncratic drug-induced liver injury: long-term follow-up in a hepatotoxicity registry. Hepatology. 2006;44:1581–8.
33. Björnsson E, Kalaitzakis E, Av Klinteberg V, Alem N, Olsson R. Long-term follow-up of patients with mild to moderate drug-induced liver injury. Aliment Pharmacol Ther. 2007;26:79–85.
34. Bjornsson E, Davidsdottir L. The long-term follow-up after idiosyncratic drug-induced liver injury with jaundice. J Hepatol. 2009;50:511.
35. Glover SC, McPhie JL, Brunt PW. Cholestasis in acute alcoholic liver disease. Lancet. 1977;2(8052–8053):1305–7.
36. Chand N, Sanyal AJ. Sepsis-induced cholestasis. Hepatology. 2007;45:230–41.
37. Poelzl G, Ess M, Mussner-Seeber C, Pachinger O, Frick M, Ulmer H. Liver dysfunction in chronic heart failure: prevalence, characteristics and prognostic significance. Eur J Clin Invest. 2012;42:153–63.
38. Jain J, Jain M. Atypical manifestations of viral hepatitis A and E. Trop Doct. 2013;43:17–8.
39. Maggio MC, Liotta A, Cardella F, Corsello G. Stevens-Johnson syndrome and cholestatic hepatitis induced by acute Epstein-Barr virus infection. Eur J Gastroenterol Hepatol. 2011;23:289.
40. Choi HC, Lee SH, Kim J, Kim SH, Hwang JH, Kim JW, Jeong SH, Kim H. A case of acute Q fever with severe acute cholestatic hepatitis. Gut Liver. 2009;3:141–4.
41. Ratnayake EC, Shivanthan C, Wijesiriwardena BC. Cholestatic hepatitis in a patient with typhoid fever—a case report. Ann Clin Microbiol Antimicrob. 2011;10:35.
42. Breidert M, Offensperger S, Blum HE, Fischer R. Weight loss and severe jaundice in a patient with hyperthyroidism. Z Gastroenterol. 2011;49:1267–9.
43. Larrey D, Vial T, Micaleff A, Babany G, Morichau-Beauchant M, Michel H, Benhamou JP. Hepatitis associated with amoxycillin-clavulanic acid combination report of 15 cases. Gut. 1992;33:368–71.
44. http://livertox.nlm.nih.gov
45. Hautekeete ML, Horsmans Y, Van Waeyenberge C, et al. HLA association of amoxicillin-clavulanate-induced hepatitis. Gastroenterology. 1999;117:1181–6.
46. O'Donohue J, Oien KA, Donaldson P, et al. Co-amoxiclav jaundice: clinical and histological features and HLA class II association. Gut. 2000;47:717–20.
47. Andrade RJ, Lucena MI, Alonso A, et al. HLA class II genotype influences the type of liver injury in drug-induced idiosyncratic liver disease. Hepatology. 2004;39:1603–12.
48. Daly AK, Donaldson PT, Bhatnagar P, et al. HLA-B*5701 genotype is a major determinant of drug-induced liver injury due to flucloxacillin. Nat Genet. 2009;41:816–21.
49. Meier Y, Zodan T, Lang C, Zimmermann R, Kullak-Ublick GA, Meier PJ, Stieger B, Pauli-Magnus C. Increased susceptibility for intrahepatic cholestasis of pregnancy and contraceptive-induced cholestasis in carriers of the 1331T>C polymorphism in the bile salt export pump. World J Gastroenterol. 2008;14:38–45.

50. Bachs L, Pares A, Elena M, et al. Effects of long-term rifampicin administration in primary biliary cirrhosis. Gastroenterology. 1992;102:2077–80.
51. Prince MI, Burt AD, Jones DE. Hepatitis and liver dysfunction with rifampicin therapy for pruritus in primary biliary cirrhosis. Gut. 2002;50:436–9.
52. Lindberg MC. Hepatobiliary complications of oral contraceptives. J Gen Intern Med. 1992;7:199–209.
53. Leevy CB, Koneru B, Klein KM. Recurrent familial prolonged intrahepatic cholestasis of pregnancy associated with chronic liver disease. Gastroenterology. 1997;113:966–72.
54. Lucena MI, Andrade RJ, Kaplowitz N, et al. Phenotypic characterization of idiosyncratic drug-induced liver injury: the influence of age and gender. Hepatology. 2009;49:2001–9.
55. Lucena MI, Andrade RJ, Rodrigo L, Salmer6n J, Alvarez A, Lopez-Garrido MJ, Camargo R, Alcantára R. Trovafloxacin-induced acute hepatitis. Clin Infect Dis. 2000;30:400–1.
56. Lammert C, Bjornsson E, Niklasson A, Chalasani N. Oral medications with significant hepatic metabolism at higher risk for hepatic adverse events. Hepatology. 2010;51:615–20.
57. Chen M, Borlak J, Tong W. High lipophilicity and high daily dose of oral medications are associated with significant risk for drug-induced liver injury. Hepatology. 2013;58:388–96.
58. Gibson GG, Skett P. Introduction to drug metabolism. 3rd ed. Cheltenham: Nelson Thornes; 2001.
59. Ho RH, Kim RB. Transporters and drug therapy: implications for drug disposition and disease. Clin Pharmacol Ther. 2005;78:260–77.
60. Pauli-Magnus C, Meier PJ. Hepatobiliary transporters and drug-induced cholestasis. Hepatology. 2006;44:778–87.
61. Pauli-Magnus C, Stieger B, Meier Y, et al. Enterohepatic transport of bile salts and genetics of cholestasis. J Hepatol. 2005;43:342–57.
62. Vavricka SR, Van Montfoort J, Ha HR, et al. Interactions of rifamycin SV and rifampicin with organic anion uptake systems of human liver. Hepatology. 2002;36:164–72.
63. Lakehal F, Dansette PM, Becquemont L, et al. Indirect cytotoxicity of flucloxacillin toward human biliary epithelium via metabolite formation in hepatocytes. Chem Res Toxicol. 2001;14:694–701.
64. Iverson SL, Uetrecht JP. Identification of a reactive metabolite of terbinafine: insights into terbinafine-induced hepatotoxicity. Chem Res Toxicol. 2001;14:175–81.
65. Bolder U, Trang NV, Hagey LR, et al. Sulindac is excreted into bile by a canalicular bile salt pump and undergoes a cholehepatic circulation in rats. Gastroenterology. 1999;117:962–71.
66. Fattinger K, Funk C, Pantze M, et al. The endothelin antagonist bosentan inhibits the canalicular bile salt export pump: a potential mechanism for hepatic adverse reactions. Clin Pharmacol Ther. 2001;69:223–31.
67. Leslie EM, Watkins PB, Kim RB, et al. Differential inhibition of rat and human Na^+-dependent taurocholate cotransporting polypeptide (NTCP/SLC10A1) by bosentan: a mechanism for species differences in hepatotoxicity. J Pharmacol Exp Ther. 2007;321:1170–8.
68. Lang C, Meier Y, Stieger B, et al. Mutations and polymorphisms in the bile salt export pump and the multidrug resistance protein 3 associated with drug-induced liver injury. Pharmacogenet Genomics. 2007;17:47–60.
69. Trauner M, Meier PJ, Boyer JL. Molecular pathogenesis of cholestasis. N Engl J Med. 1998;339:1217–27.
70. Turner IB, Eckstein RP, Riley JW, Lunzer MR. Prolonged hepatic cholestasis after flucloxacillin therapy. Med J Aust. 1989;151:701–5.
71. Fairley CK, McNeil JJ, Desmond P, Smallwood R, Young H, Forbes A, Purcell P, Boyd I. Risk factors for development of flucloxacillin associated jaundice. BMJ. 1993;306:233–5.
72. Hussaini SH, O'Brien CS, Despott EJ, Dalton HR. Antibiotic therapy: a major cause of drug-induced jaundice in southwest England. Eur J Gastroenterol Hepatol. 2007;19:15–20.
73. Polson JE. Hepatotoxicity due to antibiotics. Clin Liver Dis. 2007;11:549–61.
74. Andrade RJ, Guilarte J, Salmer6n FJ, Lucena MI, Bellot V. Benzylpenicillin-induced prolonged cholestasis. Ann Pharmacother. 2001;35:783–4.

75. Lucena MI, Andrade RJ, Fernández MC, Pachkoria K, Pelaez G, Durán JA, et al. Determinants of the clinical expression of amoxicillin-clavulanate hepatotoxicity: a prospective series from Spain. Hepatology. 2006;44:850–6.
76. García Rodríguez LA, Stricker BH, Zimmerman HJ. Risk of acute liver injury associated with the combination of amoxicillin and clavulanic acid. Arch Intern Med. 1996;156:1327–32.
77. Fontana RJ, Shakil AO, Greenson JK, Boyd I, Lee WM. Acute liver failure due to amoxicillin and amoxicillin/clavulanate. Dig Dis Sci. 2005;50:1785–90.
78. Anon. Tetracycline hepatotoxicity. Br Med J. 1964; 2(5424):1545-6.
79. Björnsson E, Lindberg J, Olsson R. Liver reactions to oral low-dose tetracyclines. Scand J Gastroenterol. 1997;32:390–5.
80. Heaton PC, Fenwick SR, Brewer DE. Association between tetracycline or doxycycline and hepatotoxicity: a population based case-control study. J Clin Pharm Ther. 2007;32:483–7.
81. Mainra RR, Card SE. Trimethoprim-sulfamethoxazole-associated hepatotoxicity-part of a hypersensitivity syndrome. Can J Clin Pharmacol. 2003;10:175–8.
82. Björnsson E, Kalaitzakis E, Olsson R. The impact of eosinophilia and hepatic necrosis on prognosis in patients with drug-induced liver injury. Aliment Pharmacol Ther. 2007;25:1411–21.
83. Brown BA, Wallace Jr RJ, Griffith DE, Girard W. Clarithromycin-induced hepatotoxicity. Clin Infect Dis. 1995;20:1073–4.
84. Lockwood AM, Cole S, Rabinovich M. Azithromycin-induced liver injury. Am J Health Syst Pharm. 2010;67:810–4.
85. Zapata Garrido AJ, Romo AC, Padilla FB. Terbinafine hepatotoxicity. A case report and review of literature. Ann Hepatol. 2003;2:47–51.
86. Agarwal K, Manas DM, Hudson M. Terbinafine and fulminant hepatic failure. N Engl J Med. 1999;340:1292–3.
87. Hautekeete ML, Kockx MM, Naegels S, Holvoet JK, Hubens H, Kloppel G. Cholestatic hepatitis related to quinolones: a report of two cases. J Hepatol. 1995;23:759–60.
88. Bataille L, Rahier J, Geubel A. Delayed and prolonged cholestatic hepatitis with ductopenia after long-term ciprofloxacin therapy for Crohn's disease. J Hepatol. 2002;37:696–9.
89. Skoog SM, Smyrk TC, Talwalkar JA. Cephalexin-induced cholestatic hepatitis. J Clin Gastroenterol. 2004;38:833.
90. Alqahtani S, Hoofnagle JH, Ghabril M, Chalasani N, Rockey DC. Cephalosporin induced liver injury: clinical and biochemical features. Hepatology. 2011;54:516A.
91. Romagnuolo J, Sadowski DC, Lalor E, Jewell L, Thomson AB. Cholestatic hepatocellular injury with azathioprine: a case report and review of the mechanisms of hepatotoxicity. Can J Gastroenterol. 1998;12:479–83.
92. Ben Salem C, Ben Salah L, Belajouza C, Bouraoui K. Azathioprine-induced severe cholestatic hepatitis in patient carrying TPMT*3C polymorphism. Pharm World Sci. 2010;32:701–3.
93. Roda G, Caponi A, Belluzzi A, Roda E. Severe cholestatic acute hepatitis following azathioprine therapy in a patient with ulcerative pancolitis. Dig Liver Dis. 2009;41:914–5.
94. Bastida G, Nos P, Aguas M, et al. Incidence, risk factors and clinical course of thiopurine-induced liver injury in patients with inflammatory bowel disease. Aliment Pharmacol Ther. 2005;22:775–82.
95. Gisbert JP, González-Lama Y, Maté J. Thiopurine-induced liver injury in patients with inflammatory bowel disease: a systematic review. Am J Gastroenterol. 2007;102:1518–27.
96. Krebs S, Dormann H, Muth-Selbach U, Hahn EG, Brune K, Schneider HT. Risperidone-induced cholestatic hepatitis. Eur J Gastroenterol Hepatol. 2001;13:67–9.
97. Wright TM, Vandenberg AM. Risperidone- and quetiapine-induced cholestasis. Ann Pharmacother. 2007;41:1518–23.
98. Vuppalanchi R, Hayashi PH, Chalasani N, Fontana RJ, Bonkovsky H, Saxena R, Kleiner D, Hoofnagle JH. Duloxetine hepatotoxicity: a case-series from the drug-induced liver injury network. Aliment Pharmacol Ther. 2010;32:1174–83.

99. Servoss JC, Kitch DW, Andersen JW, Reisler RB, Chung RT, Robbins GK. Predictors of antiretroviral-related hepatotoxicity in the adult AIDS Clinical Trial Group (1989-1999). J Acquir Immune Defic Syndr. 2006;43:320–3.
100. Akhtar AJ, Shaheen M. Jaundice in African-American and Hispanic patients with AIDS. J Natl Med Assoc. 2007;99:825–9.
101. Björnsson E, Olsson R. Suspected drug-induced liver fatalities reported to the WHO database. Dig Liver Dis. 2006;38:33–8.
102. Schiano TD, Kotler DP, Ferran E, Fiel MI. Hepatoportal sclerosis as a cause of noncirrhotic portal hypertension in patients with HIV. Am J Gastroenterol. 2007;102:2536–40.
103. Saifee S, Joelson D, Braude J, Shrestha R, Johnson M, Sellers M, Galambos MR, Rubin RA. Noncirrhotic portal hypertension in patients with human immunodeficiency virus-1 infection. Clin Gastroenterol Hepatol. 2008;6:1167–9.
104. Kovari H, Ledergerber B, Peter U, Flepp M, Jost J, Schmid P, Calmy A, Mueller NJ, Muellhaupt B, Weber R. Association of noncirrhotic portal hypertension in HIV-infected persons and antiretroviral therapy with didanosine: a nested case-control study. Clin Infect Dis. 2009;49:626–35.
105. Cachay ER, Peterson MR, Goicoechea M, Mathews WC. Didanosine exposure and noncirrhotic portal hypertension in a HIV clinic in North America: a follow-up Study. Br J Med Med Res. 2011;1:346–55.
106. Dourakis SP, Tolis G. Sex hormonal preparations and the liver. Eur J Contracept Reprod Health Care. 1998;3:7–16.
107. Lindgren A, Olsson R. Liver damage from low-dose oral contraceptives. J Intern Med. 1993;234:287–92.
108. Kafrouni MI, Anders RA, Verma S. Hepatotoxicity associated with dietary supplements containing anabolic steroids. Clin Gastroenterol Hepatol. 2007;5:809–12.
109. Navarro VJ. Herbal and dietary supplement hepatotoxicity. Semin Liver Dis. 2009;29:373–82.
110. Lee WM, Hynan LS, Rossaro L, Fontana RJ, Stravitz RT, Larson AM, Davern II TJ, Murray NG, McCashland T, Reisch JS, Robuck PR. Intravenous N-acetylcysteine improves transplant-free survival in early stage non-acetaminophen acute liver failure. Gastroenterology. 2009;137:856–64.
111. Papay JI, Clines D, Rafi R, Yuen N, Britt SD, Walsh JS, Hunt CM. Drug-induced liver injury following positive drug rechallenge. Regul Toxicol Pharmacol. 2009;54:84–90.

Chapter 3
Primary Biliary Cirrhosis

Marina G. Silveira

Abbreviations

AASLD	American Association for the Study of Liver Diseases
ALT	Alanine aminotransferase
AlkPhos	Alkaline phosphatase
AMA	Anti-mitochondrial antibodies
AST	Aspartate aminotransferase
ELISA	Enzyme-linked immune assay
FDA	Food and Drug Administration
LT	Liver Transplantation
MRS	Mayo risk score
PBC	Primary biliary cirrhosis
UDCA	Ursodeoxycholic acid
ULN	Upper limits of normal

Introduction

Primary biliary cirrhosis (PBC) is a relatively rare but important cause of chronic cholestatic liver disease that affects predominantly middle-aged women [1]. Small and medium-sized bile ducts are destroyed by an inflammatory process, presumably autoimmune in nature, resulting in cholestasis, advanced fibrosis, cirrhosis, and liver failure if untreated. Most patients are asymptomatic at presentation, likely as a result of widespread use of screening biochemical tests and the specific

M.G. Silveira, M.D. (✉)
Gastroenterology and Hepatology, 10701 East Blvd 111E (W),
Cleveland, OH 44106, USA
e-mail: marina.silveira@va.gov

E.J. Carey and K.D. Lindor (eds.), *Cholestatic Liver Disease*, Clinical Gastroenterology,
DOI 10.1007/978-1-4939-1013-7_3,

anti-mitochondrial antibody (AMA) assay. Symptomatic patients usually present with either fatigue or pruritus. Ursodeoxycholic acid (UDCA) is the only established treatment for PBC and may improve survival in selected patients. However, some patients do not respond adequately to UDCA and might need alternative therapeutic approaches.

Pathogenesis

PBC is considered a prototypical autoimmune disease because of the well-defined nature of the autoantigen, its homogeneous clinical expression, and its overwhelming predominance in females [2]. Similar to other complex diseases, the combination of a susceptible genetic background and exposure to environmental triggers is needed to initiate and promote the disorder.

Pathologically, PBC includes chronic small bile duct cholangitis, probably mediated by a multilineage humoral and cellular adaptive response, but may also include innate immune responses against biliary epithelial cells [3, 4]. The autoimmune nature of PBC is characterized by a distinctive loss of tolerance to a series of ubiquitous mitochondrial autoantigens, the E2 subunits of the oxo-dehydrogenase pathway of phosphorylation, which appears to be an early event and could be independent of the development of liver disease [3]. This response to mitochondrial autoantigens appears to be integrally related to bile duct loss that progresses through lymphocytic cholangitis to progressive ductopenia, associated cholestasis, and resultant fibrosis.

Several studies support the importance of genetic susceptibility factors in the pathogenesis of PBC. Immune-related genetic polymorphisms are increased in frequency in PBC [5, 6]. The interleukin (IL)-12 signaling axis has been identified as a critical focus in modulating disease activity, both in animal models [7] and in genome-wide association studies in humans [6, 8]. Also, the concordance rate of PBC among monozygotic twins is significantly higher than among dizygotic twins [9], as high or higher than that observed in any autoimmune diseases believed to have an autoimmune component. Several studies have shown that the prevalence of PBC within families of affected individuals is significantly higher than in the general population [10–12].

Findings of epidemiological studies and animal models suggest a possible role for exogenous chemical and infectious agents through molecular mimicry. Differences in geographical distribution and clustering of cases of PBC suggest that exposure to environmental agents plays a role in the etiology of disease [13]. In the first study to identify geographic factors in the USA, cases of PBC were found to cluster after superfund toxic waste sites [14], providing more evidence for environmental factors. Space-time clustering in northeast England provides epidemiological evidence for a role of chemical, infectious agents, or both [15]. Additional data that lend support to a role for infections in disease development include the significantly higher prevalence than usual of recurrent urinary tract infections in patients with PBC [16, 17] and experimental findings of sequence similarity between the E2 enzyme of the pyruvate dehydrogenase complex recognized by autoantibodies and bacterial proteins [18, 19]. Smoking has also been identified as a risk factor for development [17] and progression of disease [20] in PBC.

Epidemiology

PBC is primarily a disease of middle-aged women, affecting women more often than men. The peak incidence occurs in the fifth decade of life, and it is uncommon in patients less than 25 years of age [21]. Large geographic variations in the incidence and prevalence of PBC have been reported. Earlier epidemiological studies report an annual incidence ranging from 2.27 to 32 per million [22, 23] with a female to male gender ratio averaging approximately 10:1 [13], although over the last decade the disease is reported more frequently [24], perhaps at least in part due to greater disease awareness [25]. PBC occurs in all races and ethnicities, the highest rates of prevalence and incidence have been within Caucasian populations from Scandinavia (prevalence 151 cases per million, incidence 13 cases per million) [26], Spain (prevalence 195 cases per million, incidence 17 cases per million) [27], Canada (prevalence 227 cases per million, incidence 30 cases per million) [28], the UK (prevalence 392 cases per million, incidence 58 cases per million) [22, 25], and Minnesota (prevalence 402 cases per million, incidence 27 cases per million) [29], and it is infrequently reported in Africa and the Indian subcontinent.

Diagnosis

Clinical Features

The majority of patients is asymptomatic at presentation [29, 30] and is diagnosed as a result of widespread use of screening biochemical tests and the specific AMA assay. The most common presenting symptoms in patients who have PBC are fatigue and pruritus [31]. The cumulative risk for developing fatigue over a 5–10-year period is substantial at 44–56 % [30]. Fatigue has been noted in up to 80 % of patients in some studies and can be a significant cause of disability [32]. Studies indicate that patients report an impaired quality of life that is independent of the severity or stage of the disease but is significantly associated with the presence of fatigue and to a lesser extent of pruritus [32–36]. The degree of severity of the fatigue is independent of the degree of severity of the liver disease when assessed with classical markers of disease severity such as histological stage, patient age, serum bilirubin and albumin levels, and the prothrombin time [37]. Nonetheless, it has been reported that the presence of fatigue in PBC is independently associated with a significantly increased risk of liver-related death [33, 38, 39] and death in general [33], though these findings have not been confirmed in all patient populations [40]. No specific treatment for fatigue is available. Pruritus has been reported to affect up to 69 % of patients with PBC [41]. Similarly to fatigue, the presence of pruritus can have a significant negative impact in the quality of life of patients with PBC. Treatment options include cholestyramine, rifampin, anti-histamines, opioid antagonists, and sertraline. In some patients with refractory pruritus, liver transplantation may be the only effective treatment. Treatment with UDCA has been reported to precipitate pruritus in some patients and this effect can usually be avoided by initiating UDCA gradually over a few weeks [42].

Other important disease-related complications of PBC include vitamin deficiencies and metabolic bone disease. Risk factors for osteoporosis in PBC are older age, lower body mass index, severity of cholestasis, and advanced histologic stage. Reduced bone formation is considered the primary explanation for osteoporosis in at-risk individuals with PBC [1]. Bilirubin has been shown to inhibit osteoblast function in vitro and this osteoblast dysfunction may play a role in the low bone formation rate seen in PBC. Patients who have advanced stage PBC have a fivefold increase in risk for developing osteoporosis than those who have early-stage disease [43]. Although most patients with PBC do not have malabsorption and significant fat-soluble vitamin deficiencies, supplementation with calcium and vitamin D and weight bearing exercises are generally recommended. Therapy with bisphosphonates has been shown to be effective in the treatment of osteoporosis in patients with PBC [44–46].

The association with extrahepatic autoimmune diseases is commonly seen in patients with PBC. The most frequently associated disease is Sjogren's syndrome, reported in up to approximately 70–80 % of cases when sought with specific testing [47]. Autoimmune thyroid diseases such as Hashimoto's thyroiditis, euthyroid goiter, and, less commonly, Grave's disease, have been described in approximately 15–20 % of cases [48]. Other associated diseases include rheumatoid arthritis and scleroderma and variants such as Raynaud's phenomenon and CREST syndrome, pernicious anemia, celiac disease, inflammatory bowel disease, and pulmonary fibrosis, and autoimmune thyroid disease. Autoimmune comorbidities do not modify the natural history or clinical presentation of PBC, with the exception of a reported slower progression of liver fibrosis in patients with scleroderma [49].

Biochemical and Serologic Features

Elevations in serum alkaline phosphatase (AlkPhos) levels are the biochemical hallmark of PBC. In this context, the best diagnostic tool for PBC is the measurement of anti-mitochondrial antibodies (AMAs), which are characteristic of PBC and are present in at least 90 % of the cases [21]. AMAs are directed against a highly specific epitope within the lipoic acid binding domain of the pyruvate dehydrogenase-E2 subunit (PDC-E2) [50]. There are several methodologies for determining AMA, including indirect immunofluorescence and enzyme-linked immunosorbent assay

(ELISA). ELISA is recognized as more sensitive, but perhaps not as specific [51]. Detection of AMA by any method is acceptable for diagnosis. The presence of antibody, rather than the magnitude of antibody level, establishes AMA-positivity.

Autoantibodies are common in autoimmune liver disease, but typically lack disease-specificity, and per se do not establish a diagnosis [52], except perhaps AMAs. Antinuclear antibodies (ANAs) are the most commonly assessed, but least specific, serologic markers of autoimmunity in acute and chronic liver disease [53]. ANAs are found in approximately 50 % of patients with PBC, and often in patients who do have anti-mitochondrial antibodies [21]. The ANA reactivity in PBC, unlikely other autoimmune disorders, tends to be very specific. Some of the antigens specific for PBC include nuclear body speckled 100 kDa (Sp100), promyelocytic leukemia (PML) cells, glycoprotein 120 (gp120), and nucleoporin 62 (p62) [54]. PBC-specific indirect immunofluorescent patterns include nuclear rim, identified on the basis of the autoantibodies' recognition of gp210 and p62, and multiple nuclear dots, identified on the basis of reactivity with sp100, PML cells, and sp140 (nuclear body proteins). Also, small ubiquitin-like modifiers bound to both sp100 and PML cells may be independent, PBC-specific antigens [55]. The presence of ANA in PBC is clinically significant in the diagnosis of patients who are AMA negative, and prognostically with regard to the risk of portal hypertension and liver failure [56, 57].

Histologic Features

Histologically, PBC is characterized by chronic portal inflammation with infiltration, destruction, and loss of the epithelial cells in the small- and medium-sized bile ducts [58]. The characteristic lesion of PBC is the "florid duct lesion" or chronic non-suppurative destruction of the interlobular bile ducts. Eosinophils and granulomas are also characteristic but not diagnostic of PBC.

Histologic staging systems have been developed by Rubin et al. [59], Scheuer [60], Popper and Schaffner, and Ludwig et al. [61], which evaluate features of inflammation and biliary damage (e.g., lymphocytic cholangitis, duct injury and destruction, ductopenia, portal lymphoplasmacytic inflammation, periportal or interface activity, and periportal ductular proliferation) along with fibrosis (portal, periportal, bridging, cirrhosis) together in three-tiered or four-tiered staging systems (summarized in Table 3.1). Most pathologists in current practice use a four stage system (stages I–IV) that follows the histological system of Ludwig et al. [61] or of Scheuer [60], ranging from portal-tract inflammation with predominantly lymphoplasmacytoid infiltrates and septal and interlobular bile-duct loss (stage I) to frank cirrhosis (stage IV). When two or more stages manifest within the same liver sample, the patients is classified as belonging to the more severe stage.

Liver biopsy is not required for clinical diagnosis in PBC, as the presence of AMA and cholestatic enzymes in a middle aged woman reportedly have a 98 % positive predictive value for the presence of PBC [62], obviating the need for a liver

Table 3.1 Histologic features among different staging systems

	Stage 1	Stage 2	Stage 3	Stage 4
Rubin et al. [59]	Portal inflammation and bile duct injury	Proliferation and destruction of bile ductules	Cirrhosis	
Scheuer [60]	Florid duct lesion (portal hepatitis)	Ductular proliferation (periportal hepatitis)	Scarring (ductopenia and bridging fibrosis)	Nodular cirrhosis
Ludwig et al. [61]	Portal inflammation (portal stage)	Periportal inflammation with or without bile duct loss (periportal stage)	Bridging fibrosis (septal stage)	Cirrhosis

biopsy for diagnostic purposes in most cases. Biopsy is still essential for diagnosis in cases where the AMA is negative or in low titer, or if the patient has a biochemical picture with prominent elevation of the transaminase levels, i.e., *hepatitic*, or has been taking potentially hepatotoxic drugs [63]. Diagnosis of concurrent pathological processes is an invaluable consideration for liver biopsy; steatohepatitis has been documented in up to 5 % of other forms of chronic liver disease [64], and the presence of "overlap" features of autoimmune hepatitis are best documented by liver biopsy findings. Up to 20 % of otherwise typical PBC could be given a diagnosis of "probable" autoimmune hepatitis, according to the revised Autoimmune Hepatitis Group scoring system [65] and were thus considered as having PBC-autoimmune hepatitis overlap. The histological finding of interface hepatitis in biopsy was one of five features that distinguished between overlap and non-overlap patients. After six years of follow-up, the patients with overlap had significantly worse clinical outcomes than the non-overlap PBC patients, thus confirming the potential importance of using liver biopsy to establish the correct diagnosis [66]. Moreover, patients whose liver biopsies have interface hepatitis may have a more rapidly progressive disease than patients without this histologic feature [67], thus interface hepatitis is an important prognostic parameter. Other histological factors may also have prognostic significance, such as the degree of ductopenia [68].

Natural History and Prognosis

PBC is a slowly progressive disease that causes substantial loss of intrahepatic bile ducts, ultimately resulting in cholestasis, advanced fibrosis, cirrhosis, and liver failure. As such, PBC is an important indication for liver transplantation [1]. Cirrhosis may also lead to hepatocellular carcinoma in PBC, particularly in male patients and those with advanced histologic stages and evidence of portal hypertension [69, 70].

Progression of disease occurs at different rates and with varying degrees of severity in different patients [21]. The natural history of PBC can be divided in four phases. The *silent* or *preclinical phase* is characterized by isolated AMA positivity and normal serum biochemistries [71]; this phase may last many years. The next phase is characterized by gradual elevation of the serum AlkPhos levels. The vast majority of newly diagnosed patients with PBC presents without symptoms attributable to liver disease and are in this *asymptomatic phase*. Although this phase may last up to 20 years, only 30–50 % of patients remain asymptomatic after 5 years of follow-up [72]. As PBC is diagnosed increasingly earlier, this percentage may be increasing. Patients in the *symptomatic phase* will most often complain of fatigue and/or pruritus, but may also report abdominal pain. Symptoms related to portal hypertension usually appear later, with 20 % developing ascites and 10 % developing bleeding varices within a 10-year period [30]. Most patients who develop portal hypertension are often either anicteric or mildly jaundiced. If untreated, median survival ranges from 6 to 10 years, with an accelerated course after development of ascites and hepatic encephalopathy. Once progressive jaundice develops, patients enter a *pre-terminal phase*, which can last up to 4 years [30, 73]. Mean survival once the bilirubin is 2.0 mg/dL is 4 years, and when the bilirubin reaches 6.0 mg/dL, mean survival is only 2 years [74].

Natural history studies have identified numerous markers of progressive disease in PBC, including but not limited to: response to UDCA [75–78], histology (degree of interface hepatitis and features of overlap with autoimmune hepatitis) [66, 67], biochemical markers (serum bilirubin, albumin, and prothrombin time) [79], presence and/or degree of portal hypertension [80], certain genetic polymorphisms (apolipoprotein A, tumor necrosis factor [TNF]-alpha), specific autoantibodies (anti-gp210, anti-promyelocytic leukemia protein [PML], anti-sp100, anti-centromere) [56, 57], and serum markers of fibrosis (hyaluronic acid, procollagen III, tissue inhibitor metalloproteinase) [81].

Models using time-fixed Cox proportional hazards regression analysis have been developed to predict survival in PBC. Among several well-validated models (European, Mayo, Oslo, Barcelona, Newcastle) [30, 79, 82, 83], the Mayo risk score is the most widely used, at least in the USA, and includes the following variables: age, total bilirubin, prothrombin time, albumin and presence/absence of peripheral edema, and response to diuretics [79]. This model has been used as a historical control to estimate the benefits of treatment, including pharmacological therapy and liver transplantation [84], as well as in everyday practice to counsel patients and help make clinical management decisions. This model has the disadvantage of overestimating the survival in patients with poor short-term survival.

Of all the serum markers studied to date, serum bilirubin is the best independent predictor of survival [74, 85, 86], but it only becomes abnormal in late stages of the disease and therefore is less useful in assessing improvement in patients with mild-moderate disease. Response of AlkPhos to therapy has been shown to be a good correlate of both survival [76] and liver histology [62] in PBC and is used globally in clinical practice to predict the progression of the disease; it is therefore an acceptable therapeutic criterion to monitor PBC treatment. Analysis of UDCA trials demonstrated that normalization of AlkPhos, when assessing a large group, was associated with better survival than expected [75, 77].

Treatment

UDCA has been the drug most widely evaluated in the treatment of PBC. At least four mechanisms of action are involved in the beneficial therapeutic effects of UDCA in PBC, including an increased hydrophilicity index of the circulating bile acid pool, stimulation of hepatocellular and ductular secretions, cytoprotection against bile acid and cytokine-induced injury, and immunomodulation and anti-inflammatory effects [87]. Currently, treatment with UDCA in a dose of 13–15 mg/kg/day is recommended as therapy for PBC by the American Association for the Study of Liver Diseases (AASLD) [88] and is approved for this indication by the US Food and Drug Administration (FDA).

Early trials have clearly shown that UDCA improves serum liver tests including bilirubin and other markers of cholestasis [89–93]. Long-term follow-up studies show that improvement in liver biochemistries can be sustained, however, interruption of UDCA therapy is associated with a deterioration in liver biochemistries, indicating that the treatment is needed indefinitely [94]. Biochemical response to UDCA at one year is a strong predictor of long-term prognosis [75–78]. Indeed, patients with PBC who have achieved a biochemical response to UDCA have been shown to survive just as long as the normal population [95]. Biochemical response has been be defined by numerous criteria (summarized in Table 3.2): the Mayo criteria [75] (AlkPhos <2 times the upper limits of normal [ULN]), the French criteria [77] (AlkPhos<3 times ULN, aspartate aminotransferase [AST] <2 times ULN, and bilirubin <1.0 mg/dL), the Spanish criteria [76] (decline in AlkPhos of more than 40 % of baseline or to a normal value), or the Dutch (Rotterdam) criteria [78] (normalization of bilirubin and/or albumin after treatment if one or both were abnormal at baseline) have been most commonly used. Around 50 % of patients fulfill at least one criterion of incomplete biochemical response to USDA. These patients have an increased risk of adverse events during the course of their disease.

None of the studies that evaluated the effect of UDCA treatment on the symptoms of fatigue and pruritus [90–93, 96, 97] showed any significant effect on fatigue and only one study reported a significant reduction of pruritus in the UDCA group compared with the placebo group [96]. There was no effect of UDCA on autoimmune conditions [98] or on bone disease in PBC [99]. Therapy with UDCA appears to reduce the onset and severity of portal hypertension, including the development of ascites [90, 91, 93, 97] and esophageal varices [100].

Treatment with UDCA may delay disease progression and prolong survival free of liver transplantation [101]. No single randomized controlled trial has demonstrated a survival benefit using UDCA versus placebo. However, most of the trials of UDCA have not recruited sufficient patients to have the power to show an effect

Table 3.2 Biochemical response to treatment with ursodeoxycholic acid

Angulo et al. [75][a]	
	AlkPhos < 2 times ULN
Pares et al. [76][b]	
	AlkPhos < 40 % from baseline or to normal value
Corpechot et al. [77][b]	
	AlkPhos < 3 times ULN
	AST < 2 times ULN
	Bilirubin < 1.0 mg/dL
Kuiper et al. [78][b]	
	Normal bilirubin and albumin (if one or both were abnormal before treatment)
	Normal bilirubin or albumin (if both were abnormal before treatment)
Kumagi et al. [134][c]	
	AlkPhos ≤ 1.67 times ULN
	Bilirubin < 1.0 mg/dL
Momah et al. [135][b]	
	AlkPhos ≤ 1.67 times ULN
	Bilirubin < 1.0 mg/dL

AlkPhos alkaline phosphatase, *AST* aspartate aminotransferase, *ULN* upper limits of normal
[a]At 6 months of therapy
[b]At 12 months of therapy
[c]At 24 months of therapy

of therapy on survival. Therefore, the evidence that UDCA inhibits the progression of the disease has been delayed until long after the completion of the trials that demonstrated improvement in markers of cholestasis. Analysis of the combined data from three large, well-designed, controlled trials that used adequate UDCA doses up to four years, including a total of 548 patients, showed that UDCA significantly reduced the likelihood of liver transplantation or death [101]. Several studies evaluating long-term survival of patients have been published and uniformly they indicate that those who demonstrated biochemical response to adequate doses of UDCA for prolonged periods of time have longer survival free of liver transplantation and longer overall survival [75–78]. Additional indirect support for a long-term beneficial effect of UDCA in PBC might come from retrospective studies of transplantation trends among patients with PBC [102]. Several studies evaluating large series of patients in Europe and in the USA indicate that the proportion and the absolute number of patients transplanted for PBC are decreasing [102–104] while the incidence of the disease appears to be stable [105] and the prevalence, rising [106].

A variety of immunosuppressive medications have been used alone or with UDCA in patients with PBC, particularly those with incomplete response to UDCA monotherapy. Medications evaluated include azathioprine, budesonide, chlorambucil, cyclosporine, methotrexate, mycophenolate mofetil, prednisone, prednisolone, and tacrolimus. Some small studies have suggested that combination therapy may be superior to UDCA monotherapy [107–109], but further studies are necessary.

At present, there are insufficient data to support the use of immunosuppressive therapy for PBC [110].

Additional treatments are needed for patients who have an incomplete response to UDCA. Drugs that are directed at reducing the presence of autoantibodies, such as rituximab, have led to some benefit in two small studies [111, 112]. New therapies are being directed at NF-κB using various activators of peroxisome proliferator-activated receptor (PPAR) α including the fibrates with some evidence of benefit [113–117], but larger studies are needed. Preliminary phase II studies of obeticholic acid, a farnesoid X receptor, in patients with PBC have demonstrated marked biochemical improvement in patients with PBC when administered in combination with UDCA and alone [118, 119], and is a promising agent for treatment for PBC. Pruritus is the most common side effect, limiting treatment when obeticholic acid is administered at higher doses. The discovery that mutations in the interleukin 12 (IL-12) pathway are associated with PBC [5] may lead to immunotherapy directed at this pathway.

Liver Transplantation

As patients with PBC progress to end-stage liver disease, liver transplantation (LT) remains their only therapeutic option. PBC is one of the top six indications for LT in the USA and Europe. To date, over 6,000 liver transplants have been performed for PBC in both regions combined [120]. Over time, however, a notable decline in the number of liver transplantations and waiting list additions for PBC has been observed [103, 121, 122]. Patient and graft survival for PBC are excellent compared to other indications. One, five, and ten-year survival rates for PBC are estimated at 83 %, 77 %, and 69 %, respectively [120]. At selected centers, the 1 and 5-year survival rates may exceed 90 % and 80 %, respectively [123, 124].

With prolonged survival, recurrent disease becomes a major problem in this patient population. The prevalence rates for recurrent PBC reported by individual LT programs range between 9 and 35 % [103, 125–131]. The cumulative incidence rate, which better describes the risk of recurrent disease, varies between 21 and 37 % at 10 years [103, 125, 130], and maybe as high as 43 % at 15 years [130]. Among centers with over 100 patients transplanted for PBC, the average time to recurrence ranges between 3 and 5.5 years [103, 125, 127, 130, 132]. Though an increased risk for advanced liver disease in patients with recurrent PBC has been described—cirrhosis was observed in 25 % of patients in one study [128], and hepatic retransplantation or death due to organ dysfunction related to recurrent PBC remains an uncommon scenario [133].

No standard approach exists for the treatment of recurrent PBC. Dose modification or re-institution of corticosteroids, azathioprine, and/or mycophenolate mofetil has not been formally reported as an interventional strategy. Given the near universal presence of early stage disease at diagnosis, a potential role for UDCA therapy exists [103, 127, 128, 130, 132]. Though improvements in serum liver biochemistries are reported in patients with recurrent PBC treated with UDCA [129, 130], significant differences in histologic progression rate or the probability of death or liver retransplantation for patients treated with UDCA when compared to untreated patients have not been described.

References

1. Talwalkar JA, Lindor KD. Primary biliary cirrhosis. Lancet. 2003;362(9377):53–61. PubMed PMID: 12853201.
2. Hirschfield GM, Gershwin ME. The immunobiology and pathophysiology of primary biliary cirrhosis. Annu Rev Pathol. 2013;8:303–30. PubMed PMID: 23347352.
3. Selmi C, Bowlus CL, Gershwin ME, Coppel RL. Primary biliary cirrhosis. Lancet. 2011;377(9777):1600–9. PubMed PMID: 21529926.
4. Gershwin ME, Mackay IR. The causes of primary biliary cirrhosis: convenient and inconvenient truths. Hepatology. 2008;47(2):737–45. PubMed PMID: 18098322.
5. Hirschfield GM, Liu X, Xu C, Lu Y, Xie G, Lu Y, et al. Primary biliary cirrhosis associated with HLA, IL12A, and IL12RB2 variants. N Engl J Med. 2009;360(24):2544–55. PubMed PMID: 19458352; Pubmed Central PMCID: 2857316.
6. Hirschfield GM, Xie G, Lu E, Sun Y, Juran BD, Chellappa V, et al. Association of primary biliary cirrhosis with variants in the CLEC16A, SOCS1, SPIB and SIAE immunomodulatory genes. Genes Immun. 2012;13(4):328–35. PubMed PMID: 22257840. Pubmed Central PMCID: 3360983.
7. Yoshida K, Yang GX, Zhang W, Tsuda M, Tsuneyama K, Moritoki Y, et al. Deletion of Interleukin-12p40 suppresses autoimmune cholangitis in dominant negative transforming growth factor beta receptor Type II Mice. Hepatology. 2009;50(5):1494–500. PubMed PMID: WOS:000271565600021. English.
8. Liu XD, Invernizzi P, Lu Y, Kosoy R, Lu Y, Bianchi I, et al. Genome-wide meta-analyses identify three loci associated with primary biliary cirrhosis. Nat Genet. 2010;42(8):658–60. PMID: WOS:000280524000007. English.
9. Selmi C, Mayo MJ, Bach N, Ishibashi H, Invernizzi P, Gish RG, et al. Primary biliary cirrhosis in monozygotic and dizygotic twins: genetics, epigenetics, and environment. Gastroenterology. 2004;127(2):485–92. PubMed PMID: 15300581.
10. Jones DE, Watt FE, Metcalf JV, Bassendine MF, James OF. Familial primary biliary cirrhosis reassessed: a geographically-based population study. J Hepatol. 1999;30(3):402–7. PubMed PMID: 10190721.
11. Bach N, Schaffner F. Familial primary biliary cirrhosis. J Hepatol. 1994;20(6):698–701. PubMed PMID: 7930467.
12. Lazaridis KN, Juran BD, Boe GM, Slusser JP, de Andrade M, Homburger HA, et al. Increased prevalence of antimitochondrial antibodies in first-degree relatives of patients with primary biliary cirrhosis. Hepatology. 2007;46(3):785–92. PubMed PMID: 17680647.
13. Selmi C, Invernizzi P, Zuin M, Podda M, Gershwin ME. Genetics and geoepidemiology of primary biliary cirrhosis: following the footprints to disease etiology. Semin Liver Dis. 2005;25(3):265–80. PubMed PMID: 16143943. English.
14. Ala A, Stanca CM, Bu-Ghanim M, Ahmado I, Branch AD, Schiano TD, et al. Increased prevalence of primary biliary cirrhosis near Superfund toxic waste sites. Hepatology. 2006;43(3):525–31. PubMed PMID: 16496326.
15. McNally RJ, Ducker S, James OF. Are transient environmental agents involved in the cause of primary biliary cirrhosis? Evidence from space-time clustering analysis. Hepatology. 2009;50(4):1169–74. PubMed PMID: 19711423.

16. Burroughs AK, Rosenstein IJ, Epstein O, Hamilton-Miller JM, Brumfitt W, Sherlock S. Bacteriuria and primary biliary cirrhosis. Gut. 1984;25(2):133–7. PubMed PMID: 6363217; Pubmed Central PMCID: 1432247.
17. Parikh-Patel A, Gold EB, Worman H, Krivy KE, Gershwin ME. Risk factors for primary biliary cirrhosis in a cohort of patients from the United States. Hepatology. 2001;33(1):16–21. PubMed PMID: 11124815.
18. Padgett KA, Selmi C, Kenny TP, Leung PS, Balkwill DL, Ansari AA, et al. Phylogenetic and immunological definition of four lipoylated proteins from Novosphingobium aromaticivorans, implications for primary biliary cirrhosis. J Autoimmun. 2005;24(3):209–19. PubMed PMID: 15848043.
19. Shimoda S, Nakamura M, Ishibashi H, Kawano A, Kamihira T, Sakamoto N, et al. Molecular mimicry of mitochondrial and nuclear autoantigens in primary biliary cirrhosis. Gastroenterology. 2003;124(7):1915–25. PubMed PMID: 12806624.
20. Zein CO, Beatty K, Post AB, Logan L, Debanne S, McCullough AJ. Smoking and increased severity of hepatic fibrosis in primary biliary cirrhosis: A cross validated retrospective assessment. Hepatology. 2006;44(6):1564–71. PubMed PMID: 17133468.
21. Kaplan MM, Gershwin ME. Primary biliary cirrhosis. N Engl J Med. 2005;353(12):1261–73. PubMed PMID: 16177252.
22. Metcalf JV, Bhopal RS, Gray J, Howel D, James OF. Incidence and prevalence of primary biliary cirrhosis in the city of Newcastle upon Tyne, England. Int J Epidemiol. 1997;26(4): 830–6. PubMed PMID: 9279616. English.
23. Watson RG, Angus PW, Dewar M, Goss B, Sewell RB, Smallwood RA. Low prevalence of primary biliary cirrhosis in Victoria, Australia. Melbourne Liver Group. Gut. 1995;36(6): 927–30. PubMed PMID: 7615286. English.
24. Boonstra K, Beuers U, Ponsioen CY. Epidemiology of primary sclerosing cholangitis and primary biliary cirrhosis: a systematic review. J Hepatol. 2012;56(5):1181–8. PubMed PMID: 22245904.
25. James OF, Bhopal R, Howel D, Gray J, Burt AD, Metcalf JV. Primary biliary cirrhosis once rare, now common in the United Kingdom? Hepatology. 1999;30(2):390–4. PubMed PMID: 10421645. English.
26. Danielsson A, Boqvist L, Uddenfeldt P. Epidemiology of primary biliary cirrhosis in a defined rural population in the northern part of Sweden. Hepatology. 1990;11(3):458–64. PMID: 2312058. English.
27. Pla X, Vergara M, Gil M, Dalmau B, Cistero B, Bella RM, et al. Incidence, prevalence and clinical course of primary biliary cirrhosis in a Spanish community. Eur J Gastroenterol Hepatol. 2007;19(10):859–64. PubMed PMID: 17873609.
28. Myers RP, Shaheen AA, Fong A, Burak KW, Wan A, Swain MG, et al. Epidemiology and natural history of primary biliary cirrhosis in a Canadian health region: a population-based study. Hepatology. 2009;50(6):1884–92. PubMed PMID: 19821525.
29. Kim WR, Lindor KD, Locke III GR, Therneau TM, Homburger HA, Batts KP, et al. Epidemiology and natural history of primary biliary cirrhosis in a US community. Gastroenterology. 2000;119(6):1631–6. PubMed PMID: 11113084.
30. Prince M, Chetwynd A, Newman W, Metcalf JV, James OF. Survival and symptom progression in a geographically based cohort of patients with primary biliary cirrhosis: follow-up for up to 28 years. Gastroenterology. 2002;123(4):1044–51. PubMed PMID: 12360466. English.
31. Witt-Sullivan H, Heathcote J, Cauch K, Blendis L, Ghent C, Katz A, et al. The demography of primary biliary cirrhosis in Ontario, Canada. Hepatology. 1990;12(1):98–105. PubMed PMID: 2197212.
32. Newton JL, Bhala N, Burt J, Jones DE. Characterisation of the associations and impact of symptoms in primary biliary cirrhosis using a disease specific quality of life measure. J Hepatol. 2006;44(4):776–83. PubMed PMID: 16487619.
33. Jones DE, Bhala N, Burt J, Goldblatt J, Prince M, Newton JL. Four year follow up of fatigue in a geographically defined primary biliary cirrhosis patient cohort. Gut. 2006;55(4):536–41. PubMed PMID: 16299032.

34. Jones DE, Bhala N, Newton JL. Reflections on therapeutic trials in primary biliary cirrhosis: a quality of life oriented counter-view. Hepatology. 2006;43(3):633; author reply 4. PubMed PMID: 16496315.
35. Newton JL, Gibson GJ, Tomlinson M, Wilton K, Jones D. Fatigue in primary biliary cirrhosis is associated with excessive daytime somnolence. Hepatology. 2006;44(1):91–8. PubMed PMID: 16800007.
36. Stanca CM, Bach N, Krause C, Tandon N, Freni MA, Gutierrez JA, et al. Evaluation of fatigue in U.S. patients with primary biliary cirrhosis. Am J Gastroenterol. 2005;100(5): 1104–9. PubMed PMID: 15842585.
37. Prince MI, James OF, Holland NP, Jones DE. Validation of a fatigue impact score in primary biliary cirrhosis: towards a standard for clinical and trial use. J Hepatol. 2000;32(3):368–73. PubMed PMID: 10735604.
38. Bjornsson E, Kalaitzakis E, Neuhauser M, Enders F, Maetzel H, Chapman RW, et al. Fatigue measurements in patients with primary biliary cirrhosis and the risk of mortality during follow-up. Liver Int. 2010;30(2):251–8. PubMed PMID: 19922590.
39. Jones DE, Al-Rifai A, Frith J, Patanwala I, Newton JL. The independent effects of fatigue and UDCA therapy on mortality in primary biliary cirrhosis: results of a 9 year follow-up. J Hepatol. 2010;53(5):911–7. PubMed PMID: 20800924.
40. Zein CO, McCullough AJ. Association between fatigue and decreased survival in primary biliary cirrhosis. Gut. 2007;56(8):1165–6; author reply 6. PubMed PMID: 17625151. Pubmed Central PMCID: 1955491.
41. Crowe J, Christensen E, Doniach D, Popper H, Tygstrup N, Williams R. Early features of primary biliary cirrhosis: an analysis of 85 patients. Am J Gastroenterol. 1985;80(6):466–8. PubMed PMID: 4003376.
42. Lindor K. Ursodeoxycholic acid for the treatment of primary biliary cirrhosis. N Engl J Med. 2007;357(15):1524–9. PubMed PMID: 17928600.
43. Menon KV, Angulo P, Weston S, Dickson ER, Lindor KD. Bone disease in primary biliary cirrhosis: independent indicators and rate of progression. J Hepatol. 2001;35(3):316–23. PubMed PMID: 11592591.
44. Zein CO, Jorgensen RA, Clarke B, Wenger DE, Keach JC, Angulo P, et al. Alendronate improves bone mineral density in primary biliary cirrhosis: a randomized placebo-controlled trial. Hepatology. 2005;42(4):762–71. PubMed PMID: 16175618.
45. Treeprasertsuk S, Silveira MG, Petz JL, Lindor KD. Parenteral bisphosphonates for osteoporosis in patients with primary biliary cirrhosis. Am J Ther. 2011;18(5):375–81. PubMed PMID: 20460985.
46. Guanabens N, Monegal A, Cerda D, Muxi A, Gifre L, Peris P, et al. A randomized trial comparing monthly ibandronate and weekly alendronate for osteoporosis in patients with primary biliary cirrhosis. Hepatology. 2013;58(6):2070–8. PubMed PMID: 23686738.
47. Tsianos EV, Hoofnagle JH, Fox PC, Alspaugh M, Jones EA, Schafer DF, et al. Sjogren's syndrome in patients with primary biliary cirrhosis. Hepatology. 1990;11(5):730–4. PMID: 2347546.
48. Culp KS, Fleming CR, Duffy J, Baldus WP, Dickson ER. Autoimmune associations in primary biliary cirrhosis. Mayo Clin Proc. 1982;57(6):365–70. PubMed PMID: 6896227.
49. Rigamonti C, Shand LM, Feudjo M, Bunn CC, Black CM, Denton CP, et al. Clinical features and prognosis of primary biliary cirrhosis associated with systemic sclerosis. Gut. 2006;55(3):388–94. PubMed PMID: 16150855; Pubmed Central PMCID: 1856066.
50. Gershwin ME, Mackay IR, Sturgess A, Coppel RL. Identification and specificity of a cDNA encoding the 70 kd mitochondrial antigen recognized in primary biliary cirrhosis. J Immunol. 1987;138(10):3525–31. PubMed PMID: 3571977.
51. Miyakawa H, Tanaka A, Kikuchi K, Matsushita M, Kitazawa E, Kawaguchi N, et al. Detection of antimitochondrial autoantibodies in immunofluorescent AMA-negative patients with primary biliary cirrhosis using recombinant autoantigens. Hepatology. 2001;34(2):243–8. PubMed PMID: 11481607. English.

52. Czaja AJ, Norman GL. Autoantibodies in the diagnosis and management of liver disease. J Clin Gastroenterol. 2003;37(4):315–29. PubMed PMID: 14506390.
53. Czaja AJ, Homburger HA. Autoantibodies in liver disease. Gastroenterology. 2001;120(1):239–49. PubMed PMID: 11208733.
54. Invernizzi P, Selmi C, Ranftler C, Podda M, Wesierska-Gadek J. Antinuclear antibodies in primary biliary cirrhosis. Semin Liver Dis. 2005;25(3):298–310. PubMed PMID: 16143945.
55. Janka C, Selmi C, Gershwin ME, Will H, Sternsdorf T. Small ubiquitin-related modifiers: a novel and independent class of autoantigens in primary biliary cirrhosis. Hepatology. 2005;41(3):609–16. PubMed PMID: 15726652.
56. Zuchner D, Sternsdorf T, Szostecki C, Heathcote EJ, Cauch-Dudek K, Will H. Prevalence, kinetics, and therapeutic modulation of autoantibodies against Sp100 and promyelocytic leukemia protein in a large cohort of patients with primary biliary cirrhosis. Hepatology. 1997;26(5):1123–30. PubMed PMID: 9362351. English.
57. Nakamura M, Kondo H, Mori T, Komori A, Matsuyama M, Ito M, et al. Anti-gp210 and anti-centromere antibodies are different risk factors for the progression of primary biliary cirrhosis. Hepatology. 2007;45(1):118–27. PubMed PMID: 17187436. English.
58. Scheuer PJ. Ludwig symposium on biliary disorders—Part II. Pathologic features and evolution of primary biliary cirrhosis and primary sclerosing cholangitis. Mayo Clin Proc. 1998;73(2):179–83. PubMed PMID: 9473003.
59. Rubin E, Schaffner F, Popper H. Primary biliary cirrhosis. Chronic non-suppurative destructive cholangitis. Am J Pathol. 1965;46:387–407. PubMed PMID: 14266218.
60. Scheuer P. Primary biliary cirrhosis. Proc R Soc Med. 1967;60(12):1257–60. PubMed PMID: 6066569.
61. Ludwig J, Dickson ER, McDonald GS. Staging of chronic nonsuppurative destructive cholangitis (syndrome of primary biliary cirrhosis). Virchows Arch A Pathol Anat Histol. 1978;379(2):103–12. PubMed PMID: 150690.
62. Zein CO, Angulo P, Lindor KD. When is liver biopsy needed in the diagnosis of primary biliary cirrhosis? Clin Gastroenterol Hepatol. 2003;1(2):89–95. PubMed PMID: 15017500.
63. Heathcote EJ. Management of primary biliary cirrhosis. The American Association for the Study of Liver Diseases practice guidelines. Hepatology. 2000;31(4):1005–13. PubMed PMID: 10733559.
64. Brunt EM, Ramrakhiani S, Cordes BG, Neuschwander-Tetri BA, Janney CG, Bacon BR, et al. Concurrence of histologic features of steatohepatitis with other forms of chronic liver disease. Mod Pathol. 2003;16(1):49–56. PubMed PMID: 12527713. English.
65. Alvarez F, Berg PA, Bianchi FB, Bianchi L, Burroughs AK, Cancado EL, et al. International Autoimmune Hepatitis Group Report: review of criteria for diagnosis of autoimmune hepatitis. J Hepatol. 1999;31(5):929–38. PubMed PMID: 10580593.
66. Silveira MG, Talwalkar JA, Angulo P, Lindor KD. Overlap of autoimmune hepatitis and primary biliary cirrhosis: long-term outcomes. Am J Gastroenterol. 2007;102(6):1244–50. PubMed PMID: 17319931. English.
67. Corpechot C, Carrat F, Poupon R, Poupon RE. Primary biliary cirrhosis: incidence and predictive factors of cirrhosis development in ursodiol-treated patients. Gastroenterology. 2002;122(3):652–8. PubMed PMID: 11874998. English.
68. Vleggaar FP, van Buuren HR, Zondervan PE, ten Kate FJ, Hop WC. Jaundice in non-cirrhotic primary biliary cirrhosis: the premature ductopenic variant. Gut. 2001;49(2):276–81. PubMed PMID: 11454806. English.
69. Silveira MG, Suzuki A, Lindor KD. Surveillance for hepatocellular carcinoma in patients with primary biliary cirrhosis. Hepatology. 2008;48(4):1149–56. PubMed PMID: 18785621.
70. Tomiyama Y, Takenaka K, Kodama T, Kawanaka M, Sasaki K, Nishina S, et al. Risk factors for survival and the development of hepatocellular carcinoma in patients with primary biliary cirrhosis. Intern Med. 2013;52(14):1553–9. PubMed PMID: 23857086.
71. Metcalf JV, Mitchison HC, Palmer JM, Jones DE, Bassendine MF, James OF. Natural history of early primary biliary cirrhosis. Lancet. 1996;348(9039):1399–402. PubMed PMID: 8937278. English.

72. Springer J, Cauch-Dudek K, O'Rourke K, Wanless IR, Heathcote EJ. Asymptomatic primary biliary cirrhosis: a study of its natural history and prognosis. Am J Gastroenterol. 1999;94(1):47–53. PubMed PMID: 9934730. English.
73. Pasha TM, Dickson ER. Survival algorithms and outcome analysis in primary biliary cirrhosis. Semin Liver Dis. 1997;17(2):147–58. PubMed PMID: 9170202.
74. Shapiro JM, Smith H, Schaffner F. Serum bilirubin: a prognostic factor in primary biliary cirrhosis. Gut. 1979;20(2):137–40. PubMed PMID: 428825; Pubmed Central PMCID: 1419455.
75. Angulo P, Lindor KD, Therneau TM, Jorgensen RA, Malinchoc M, Kamath PS, et al. Utilization of the Mayo risk score in patients with primary biliary cirrhosis receiving ursodeoxycholic acid. Liver. 1999;19(2):115–21. PubMed PMID: 10220741.
76. Pares A, Caballeria L, Rodes J. Excellent long-term survival in patients with primary biliary cirrhosis and biochemical response to ursodeoxycholic Acid. Gastroenterology. 2006;130(3):715–20. PubMed PMID: 16530513.
77. Corpechot C, Abenavoli L, Rabahi N, Chretien Y, Andreani T, Johanet C, et al. Biochemical response to ursodeoxycholic acid and long-term prognosis in primary biliary cirrhosis. Hepatology. 2008;48(3):871–7. PubMed PMID: 18752324. English.
78. Kuiper EM, Hansen BE, de Vries RA, den Ouden-Muller JW, van Ditzhuijsen TJ, Haagsma EB, et al. Improved prognosis of patients with primary biliary cirrhosis that have a biochemical response to ursodeoxycholic acid. Gastroenterology. 2009;136(4):1281–7. PubMed PMID: 19208346. English.
79. Dickson ER, Grambsch PM, Fleming TR, Fisher LD, Langworthy A. Prognosis in primary biliary cirrhosis: model for decision making. Hepatology. 1989;10(1):1–7. PubMed PMID: 2737595.
80. Huet PM, Vincent C, Deslaurier J, Cote J, Matsutami S, Boileau R, et al. Portal hypertension and primary biliary cirrhosis: effect of long-term ursodeoxycholic acid treatment. Gastroenterology. 2008;135(5):1552–60. PubMed PMID: 18722374. English.
81. Mayo MJ, Parkes J, Adams-Huet B, Combes B, Mills AS, Markin RS, et al. Prediction of clinical outcomes in primary biliary cirrhosis by serum enhanced liver fibrosis assay. Hepatology. 2008;48(5):1549–57. PubMed PMID: 18846542. English.
82. Christensen E, Neuberger J, Crowe J, Altman DG, Popper H, Portmann B, et al. Beneficial effect of azathioprine and prediction of prognosis in primary biliary cirrhosis. Final results of an international trial. Gastroenterology. 1985;89(5):1084–91. PubMed PMID: 3899841.
83. Rydning A, Schrumpf E, Abdelnoor M, Elgjo K, Jenssen E. Factors of prognostic importance in primary biliary cirrhosis. Scand J Gastroenterol. 1990;25(2):119–26. PubMed PMID: 2305209. English.
84. Markus BH, Dickson ER, Grambsch PM, Fleming TR, Mazzaferro V, Klintmalm GB, et al. Efficiency of liver transplantation in patients with primary biliary cirrhosis. N Engl J Med. 1989;320(26):1709–13. PubMed PMID: 2659986.
85. Krzeski P, Zych W, Kraszewska E, Milewski B, Butruk E, Habior A. Is serum bilirubin concentration the only valid prognostic marker in primary biliary cirrhosis? Hepatology. 1999;30(4):865–9. PubMed PMID: 10498635. English.
86. Bonnand AM, Heathcote EJ, Lindor KD, Poupon RE. Clinical significance of serum bilirubin levels under ursodeoxycholic acid therapy in patients with primary biliary cirrhosis. Hepatology. 1999;29(1):39–43. PubMed PMID: 9862847. English.
87. Poupon R. Ursodeoxycholic acid and bile-acid mimetics as therapeutic agents for cholestatic liver diseases: an overview of their mechanisms of action. Clin Res Hepatol Gastroenterol. 2012;36 Suppl 1:S3–12. PubMed PMID: 23141891.
88. Lindor KD, Gershwin ME, Poupon R, Kaplan M, Bergasa NV, Heathcote EJ. Primary biliary cirrhosis. Hepatology. 2009;50(1):291–308. PubMed PMID: 19554543. English.
89. Poupon R, Chretien Y, Poupon RE, Ballet F, Calmus Y, Darnis F. Is ursodeoxycholic acid an effective treatment for primary biliary cirrhosis? Lancet. 1987;1(8537):834–6. PubMed PMID: 2882236.

90. Lindor KD, Dickson ER, Baldus WP, Jorgensen RA, Ludwig J, Murtaugh PA, et al. Ursodeoxycholic acid in the treatment of primary biliary cirrhosis. Gastroenterology. 1994;106(5):1284–90. PubMed PMID: 8174890.
91. Poupon RE, Balkau B, Eschwege E, Poupon R. A multicenter, controlled trial of ursodiol for the treatment of primary biliary cirrhosis. UDCA-PBC Study Group. N Engl J Med. 1991;324(22):1548–54. PubMed PMID: 1674105.
92. Heathcote EJ, Cauch-Dudek K, Walker V, Bailey RJ, Blendis LM, Ghent CN, et al. The Canadian Multicenter Double-blind Randomized Controlled Trial of ursodeoxycholic acid in primary biliary cirrhosis. Hepatology. 1994;19(5):1149–56. PubMed PMID: 8175136.
93. Combes B, Carithers Jr RL, Maddrey WC, Lin D, McDonald MF, Wheeler DE, et al. A randomized, double-blind, placebo-controlled trial of ursodeoxycholic acid in primary biliary cirrhosis. Hepatology. 1995;22(3):759–66. PubMed PMID: 7657280.
94. Jorgensen R, Angulo P, Dickson ER, Lindor KD. Results of long-term ursodiol treatment for patients with primary biliary cirrhosis. Am J Gastroenterol. 2002;97(10):2647–50. PubMed PMID: 12385454.
95. ter Borg PC, Schalm SW, Hansen BE, van Buuren HR. Prognosis of ursodeoxycholic Acid-treated patients with primary biliary cirrhosis. Results of a 10-yr cohort study involving 297 patients. Am J Gastroenterol. 2006;101(9):2044–50. PubMed PMID: 16848809.
96. Vuoristo M, Farkkila M, Karvonen AL, Leino R, Lehtola J, Makinen J, et al. A placebo-controlled trial of primary biliary cirrhosis treatment with colchicine and ursodeoxycholic acid. Gastroenterology. 1995;108(5):1470–8. PubMed PMID: 7729640.
97. Pares A, Caballeria L, Rodes J, Bruguera M, Rodrigo L, Garcia-Plaza A, et al. Long-term effects of ursodeoxycholic acid in primary biliary cirrhosis: results of a double-blind controlled multicentric trial. UDCA-Cooperative Group from the Spanish Association for the Study of the Liver. J Hepatol. 2000;32(4):561–6. PubMed PMID: 10782903.
98. Zukowski TH, Jorgensen RA, Dickson ER, Lindor KD. Autoimmune conditions associated with primary biliary cirrhosis: response to ursodeoxycholic acid therapy. Am J Gastroenterol. 1998;93(6):958–61. PubMed PMID: 9647028.
99. Lindor KD, Janes CH, Crippin JS, Jorgensen RA, Dickson ER. Bone disease in primary biliary cirrhosis: does ursodeoxycholic acid make a difference? Hepatology. 1995;21(2):389–92. PubMed PMID: 7843710.
100. Lindor KD, Jorgensen RA, Therneau TM, Malinchoc M, Dickson ER. Ursodeoxycholic acid delays the onset of esophageal varices in primary biliary cirrhosis. Mayo Clin Proc. 1997;72(12):1137–40. PubMed PMID: 9413293.
101. Poupon RE, Lindor KD, Cauch-Dudek K, Dickson ER, Poupon R, Heathcote EJ. Combined analysis of randomized controlled trials of ursodeoxycholic acid in primary biliary cirrhosis. Gastroenterology. 1997;113(3):884–90. PubMed PMID: 9287980.
102. Corpechot C, Poupon R. Geotherapeutics of primary biliary cirrhosis: Bright and sunny around the Mediterranean but still cloudy and foggy in the United Kingdom. Hepatology. 2007;46(4):963–5. PubMed PMID: 17894325.
103. Liermann Garcia RF, Evangelista Garcia C, McMaster P, Neuberger J. Transplantation for primary biliary cirrhosis: retrospective analysis of 400 patients in a single center. Hepatology. 2001;33(1):22–7. PubMed PMID: 11124816.
104. Lee J, Belanger A, Friedman S, Bach N. Transplantation among primary biliary cirrhosis patients from 1995 to 2004. Hepatology. 2006;44(S1):A628.
105. Kim WR, Wiesner RH, Poterucha JJ, Therneau TM, Benson JT, Krom RA, et al. Adaptation of the Mayo primary biliary cirrhosis natural history model for application in liver transplant candidates. Liver Transpl. 2000;6(4):489–94. PubMed PMID: 10915173.
106. Lazaridis KN, Talwalkar JA. Clinical epidemiology of primary biliary cirrhosis: incidence, prevalence, and impact of therapy. J Clin Gastroenterol. 2007;41(5):494–500. PubMed PMID: 17450033.
107. Wolfhagen FH, van Hoogstraten HJ, van Buuren HR, van Berge-Henegouwen GP, ten Kate FJ, Hop WC, et al. Triple therapy with ursodeoxycholic acid, prednisone and azathioprine in

primary biliary cirrhosis: a 1-year randomized, placebo-controlled study. J Hepatol. 1998;29(5):736–42. PubMed PMID: 9833911.
108. Leuschner M, Maier KP, Schlichting J, Strahl S, Herrmann G, Dahm HH, et al. Oral budesonide and ursodeoxycholic acid for treatment of primary biliary cirrhosis: results of a prospective double-blind trial. Gastroenterology. 1999;117(4):918–25. PubMed PMID: 10500075.
109. Rautiainen H, Karkkainen P, Karvonen AL, Nurmi H, Pikkarainen P, Nuutinen H, et al. Budesonide combined with UDCA to improve liver histology in primary biliary cirrhosis: a three-year randomized trial. Hepatology. 2005;41(4):747–52. PubMed PMID: 15754377.
110. Ishibashi H, Komori A, Shimoda S, Gershwin ME. Guidelines for therapy of autoimmune liver disease. Semin Liver Dis. 2007;27(2):214–26. PubMed PMID: 17520519.
111. Myers R, Shaheen A, Swain M, Lee S, Cole S, Coffey-Williamson S, et al. Rituximab for primary biliary cirrhosis refractory to ursodeoxycholic acid. Hepatology. 2007;46(S1):550A.
112. Tsuda M, Moritoki Y, Lian ZX, Zhang W, Yoshida K, Wakabayashi K, et al. Biochemical and immunologic effects of rituximab in patients with primary biliary cirrhosis and an incomplete response to ursodeoxycholic acid. Hepatology. 2012;55(2):512–21. PubMed PMID: 22006563.
113. Nakai S, Masaki T, Kurokohchi K, Deguchi A, Nishioka M. Combination therapy of bezafibrate and ursodeoxycholic acid in primary biliary cirrhosis: a preliminary study. Am J Gastroenterol. 2000;95(1):326–7. PubMed PMID: 10638623. English.
114. Kurihara T, Niimi A, Maeda A, Shigemoto M, Yamashita K. Bezafibrate in the treatment of primary biliary cirrhosis: comparison with ursodeoxycholic acid. Am J Gastroenterol. 2000;95(10):2990–2. PubMed PMID: 11051391. English.
115. Kanda T, Yokosuka O, Imazeki F, Saisho H. Bezafibrate treatment: a new medical approach for PBC patients? J Gastroenterol. 2003;38(6):573–8. PubMed PMID: 12825134. English.
116. Levy C, Peter JA, Nelson DR, Keach J, Petz J, Cabrera R, et al. Pilot study: fenofibrate for patients with primary biliary cirrhosis and an incomplete response to ursodeoxycholic acid. Aliment Pharmacol Ther. 2011;33(2):235–42. PubMed PMID: 21083674.
117. Dohmen K, Mizuta T, Nakamuta M, Shimohashi N, Ishibashi H, Yamamoto K. Fenofibrate for patients with asymptomatic primary biliary cirrhosis. World J Gastroenterol. 2004;10(6):894–8. PubMed PMID: 15040040.
118. Mason A, Luketic V, Lindor K, Hirschfield G, Gordon S, Mayo M, et al. Farnesoid-X receptor agonists: a new class of drugs for the treatment of PBC? An international study evaluating the addition of INT-747 to ursodeoxycholic acid. J Hepatol. 2010;52 Suppl 1:S1.
119. Kowdley KV, Jones D, Luketic V, Chapman R, Burroughs A, Hirschfield G, et al. An international study evaluating the farnesoid X receptor agonist obeticholic acid as monotherapy in PBC. J Hepatol. 2011;54 Suppl 1:S28.
120. Neuberger J. Liver transplantation for primary biliary cirrhosis. Autoimmun Rev. 2003;2(1):1–7. PubMed PMID: 12848968. English.
121. Lee J, Belanger A, Doucette JT, Stanca C, Friedman S, Bach N. Transplantation trends in primary biliary cirrhosis. Clin Gastroenterol Hepatol. 2007;5(11):1313–5. PubMed PMID: 17900996.
122. Kuiper EM, Hansen BE, Metselaar HJ, de Man RA, Haagsma EB, van Hoek B, et al. Trends in liver transplantation for primary biliary cirrhosis in the Netherlands 1988-2008. BMC Gastroenterol. 2010;10:144. PubMed PMID: 21172005; Pubmed Central PMCID: 3020176.
123. Kim WR, Wiesner RH, Therneau TM, Poterucha JJ, Porayko MK, Evans RW, et al. Optimal timing of liver transplantation for primary biliary cirrhosis. Hepatology. 1998;28(1):33–8. PubMed PMID: 9657093. English.
124. Neuberger J. Liver transplantation for primary biliary cirrhosis: indications and risk of recurrence. J Hepatol. 2003;39(2):142–8. PubMed PMID: 12873808. English.
125. Abu-Elmagd K, Demetris J, Rakela J, et al. Transplantation for primary biliary cirrhosis: disease recurrence and outcome in 421 patients. Hepatology. 1997;26:176A.
126. Sebagh M, Farges O, Dubel L, Samuel D, Bismuth H, Reynes M. Histological features predictive of recurrence of primary biliary cirrhosis after liver transplantation. Transplantation. 1998;65(10):1328–33. PubMed PMID: 9625014.

127. Sanchez EQ, Levy MF, Goldstein RM, Fasola CG, Tillery GW, Netto GJ, et al. The changing clinical presentation of recurrent primary biliary cirrhosis after liver transplantation. Transplantation. 2003;76(11):1583–8. PubMed PMID: 14702528.
128. Khettry U, Anand N, Faul PN, Lewis WD, Pomfret EA, Pomposelli J, et al. Liver transplantation for primary biliary cirrhosis: a long-term pathologic study. Liver Transpl. 2003;9(1):87–96. PubMed PMID: 12514778.
129. Levitsky J, Hart J, Cohen SM, Te HS. The effect of immunosuppressive regimens on the recurrence of primary biliary cirrhosis after liver transplantation. Liver Transpl. 2003; 9(7):733–6. PMID: 12827561.
130. Charatcharoenwitthaya P, Pimentel S, Talwalkar JA, Enders FT, Lindor KD, Krom RA, et al. Long-term survival and impact of ursodeoxycholic acid treatment for recurrent primary biliary cirrhosis after liver transplantation. Liver Transpl. 2007;13(9):1236–45. PubMed PMID: 17763401.
131. Jacob DA, Bahra M, Schmidt SC, Schumacher G, Weimann A, Neuhaus P, et al. Mayo risk score for primary biliary cirrhosis: a useful tool for the prediction of course after liver transplantation? Ann Transplant. 2008;13(3):35–42. PubMed PMID: 18806733. English.
132. Jacob DA, Neumann UP, Bahra M, Klupp J, Puhl G, Neuhaus R, et al. Long-term follow-up after recurrence of primary biliary cirrhosis after liver transplantation in 100 patients. Clin Transplant. 2006;20(2):211–20. PubMed PMID: 16640529.
133. Manousou P, Arvaniti V, Tsochatzis E, Isgro G, Jones K, Shirling G, et al. Primary biliary cirrhosis after liver transplantation: influence of immunosuppression and HLA locus disparity. Liver Transpl. 2010;16(1):64–73. PubMed PMID: 19866449. English.
134. Kumagi T, Guindi M, Fischer SE, Arenovich T, Abdalian R, Coltescu C, et al. Baseline ductopenia and treatment response predict long-term histological progression in primary biliary cirrhosis. Am J Gastroenterol. 2010;105(10):2186–94. PubMed PMID: 20502446.
135. Momah N, Silveira MG, Jorgensen R, Sinakos E, Lindor KD. Optimizing biochemical markers as endpoints for clinical trials in primary biliary cirrhosis. Liver Int. 2012;32(5):790–5. PubMed PMID: 22136310.

Chapter 4
Primary Sclerosing Cholangitis

Meredith Borman and Bertus Eksteen

Introduction

Primary sclerosing cholangitis (PSC) is a chronic immune-mediated cholestatic liver disease of unknown aetiology that results in progressive fibro-stenotic strictures of the entire biliary tree leading eventually to liver cirrhosis and end stage liver disease. PSC stands out amongst other forms of liver disease due to its close association with inflammatory bowel disease (IBD). It is clear that between 2.5 and 7.5 % of individuals with inflammatory bowel disease will eventually develop PSC and conversely between 60 and 70 % of patients with PSC will develop inflammatory bowel disease. This association is discontinuous as PSC can arise many years after initial diagnosis of IBD or even in some instances, after a curative colectomy for ulcerative colitis has been performed. It is also well recognised that IBD can arise de novo after a successful liver transplant for PSC, thus suggesting a very close relationship and shared pathogenesis between PSC and IBD [1, 2].

PSC used to be regarded as an exceedingly rare disease after its first description by Delbet in France in 1924 as an irregular fibrotic and stenotic disease of the biliary tree. Until the introduction of endoscopic cholangiography in the second half of the 1970s, there were less than 100 cases reported in the Western literature. As the awareness of PSC has grown, combined with non-invasive means of imaging the biliary tree, it has become clear that PSC is not a rare disease and accounts for roughly 10 % of all liver transplants performed each year. PSC remains an orphan disease for which there is yet

M. Borman, M.D., Ph.D., F.R.C.P.C.
Snyder Institute for Chronic Diseases, University of Calgary, Calgary, AB, Canada

Division of Hepatology and Gastroenterology, University of Calgary, Calgary, AB, Canada

B. Eksteen, M.B.Ch.B., Ph.D., F.R.C.P. (✉)
Snyder Institute for Chronic Diseases, Division of Hepatology and Gastroenterology,
University of Calgary, 4AC66 HRIC, 3280 Hospital Drive NW, Calgary,
AB, Canada T2N 4N1
e-mail: b.eksteen@ucalgary.ca

E.J. Carey and K.D. Lindor (eds.), *Cholestatic Liver Disease*, Clinical Gastroenterology,
DOI 10.1007/978-1-4939-1013-7_4, © Springer Science+Business Media New York 2014

no effective treatment apart from liver transplantation which provides a temporary solution as this disease often recurs subsequently. Throughout the Western world, there has been an increase in inflammatory bowel disease as well as in the emerging economies. This also led to similar increases in the incidence of PSC globally. The clinical presentation of PSC has evolved through time from a largely fibrotic cholestatic disease to often milder phenotypes associated with modest liver inflammation in the setting of IBD. This heterogeneity in presentation is reflected in recent work that has defined multiple pathways as defined by disease susceptibility genes. Further complexity arises from the fact that PSC carries an excess risk of cholangiocarcinoma and colorectal carcinoma which appears to be unrelated to the severity or stage of the disease. The advent of widespread genome-wide association studies and gene expression arrays have increased our ability to understand the fundamental processes that underpin this difficult to treat disease and to develop rational therapies.

Epidemiology

PSC predominantly affects males with a median presentation in the third and fourth decades of life. Sufferers of PSC are almost universally non-smokers and not associated with lower economic status. Although traditionally, the male to female ratio has been in the order of 7:1, this has evolved with the most recent studies suggesting a 2:1 ratio. This is reflective of the evolution of IBD which has also seen an increase in female sufferers. It is also clear that PSC has a specific presentation in children and young adults as well as a delayed phenotype of mild non-progressive disease beyond the sixth decade of life. The exact incidence of PSC is largely unknown and is extrapolated from IBD data. A systematic review reports significant variation geographically with a mean incidence of 1.3 per 100,000 patient years. However, in some populations, this is reported to be as high as seven cases per 100,000 population. This variation is reflective of the variation in ulcerative colitis, the incidence of which similarly ranges from 40 to 225 cases per 100,000 population. This is likely an underestimation as there is a significant association between PSC and Crohn's disease as well as a failure to capture PSC as a diagnosis in administrative databases because of a lack of a specific disease code [3]. The prevalence of PSC ranges from 16.2 per 100,000 to 20.9 per 100,000 in Western populations. It is likely that both the incidence and prevalence of PSC is grossly underestimated as PSC can present as a subclinical disease with normal liver tests, thus avoiding diagnosis and in 20–30 % of individuals will not occur with coexisting IBD. Another confounding factor is the availability of biliary imaging and variability in local protocols to assess newly diagnosed inflammatory bowel disease patients for coexisting PSC. The majority of the published data in PSC related to Northern European and North American populations. However, it is clear that Southern European and Asian populations suffer with less coexisting IBD (approximately 30–50 %) and that the ratio of ulcerative colitis to Crohn's colitis varies significantly. Initial reports suggest that over 90 % of IBD in PSC consisted of ulcerative colitis. However, most recent reports suggest that Crohn's colitis now accounts for 1/3 of the IBD in PSC patients [4, 5].

Clinical Presentation

PSC represents a syndrome with great variation in clinical phenotypes with divergent outcomes. Traditional large duct PSC typically presents in men between the ages of 25 and 45 with symptoms of cholestasis (jaundice, pruritis) or acute bacterial cholangitis (jaundice, fever, rigours). This represents a progressive disease with increasing biliary stricture formation, recurrent bacterial cholangitis and eventually biliary cirrhosis leading to end stage liver disease over a mean period of 11–13 years. Typically during this period, these individuals will suffer from a pancolitis (both ulcerative colitis and Crohn's colitis) that typically has an indolent cause with predominantly right colonic inflammation. Both cholangiocarcinoma and colorectal cancer are increased in these individuals and require annual surveillance. A proportion of PSC patients will present with a small duct variant. These individuals typically have elevations in their alkaline phosphatase and GGT without biliary changes as defined by ERCP or MRCP. A liver biopsy is usually diagnostic in these individuals and demonstrates a pericholangitis with portal inflammation and concentric fibrosis surrounding the biliary tree. The incidence of coexisting IBD is less in this subtype. The long-term outlook is significantly better when compared to traditional large duct PSC as less than 20 % of these individuals will eventually progress to the large duct variant and ultimately end stage liver disease (Fig. 4.1). PSC can present in childhood with end stage liver disease by age 6 and a requirement for liver transplantation before age 8. In these cases, the IBD is often severe and leads to early colectomy. PSC in teenagers and young adults often starts as an autoimmune hepatitis with features of autoimmune pericholangitis. In these cases, the external

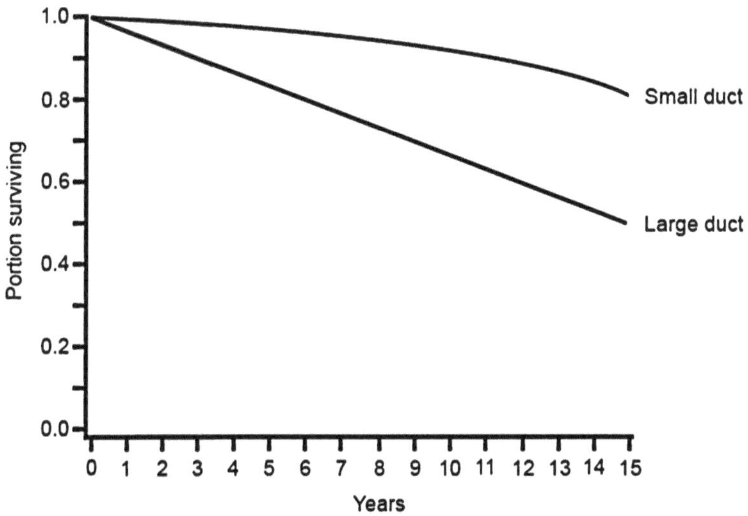

Fig. 4.1 Survival in patients with small-duct and large-duct PSC. Survival free of liver transplantation is significantly longer in patients with small-duct PSC. Modified from Bjornsson et al. Gastroenterology 2008;134(4)

biliary tree is often spared and disease remission is achieved with standard immunosuppressive drugs. However, as these individuals progress to their 20s, the elements of autoimmune hepatitis and responsiveness to immunosuppressive drugs are often lost and an evolution is seen towards a typical large duct PSC variant with progressive liver disease and biliary fibrosis. PSC can also exist in isolation without coexisting IBD and be diagnosed in individuals beyond their sixth decade of life. In these elderly individuals, the disease often has a large duct phenotype but appears to be non-progressive with very few developing symptomatic liver disease [1, 6].

Extended PSC Phenotypes and Associated Syndromes

Autoimmune Hepatitis Overlap Syndromes

Two to four percentage of individuals with PSC will suffer from coexisting autoimmune hepatitis, termed as a PSC–autoimmune hepatitis overlap syndrome. Unlike individuals with isolated PSC, these individuals will fulfil the criteria for autoimmune hepatitis diagnosis. These individuals typically have transaminase levels greater than five times the upper limit of normal, IgG levels 1.5–2 times the upper limit of normal, high titre antibodies (antinuclear antibodies, anti-smooth muscle antibodies) and on liver biopsy demonstrate an excess of plasma cell infiltration with interface hepatitis. This should be treated by standard immunosuppressive therapies for autoimmune hepatitis such as induction with corticosteroids and maintenance with azathioprine or mycophenolate mofetil. However, unlike isolated autoimmune hepatitis, these individuals never normalise transaminase levels completely which is indicative of underlying PSC. Therefore, the treatment aim should be normalisation of IgG levels and an improvement of interface hepatitis on liver biopsy. This overlap of PSC would be distinct from the variant syndromes that are seen in paediatric populations where autoimmune sclerosing cholangitis (ASC) and autoimmune hepatitis are associated with significantly better outcomes when compared to PSC. This is in contrast to adult populations where PSC–autoimmune hepatitis is associated with accelerated disease, and earlier need for transplantation and higher rates of recurrent disease post-liver transplantation [7].

IgG4 Disease

A proportion of individuals will present with features consistent with PSC and extensive biliary changes; however, they will suffer from a closely related condition termed IgG4 related disease which is a distinct entity characterised by dense lymphoplasmacytic infiltrates that are rich in IgG positive plasma cells. This disease can affect virtually every organ system and lead to intense fibrosis, autoimmune destruction and at times, the formation of inflammatory pseudotumours that can mimic cholangiocarcinoma. Individuals with IgG4 disease typically suffer not only from biliary disease but often autoimmune pancreatitis which often dominates their

Table 4.1 Classification of sclerosing cholangitis

Primary sclerosing cholangitis
Small duct disease
Large duct disease
Autoimmune cholangiopathy
Overlap syndromes
PSC/AIH
PSC/PBC
Secondary sclerosing cholangitis
Choledocholithiasis
HIV
Recurrent pygenic cholangitis
Caroli's disease
Cholangiocarcinoma
Autoimmune pancreatitis
Biliary trauma
Ischemia
Primary immune deficiency (CD40 ligand deficiency)
IgG4 disease

presentation and a relative absence of coexisting IBD although some cases have been reported. Infiltration with IgG4-secreting plasma cells is pathognomonic of this disease, and it can occur not only in the biliary tree and pancreas but also in the salivary glands, periorbital tissues, kidneys, lungs, lymph nodes, meninges, aorta, breast, prostate, thyroid, pericardium and the skin and has some similarity to sarcoidosis and its disease distribution. Although this disease can present with multiple liver masses and biliary changes suggestive of cholangiocarcinoma, these are mostly inflammatory pseudotumours that respond and disappear with immunosuppressive therapies. The mainstay of treatment for this disease is immunosuppression with corticosteroids and azathioprine with a high risk of relapse when discontinued [8].

Secondary Causes of Sclerosing Cholangitis

The biliary tree is limited in its ability to respond to dithering insults and as such, a wide range of diseases affecting the biliary tree can lead to cholestasis and eventual fibrostenotic changes (Table 4.1). All of these diseases can have typical radiological changes associated with PSC and include recurrent gallstone disease, congenital ductal plate malformations such as Caroli's disease, biliary tract trauma following cholecystectomy, cholangiocarcinoma, recurrent bacterial biliary infection, AIDS related cholangiopathy secondary to Cryptosporidium infection, portal vein thrombosis with portal venous cholangiopathy, hepatic arterial insufficiency with biliary structuring, immunodeficiency (most notably X-linked Hyper IgM syndrome) with recurrent Cryptosporidium infection and progressive cholangiopathy and associated cholangiocarcinoma. In addition to these causes, direct drug-induced effects and prolonged intensive care unit stay has also been associated with biliary stricturing as have a variety of micro-organisms which include HIV and cytomegalovirus [9].

Table 4.2 Frequency of autoimmune diseases associated with PSC

Autoimmune disease	%
Inflammatory bowel disease (IBD)	
Ulcerative colitis	58
Crohn's disease	11
Indeterminate IBD	3
Thyroid disease	6.1
Type 1 diabetes	2.6
Rheumatoid arthritis	2.5
Celiac disease	1.9
Psoriasis	1.7
Sarcoidosis	1.4
Sacroiliitis	0.7
Sjögren's	0.4
Other	2.2

Modified from Liu et al. Nature Genetics 2013;45(6)

Associated Autoimmune Diseases

Up to 20 % of patients with PSC will suffer with autoimmune diseases other than IBD. A recent study found significant association with coeliac disease, psoriasis, rheumatoid arthritis, sarcoidosis, sacroiliitis, Sjogren's syndrome, type 1 diabetes and thyroid disease. This data is summarised in Table 4.2. The mere presence of these diseases is associated with increased mortality in patients with PSC. IBD is however the most dominant associated disease which occurs in roughly 70 % of PSC sufferers at a ratio of 6:1 ulcerative colitis to Crohn's disease. IBD in PSC often precedes the diagnosis of PSC by a mean of 10–14 years and typically presents as a pancolitis. This can be asymptomatic with relative rectal sparing and predominantly right-sided inflammation. PSC-IBD has an increase in backwash ileitis but isolated small bowel IBD is uncommon [10]. A proportion of individuals with PSC will proceed to end stage liver disease and liver transplant only to develop de novo IBD following transplantation. This disease can often be aggressive and unresponsive to immunosuppressive drugs as it already occurs in the presence of potent immunosuppressive drugs required for the liver allograft. Thirty percentage of individuals with PSC appear not to suffer from IBD. It is unclear whether these individuals truly have no gut inflammation or whether this is a failure to detect subclinical inflammation by standard means as virtually all PSC patients will describe some degree of changes in their bowel habit and diarrhoea at some stage. Surgery for IBD in PSC is complicated by higher than expected rates of pouchitis when compared to patients with IBD alone. The rates of pouchitis in this population vary tremendously from 60 % to almost 100 % in some case series. There is accumulation of risk at 1, 2, 5 and 10 years following ileal pouch anal anastomosis of 22, 43, 61 and 79 % respectively for patients with PSC. Pouchitis in the setting of PSC is associated with poorer treatment responses compared to individuals without PSC and higher rate of subsequent pouch removal [11].

Pathogenesis of PSC

The aetiology of PSC is unknown. Similar to IBD, it is likely that PSC occurs in genetically susceptible individuals in response to an environmental factor, possibly their own gut microbiota that also triggers IBD. A proportion of these IBD patients will have additional genetic or possibly immunological alterations which leaves their livers susceptible to inappropriate inflammation and subsequent development of PSC. Several mechanisms that could contribute to such a model have been proposed and are summarised below [9].

Environmental Risk Factors

There is very little data on environmental risk factors for PSC. Possibly the strongest data is a negative association with cigarette smoking. In one study of 184 patients with PSC and age/sex matched controls, only 4.9 % of PSC cases smoked compared to 26.1 % of controls. 69.65 % had never smoked compared to 46.7 % of controls. These differences have since been replicated and although the absolute smoking percentages vary based on the population prevalence of smoking, these striking differences between PSC and controls remains. Some data would suggest that those with PSC that have smoked but subsequently stopped have a later onset of disease.

Less pronounced but equally significant is the negative association with coffee consumption. Seventy-six percentage of PSC cases versus 86 % of population controls (odds ratio 0.52) consumed coffee by age 18. These effects were largely restricted to male patients. Female patients with PSC reported less use of hormonal contraception use than controls. This potential interaction with female sex hormones is further underlined by the observation that female patients with multiple pregnancies develop PSC at a later age [12].

Genetics

The majority of the genetic susceptibility to PSC is strongly clustered to chromosome 6 and the human leukocyte antigen (HLA) complex. The first association with this HLA complex was reported in 1982 where it was shown that HLA-B8 and HLA-DR3 were found in 80 % of patients with PSC and ulcerative colitis. The association with HLA-B8 was subsequently replicated in a further cohort where 60 % of PSC patients compared to 25 % in controls carried this risk allele. This provided the first evidence of a heritable component to PSC which was subsequently confirmed in a Swedish study of 678 PSC patients and 6,347 healthy controls which demonstrated a substantially increased risk of PSC in first-degree relatives of PSC

Table 4.3 HLA haplotypes associated with PSC. Multiple HLA haplotypes carry a risk of PSC while others afford protection

PSC risk loci
B*08:01
DRB1*03:01-DQA1*05:01-DQB1*02:01
DRB1*13:01-DQA1*01:03-DQB1*06:03
DRB1*15:01-DQA1*01:02-DQB1*06:02
DRB1*01:01-DQA1*01:01
Protective
DRB4*01:03-DRB1*04:01-DQA1*03-DQB1*03:02
DRB4*01:03-DRB1*07:01-DQA1*02:01-DQB1*03:03
DRB4*02:02-DRB1*11:01-DQA1*05:01-DQB1*03:01
MICA*002

patients with hazard ratios of 11.5 for the offspring. Despite this compelling data, familial patterns of PSC inheritance remain rare with only five patients in this cohort having first degree relatives with PSC (3.4 %). Thus the prevalence of PSC amongst first-degree relatives was 0.7 % with a prevalence in siblings of 1.5 %.

Genetic studies in PSC have largely focused on risk alleles that increase genetic susceptibility to the disease and have expanded the HLA haplotypes associated with PSC. The initial haplotype associated with PSC were B8, DR3 and D2 as well as A1, B8 and DR3. This was expanded to include HLA-DRW52A (DRB3*0101) which has an association with PSC between 55 and 100 % depending on the cohort. Subsequently, DR6 was added as a risk haplotype and strong association reported with DRB1*1301, DQA1*1301 and DQB1*0603. Much of the difficulty in deciphering the HLA has come from the relative homogenous genetic background of the study populations which in most studies only include Caucasians from Scandinavia and North Western Europe. The recent Immunochip experiment in PSC sequenced 3,789 PSC cases using a high resolution SNP chip. This experiment replicated the previous HLA alleles and demonstrated that the majority of PSC risk resides in HLA-B and HLA-DRB1. The study showed strong linkage disequilibrium with the HLA-B*08:01 haplotype which is part of the ancestral HLAB*08:01-DRB1*03:01 haplotype (AH8.1) which is an ancestral haplotype associated with multiple autoimmune diseases. This study added HLA-B*08:01, HLA-DQA*01:03, HLA-DQA*05:01, DRB1*15:01 and DQA*01:01 to the current list of risk haplotypes for PSC. It is clear that certain HLA haplotypes carry a risk of PSC whereas others afford protection to this disease and is summarised in Table 4.3 [13, 14].

The relationship between the HLA and disease cause has been explored with HLA-DR52A, patients reportedly developing more severe disease and earlier mortality. Similarly, HLA-DR4, DR3, DQ2 heterozygosity has been associated with rapidly progressive disease. Much more work is needed to decipher the HLA complex in PSC and also the potential association with disease progression. This is, however, a key element of PSC as the HLA class 1 and class 2 genes determine the ability of the immune system to recognise both self and non-self antigens and could be a critical part in understanding potential antigens that drive PSC.

Table 4.4 PSC susceptibility genes

Chromosome	Lead SNP	Risk allele	Common allele	Nearby gene loci
1	rs3748816	A	C	MMEL1, TNFRSF14
2	rs6720394	G	A	BCL2L11
2	rs7426056	A	C	CD28
2	rs3749171	A	G	GPR35
3	rs3197999	A	C	MST1
4	rs13140464	C	T	IL2, IL21
6	rs56258221	G	A	BACH2
10	rs4147359	A	C	IL2RA
11	rs7937682	G	T	SIK2
12	rs11168249	G	T	HDAC7
12	rs3184504	A	G	SH2B3, ATXN2
18	rs1788097	A	G	CD226
18	rs1452787	G	A	TCF4
19	rs60652743	A	G	PRKD2, STRN4
21	rs2836883	G	T	PSMG1

Modified from Liu et al. Nature Genetics 2013;45(6), and Karlsen et al. Nature Genetics 2013;45(6)

Non-HLA Risk Loci

Genome-wide association studies have defined 15 non-HLA risk loci for PSC which are summarised in Table 4.4 and demonstrate significant overlap with other autoimmune diseases including ulcerative colitis, Crohn's disease, coeliac disease, type 1 diabetes, sarcoidosis, psoriasis and rheumatoid arthritis. This is hardly surprising given the strength of the HLA association in PSC which is a common feature to other autoimmune diseases as well as the fact that clinically, patients with PSC often suffer with other autoimmune conditions as described above. Much work still need to be done to determine the biological effects of these genetic risk loci [15].

IL-2/IL-2 Receptor α Risk Locus

These risk loci are commonly shared between multiple autoimmune diseases and represents a critical axis involved in activation and programming of the adaptive immune system. Mice deficient in the IL-2 receptor α gene readily developed auto-antibodies and multi-organ autoimmune disease including biliary inflammation that resembles PBC and enterocolitis. Specific studies in PSC to assess the impact of this risk locus are lacking. However, supportive evidence comes from previous studies that demonstrated impaired T-cell responses and reduced levels of IL-2 expression following mitogen stimulation of liver derived lymphocytes from PSC patients. In parallel, decreased expression of IL-2 receptor was observed in these T-cells [15, 16].

FUT-2 Risk Locus

This locus encodes galactoside 2-α-L-fucosyltransferase 2 which is intimately involved in protein glycosylation and includes the ABH blood antigen synthesis as well as the Ca19-9 pathway. The RS601338 polymorphism gives rise to a non-functional truncated FUT-2 enzyme which results in the inability to synthesise ABH antigens on mucosal surfaces and in salivary glands and is commonly referred to as a non-secretor. Similarly FUT2 polymorphisms are associated with different base line levels of Ca19-9 in the serum. FUT-2 locus is shared between PSC and Crohn's disease. The exact role is PSC is not known but appears to alter the mucosal milieu and the composition of commensal bacteria in the biliary tree. FUT-2 homozygous risk allele carriers have reduced biliary proteobacteria and increased populations of firmicutes [17, 18].

Salt-Inducible Kinase (SIK)-2 Risk Locus

The RS79376A2SNP that confers risk for PSC is located in an intron of the SIK-2 gene which encodes salt-inducible kinase-2. This gene is reported to influence both interleukin-10 in macrophages and NUR-77 which functions as an important transcription factor in leukocytes. IL-10 is critical in maintaining immunological tolerance whilst IL-10 deficiency is associated with early onset IBD. Similarly, IL-10 deficient mice developed severe colitis and provided a rationale that led to evaluation of IL-10 as a potential treatment for IBD. In strong linkage disequilibrium with this SNP is RS11168249 which is situated within the HDAC7 gene which encodes histone deacetylase 7. This molecule is implicated in the negative selection of T-cells in the thymus, a critical process in determining the development of central immune tolerance. HDAC7 is likely to play a central role in PSC as it is also linked to an intronic site in the PRKD-2 gene which encodes serine threonine protein kinase D2. PRKD-2 phosphorylates HDAC-7 during T-cell receptor engagement with thymocytes which lead to the exclusion of HDA-7 from the nucleus and eventual negative selection of immature T-cells through apoptosis. The convergence of these three risk alleles to a single T-cell selection pathway suggests that a loss of central tolerance is at least in part involved in the pathogenesis of PSC but does require biological validation [15].

Macrophage Stimulating (MST)-1

MST-1 Is the strongest non-HLA risk locus in PSC with a p value of 2.4×10^{-26} and is a shared locus with ulcerative colitis and Crohn's disease. MST-1 is associated with macrophage differentiation and skews towards M2 (anti-inflammatory) phenotypes. It is also reported to alter leukocyte trafficking by modulating integrin-mediated adhesion and is expressed throughout the liver including the biliary epithelium. The RS3197999 risk locus for PSC predicts a hypofunctional MSP1 (macrophage stimulating protein 1) with reduced receptor affinity and hence could affect PSC either by direct alteration of its function within the liver or by a lack of tolerogenic effects on recruited leukocyte subsets such as macrophages [19].

The majority of risk loci in PSC are shared with other autoimmune diseases. However, BCL2L11, SIK-2, TCF-4 and PRKD-2 appear to be PSC-specific. Much work still remains to be done to fully understand the effects of these genes in the pathogenesis and whether they affect the course of the disease. These are not necessarily the same sets of loci as polymorphism in the MMP2 gene which has recently been linked to PSC progression but does not confer risk for the disease itself. It might well be that different genetic alleles will determine the course of PSC and remains to be investigated.

Immunological Mechanisms in PSC

Auto-antibodies

The most attractive hypothesis for development of PSC is one where the enterohepatic immune system develops cross-reactive immunity to an antigen (auto-antigen or pathogen) in the setting of reduced tolerance which leads to immune-mediated gut and biliary inflammation. This is in part supported by the strong association with the HLA which hints at specific but as of yet undefined antigen recognition in PSC. A consequence of such aberrant immunity would be manifested in the generation of auto-antibodies and T-cell responses, for which there is accumulating evidence. Total IgG levels in PSC patients are often raised, suggestive of an immune-mediated process with most attention being focused on specific antibodies such as anti-neutrophil cytoplasmic antibodies (ANCA).

Positive ANCA serology is found in 42–93 % of patients with PSC and probably relates to heterogeneity in the techniques in measuring this antibody. In comparison to the conventional cytoplasmic ANCA (cANCA) and perinuclear ANCA (pANCA), the main ANCA pattern in PSC (and ulcerative colitis) produces a broad heterogeneous, rim like staining pattern of the nuclear periphery along with multiple intranuclear fluorescence spots that correspond to invaginations of the nuclear envelope. The term, peripheral anti-neutrophil nuclear antibodies has been proposed to describe this atypical pANCA indirect immunofluorescence (IF) pattern. However, IF is a time consuming, observer dependent, low throughput test that requires highly trained personnel and hence some of the variability of ANCA in different populations could be related to these confounders.

To date there has been no correlation between disease activity and individual ANCA antigens. Traditional ANCA targets such as antigen proteinase-3 (PR3) can also be detected in the serum of PSC patients (0–44 %) and is found at similar rates in patients with ulcerative colitis. The pattern of staining is similar to that of Wegener's granulomatosis and small vessel vasculitis. Several antigens have been proposed to account for the very specific staining pattern that is seen in PSC which includes pepsin G, a chymotrypsin like proteinase as well as in the toxin binding protein of polymorphonuclear granulocytes but requires further validation. ANCA titres do not appear to reflect disease activity and it is well recognised that ANCA levels can persist following liver transplantation or panproctocolectomy for ulcerative colitis.

Cellular Immunity

The biliary epithelium not only functions by contributing to bile secretion but is an active participant in liver immunity. Biliary epithelium secretes IgA and expresses multiple pattern recognition receptors such as Toll-like receptors (TLRs) and NOD-like receptors to aid in the detection of pathogen associated molecular patterns such as lipopolysaccharide. In response to infection or inflammation, biliary epithelium secretes pro-inflammatory cytokines such as IL-6, TNFα and IL-1β to drive pro-inflammatory responses. As part of this process, chemokines such as CXCL12, CXCL16, CXCL9 to CXCL11 and CCL20 are secreted to attract pro-inflammatory CD8 T-cells to the liver. Biliary epithelium expresses ICAM-1 and VCAM-1 which furthers contributes to the accumulation of inflammatory leukocytes in the peribiliary space to take part in biliary inflammation in PSC. Although pro-inflammatory CD8 recruitment to the biliary tree dominates during PSC, biliary epithelium also secretes CCL28 which serves as an attractant for immune-regulatory T-cells which express the chemokine receptor CCR10 to try to limit biliary inflammation [20].

The biliary epithelium can shape the pattern of the inflammation by secretion of IL-6 and CCL20 which preferentially attract interleukin 17 producing CD4 cells (Th17) and creates a paracrine loop to expand these pro-inflammatory cells in situ. Expression of VCAM-1 not only helps effector T-cells to adhere to the biliary epithelium and biliary structures but also provides a survival signal to these T-cells to ensure their persistence and thus chronic inflammation. Much of these processes are generic to the biliary epithelium and can be found in related biliary conditions such as PBC [20].

However, what sets PSC apart from other liver diseases is that in addition to these generic pro-inflammatory recruitment pathways to the biliary epithelium, there is aberrant expression of gut-specific adhesion molecules such as the chemokine receptor CCL25 and the integrin ligand, MAdCAM-1. Normally, these molecules are highly restricted to the gut where they drive selective recruitment of gut-specific T- and B-cells which express the CCL25 receptor, CCR9 and the integrin combination, α4β7 which binds to MAdCAM-1. These two molecules are preferentially imprinted on T- and B-cells in mesenteric lymph nodes by CD103 expressing gut dendritic cells under the control of retinoic acid. This provides a mechanism whereby gut dendritic cells that have been exposed to enteric pathogens can program specific T- and B-cells to selectively target the gut. In PSC, this normally closely regulated mechanism of gut tropism becomes aberrant and CD8 T-cells derived from the gut are able to be recruited to the liver and potentially perpetuate biliary inflammation. The opposite is also true in that vascular adhesion protein 1

(VAP-1) is normally expressed in the uninflamed liver and during IBD is rapidly upregulated in the gut, hence providing a mechanism whereby T- and B-cells potentially traffic between the gut and the liver in PSC and IBD. This provides an important rationale how gut and liver inflammation might be linked and provides important adhesion molecule targets that could be exploited as future therapies for individuals with PSC and IBD [21, 22].

Infection as a Cause for PSC

Gut inflammation is associated with increased gut permeability and hence it has been postulated that PSC occurs because of persistent portal venous bacterial translocation. This has, however, not been borne out in several studies that have failed to show significant bacterial populations within the portal venous blood or the liver. A further complicating factor is that gut permeability in IBD is dependent on the severity of the IBD which does not translate to severity of PSC. This makes a direct pathogen translocation theory less likely. This does not, however, exclude the possibility of bacterial products from the gut being involved in PSC nor does it account for potential changes in the gut microbiota which is increasingly being linked with human disease. As described above, the FUT-2 mutation does directly affect the microbiota composition within the biliary tree with similar changes expected in the gut where FUT-2 polymorphisms are also associated with Crohn's disease. IBD is associated with very significant alterations in the gut microbiota with loss of diversity and the emergence of dominant microbial flora.

Similarly, immunodeficiency syndromes can give risc to PSC-like syndromes. Both HIV as well as X-linked hyper IgM syndrome (CD40L deficiency) lead to biliary colonisation with cryptosporidium and a progressive cholangiopathy than can lead to cholangiocarcinoma. These specific defects have not been demonstrated in PSC but might well have accelerated the phenotype as recurrent biliary infections as are seen in chronic gallstone disease also lead to a sclerosing cholangitis type liver picture [9].

Viral infections are yet to be associated with PSC. Cytomegalovirus (CMV) can give rise to severe bile duct destruction and mimic PSC but does not lead to extended fibrosis and large duct disease. The effects on the biliary tree and HIV are thought not to be directly related to the HIV virus but rather persistent cryptosporidium or microsporidial infection of the biliary system.

Fungal infections are often seen in advanced large duct PSC as secondary infections. Evidence for a primary role of fungi in the pathogenesis of the PSC remains controversial. A large proportion of PSC patients will have high levels of anti-saccharomyces cerevisiae antibodies (ASCA). This appears to be independent of the stage of PSC or their IBD phenotype. Biliary cultures in these individuals have so far failed to reliably culture this organism, casting some doubt as its role in the pathogenesis of PSC.

Altered Bile Acid Metabolism

One theory to explain PSC comes from the observation that mice deficient in the MDR2 (ABCB4) gene which is involved in cannulicular phospholipid generation develop a phenotype similar to PSC with intense peribiliary fibrosis. This has led to the hypothesis of toxic bile contributing to the development of PSC. To date, the MDR2 mutation has not been reported in humans with no evidence of polymorphisms in this locus in PSC. It is conceivable that protective mechanisms such as bicarbonate secretion is altered by inflammation or that inflammation leads to dysfunction of biliary transporters which leads to the accumulation of toxic bile acids which in turn directly interact with the cholangiocytes to drive apoptosis, fibrosis and possibly carcinogenesis. This might be a direct effect of bile acid accumulation or a secondary effect due to changes in the gut microbiota which in turn affects the enterohepatic recirculation bile acid. There is no doubt that chronic cholestasis is toxic to the biliary tree whether in advanced PSC or in secondary sclerosing cholangitis due to obstructive cholangiopathy, but evidence for a primary defect to explain PSC remains lacking.

Clinical Presentation

PSC has a wide range of clinical presentations and can affect any individual at any age of life. Practically the majority of patients will be male with peak incidence in the mid to late 30s. Traditionally, these individuals present with an episode of obstructive jaundice with increased bilirubin, pale stools, dark urine and generalised itching. A proportion will present with acute cholangitis, particularly if they suffer with advanced large duct disease with another subgroup presenting with end stage liver failure in the form of decompensated liver disease such as variceal haemorrhage or the new onset of ascites or encephalopathy. This type of presentation is becoming increasingly uncommon as the majority of individuals are now picked up at much earlier stages of disease due to abnormal liver biochemistry as part of the work-up for inflammatory bowel disease or health screening visits. Traditionally, this group of patients will have a high incidence of coexisting inflammatory bowel disease that has often preceded the diagnosis. A proportion of patients will present with persistent right hypochondrial pain that precedes significant cholestasis or liver dysfunction by several years. It is also increasingly common that individuals will be completely asymptomatic and diagnosed with PSC based on incidental MRI or ultrasound findings of abnormal bile ducts at a time when undergoing abdominal imaging for other causes such as IBD. A large proportion of these individuals can have normal liver biochemistry although it is the norm to find an increased alkaline phosphatase in the majority of these cases. As the disease progresses, PSC patients increasingly develop symptoms which are summarised in Table 4.5. Symptoms such as pruritus and jaundice can be largely predicted based on the deterioration of

Table 4.5 Most common symptoms and signs of PSC at time of diagnosis

Symptoms
Fatigue
Abdominal pain
Pruritis
Fever/night sweats
Weight loss
Asymptomatic
Signs
Jaundice
Hepatomegaly
Splenomegaly
Ascites

the external biliary tree as can episodes of ascending cholangitis. Fatigue which is a prominent feature in two-thirds of patients, is however not dependent on disease stage and is often the most disabling symptom [1].

As PSC advances, patients tend to segregate into two main groups. One group will develop severe large duct disease with multiple strictures and recurrent episodes of ascending cholangitis characterised by pain, fever and jaundice. These patients are thought to be at high risk of cholangiocarcinoma. The other group will tend to have mild large duct disease but an increasingly intrahepatic fibrotic phenotype with gradual progression to traditional cirrhosis and eventual liver decompensation. Once progression to cirrhosis has occurred, PSC will have symptoms and signs associated with most other forms of liver disease which include complications of portal hypertension such as ascites, spontaneous bacterial peritonitis, hypersplenism and variceal haemorrhage as well as the development of coagulopathy and hepatic encephalopathy. The presentation of coexisting IBD during this period is highly variable with the majority of individuals suffering a pancolitis which may have features of either an indeterminate colitis, ulcerative colitis or Crohn's colitis. The activities of these diseases are often mild and inconspicuous with predominantly right sided colonic inflammation and a high proportion suffering backwash ileitis. There is often rectal sparing and a significant number of patients will be asymptomatic. This is however not exclusively the case as some individuals will have very active IBD that will require biological treatments to target anti-TNFα. A significant proportion of patients with PSC will present with a small duct variant which predominantly presents with abnormal alkaline phosphatase measurements in the absence of large duct disease as seen by biliary imaging. These individuals are often asymptomatic and diagnosed based purely by chance. The prognosis of small duct PSC is significantly better than large duct PSC with only a small proportion of patients eventually developing large duct disease and progressing to end stage liver cirrhosis.

Apart from the peak incidence in the mid to late 30s, PSC does occur at both ends of the spectrum. A proportion of individuals will present with PSC in their 60s and 70s. These individuals often have mild large duct PSC with low rates of coexisting IBD.

These individuals are very often asymptomatic and few appear to progress to end stage liver disease. These individuals are likely to represent milder phenotype that has probably suffered with mild disease for the majority of their adult life. A particular concern in this cohort of patients is the effect of chronic mild cholestasis on calcium and vitamin D metabolism which inevitably leads to low bone density and places these individuals at a particularly high risk of metabolic bone disease and a risk of fractures in their 60s or 70s.

PSC does occur in children under the age of 10 and certainly in individuals in their teenage years. The majority of these individuals will have active IBD which is often more aggressive than the types of IBD seen in later life. Severe large duct PSC is relatively rare in these young populations as they often present with typical autoimmune hepatitis. Through time their hepatic inflammation appears to switch from mostly a hepatitic phenotype to an autoimmune cholangitis phenotype which is still responsive to immunosuppression. However, in some individuals, this disease eventually will lose its responsiveness to immunosuppression with corticosteroids or azathioprine and take on the shape of a progressive large duct PSC. It is not clear if all adult PSC has a similar progression from an autoimmune phenotype through to eventually a fibrotic biliary phenotype as is seen in the young cohorts.

Diagnosis of PSC

Biochemistry and Serology

There is no specific test for PSC but rather the diagnosis is based on the presence of a cholestatic process that occurs for greater than 6 months that predominantly involves the medium and large bile ducts of the liver in the absence of other closely related diseases such as primary biliary cirrhosis or causes of secondary sclerosing cholangitis. The majority of patients have an alkaline phosphatase that is chronically raised in conjunction with a raised gamma GT which is rather less specific. This population of individuals with early disease will have significant fluctuations of the alkaline phosphatase with periods of normality and hence a better long-term prognosis. It is important to recognise that alkaline phosphatase in the setting of IBD could also be raised from gut infection or potentially from coexisting metabolic bone disease. Serum aminotransferase levels are raised in the majority of individuals with PSC. However, this is almost always less than five times the upper limit or normal. Increases beyond this should raise significant suspicion of an overlap with autoimmune hepatitis, particularly in young individuals or the possibility of IgG4 associated cholangitis. Flares of IBD as well as episodes of ascending cholangitis can both be associated with transient increases in both the alkaline phosphatase as well as the aminotransferase levels in PSC. Serum bilirubin levels are typically normal in early disease and tend to fluctuate depending on the coexistence of ascending cholangitis or new dominant biliary strictures. The majority of the bilirubin will be conjugated with persistent elevations of bilirubin suggestive of advanced disease.

Sudden increases in bilirubin should raise suspicions of complications of PSC such as the development a new biliary stricture, impending cholangitis, development of cholangiocarcinoma or cholelithiasis. Decreases in albumin as well as increases in the prothrombin time are seen late disease as seen as part of hepatic decompensation. Serological markers in PSC are critical in distinguishing PSC from primary biliary cirrhosis (PBC). PBC patients typically will have positive ANA or AMA antibodies and should raise suspicion of a diagnosis of PBC rather than PSC. An overlap between the diseases is increasingly rare with than less than 5 % of PSC patients suffering with positive antimitochondrial antibodies. IgG levels are often mildly increased up to 1.5 times the upper limit of normal but further increases should raise a suspicion of an overlap with autoimmune cholangitis or autoimmune hepatitis. IgG4 subtype levels can be as high as twice the upper limit of normal which generally is regarded as a worse prognostic factor in PSC. However, levels in excess of this range should raise suspicion of IgG4 associated disease. As described earlier, a significant proportion of patients will have pANCA positivity which can be associated both with ulcerative colitis as well as PSC. This is by no means diagnostic but occurs in 65–90 % of individuals with PSC. A proportion of individuals will also have ASCA antibody positivity in conjunction with their IBD. Serology for viral hepatitis and HIV should be negative as well as biochemistry to suggest other forms of chronic liver disease. CA 19-9 levels may be mildly elevated in patients with PSC, particularly at the time of significant large duct disease or ascending bacterial cholangitis. However, serial increases in this maker should raise the suspicion of coexisting cholangiocarcinoma.

Radiology

Primary sclerosing cholangitis used to be exceedingly rare before the advent of biliary imaging in the form of ERCP or percutaneous transhepatic cholangiography (PTC). These modalities are still used today to make a diagnosis of large duct PSC. However, increasingly, these invasive procedures which carry significant risks of introducing ascending cholangitis into the biliary system of individuals and are being replaced with non-invasive imaging modalities. Magnetic resonance cholangiopancreatography (MRCP) is now the most common form of imaging used to diagnose PSC and to define the biliary tree (Fig. 4.2). This can be achieved without the addition of intravenous contrast and carries no risk of biliary sepsis to the patient. Typical findings at ERCP/MCRP will be the development of multifocal strictures throughout the biliary tree in the liver with areas of proximal dilatation. As the disease progresses, the biliary tree becomes pruned with loss of distal bile ducts and in some individuals, there will be the emergence of dominant strictures in the main common bile duct or left or right hepatic ducts. These may be amenable to dilatation either through endoscopic procedures such as ERCP or a transhepatic procedure using PTC. Gallbladder dysfunction is common in PSC and can range from cystic duct strictures with recurrent cholecystitis to the emergence of gallstone disease and CBD stones.

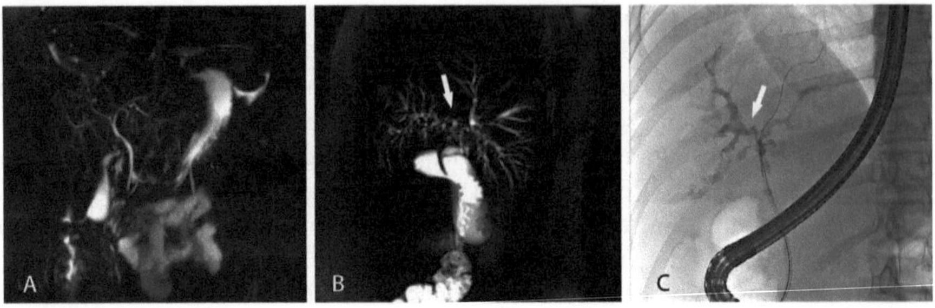

Fig. 4.2 MRCP and ERCP findings in normal and PSC liver. (**a**) Demonstrates a normal biliary tree as imaged by MRCP. (**b**) Extensive biliary changes with hilar strictures, beading and segments of dilatation (*arrow*) as imaged by MRCP. (**c**) Corresponding ERCP image of (**b**) with similar changes at the hilum involving typically the right duct system (*arrow*)

The emergence of a new stricture should, however, raise the suspicion of the development of a cholangiocarcinoma. Higher lymph nodes are often enlarged in PSC and IBD and do not necessarily signify the emergence of a neoplastic process. Endoscopic ultrasound has also been demonstrated to have an increasingly important role in evaluating the biliary tree, particularly in assessing common bile duct strictures as to determine whether they are benign or have significant mass effects to suggest a cholangiocarcinoma. Endoscopic ultrasound has the added benefit of being able to sample regional lymph nodes to exclude a neoplastic process. It is however limited in its penetration and its ability to evaluate the proximal common bile dust and intrahepatic ducts. Contrast enhanced ultrasound relies on standard transcutaneous ultrasound scanning of the liver in combination with a microaggregated bubble contrast agent which is injected intravenously to highlight the blood flow in the liver during ultrasound imaging. This procedure has the benefit of detecting inflammation within the biliary tree at a very early stage before this may become apparent on MRI scanning. Some studies have suggested that some of these early changes are not specific and that some individuals will not proceed to PSC. However, this does provide an alternative to MRI scanning and is a very useful modality in assessing new lesions to exclude the development of cholangiocarcinoma. ERCP and PTC are at present largely restricted to special circumstances where either these alternative modalities are not available or where therapeutic interventions are anticipated. It is particularly useful in the assessment of a new stricture where cytology may be obtained with endoscopic brushings or targeting the lesion with endoscopic biopsies through spyglass technologies. This involves a small endoscope that is passed through the ERCP scope into the bile duct for direct visualisation of the biliary mucosa and potential lesions. ERCP can also be used to remove sludge or biliary stones as well as to perform dilatation of strictures and rarely placement of biliary stents to ensure biliary drainage although this is extremely hazardous in PSC given the high risk of ascending cholangitis. PTC has a similar utility and is mostly applicable in the scenario in patients that have had a biliary reconstruction surgery with a Roux-en-Y anastomosis in which ERCP is particularly difficult.

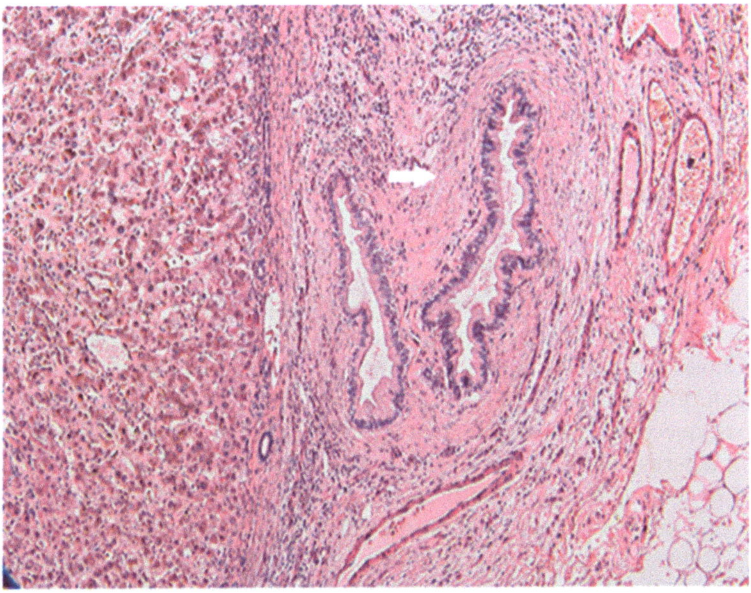

Fig. 4.3 Liver histology of PSC. Liver biopsy showing typical features of PSC including portal inflammation, concentric peribiliary fibrosis (*arrow*) and prominent oedema

Both tests rely on the administration of intrabiliary contrast agents and on radiation which is a limiting factor. Currently, endoscopic confocal imaging is being increasingly employed to assess the GI tract with probes available for placement up the biliary tree to help the diagnosis of benign versus malignant strictures but have yet to become mainstream and widely available.

Histology

A proportion of patients with PSC will have a normal cholangiogram and suffer from a predominantly intrahepatic small duct variant of PSC. In these cases, a liver biopsy is critical in making the diagnosis. However, liver biopsy may also be utilised in PSC to determine an overlap with predominantly autoimmune hepatitis or in cases where another cause of cholestasis might be considered. Liver biopsies in PSC can range from non-specific periportal inflammation with minimal abnormalities of the biliary epithelium to the typical changes that consist of bile duct proliferation, ductopaenia, peribiliary fibrosis and prominent oedema and expansion of the portal tracts (Fig. 4.3). The biliary epithelium is often surrounded by a mixed inflammatory infiltrate with intra-epithelial lymphocytes. As the disease progresses, the bile ducts become obliterated, leaving large fibrotic scars within the portal tracts. An excess of plasma cells within the infiltrate should raise suspicion of overlapping autoimmune hepatitis or IgG4 disease. Liver biopsy does have some failings in PSC as this disease is often patchy and the severity of liver fibrosis on one biopsy might not be indicative of the overall level of hepatic fibrosis.

Differential Diagnosis

As described earlier in this article, several diseases have the capacity of causing a PSC-like syndrome and should be actively excluded as part of making the diagnosis of PSC. This is particularly important in individuals that do not have coexisting IBD. Cholestasis and ductopaenia are common to multiple forms of liver disease, including drug-induced liver disease, sarcoidosis, PBC, graft-versus-host disease and liver rejection. Both autoimmune hepatitis and PBC can be excluded on the basis of a normal cholangiogram. However, as these diseases can occur in the setting of overlap syndromes, the presence of antimitochondrial antibodies should raise suspicion of PBC where high titres of IgG as well as ANA or anti-smooth muscle antibodies should trigger further consideration of autoimmune hepatitis. Other causes that lead to large duct changes on imaging such as chronic biliary infection secondary to HIV or immunodeficiency should be excluded. Similarly, chronic gallstone disease with secondary sclerosing cholangitis should be considered. Possibly the most important diagnosis to exclude in these individuals is the presence of cholangiocarcinoma which may present with an obstructive jaundice picture and biliary strictures. IgG4 disease can mimic PSC but has a high rate of coexisting pancreatic disease and a relative paucity of IBD. IgG4 levels in these individuals might be normal with the diagnosis heavily relying on histology and the determination of IgG4 immunohistochemistry staining of the samples [9].

Inflammatory Bowel Disease

Sixty to seventy percentage of individuals with PSC will develop IBD of which roughly 80 % will suffer with ulcerative colitis and a further 20 % from Crohn's colitis. The nature of the coexisting IBD is often an indeterminate colitis and it appears that the strongest association between PSC and IBD comes from disease processes that involve the colon. Over 70 % of individuals will have backwash ileitis as a feature of a disease and have a distribution that favours the proximal colon with relative rectal sparing (Fig. 4.4) [10]. Although cases of isolated small bowel Crohn's disease or perianal Crohn's disease have been described in PSC, this is particularly unusual. The range of activity of this disease is very significant with the majority of individuals at presentation suffering from mild or asymptomatic IBD. On average, the duration of IBD diagnosis precedes the diagnosis of PSC by an average of 7 years. However, it is not uncommon for this diagnosis to be made simultaneously or even many years later following a successful liver transplant for PSC. It is also not uncommon to have a curative panproctocolectomy for ulcerative colitis

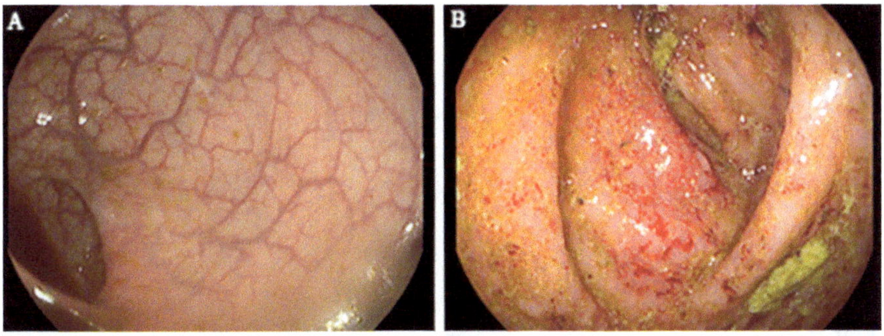

Fig. 4.4 Endoscopic images showing typical findings on colonoscopy in PSC. Colonoscopy shows rectal sparing (**a**) and diffuse right sided inflammation (**b**) frequently seen PSC

and to develop PSC subsequently. Although most patients with PSC will describe some gastrointestinal symptoms such as occasional loose stools or increased frequency, over 80 % of individuals will suffer with mild IBD. The link with IBD is, however, significantly different at the age extremes of the disease. Individuals in their teenage and young adult years often suffer with very reactive IBD and require intense immunosuppression or the initiation of biological therapies that target anti-TNFα. No direct effects have been demonstrated to suggest that anti-TNFα treatment directly affects the liver but rather indirectly by controlling IBD. It is not uncommon for these young individuals treated with these drugs to see improvements in their liver transaminases. Pouchitis is a particular concern in PSC as almost 100 % of individuals with PSC will develop pouchitis following a total proctocolectomy and the formation of an ileal pouch anal anastomosis. Great variation is reported in different studies as to the response to standard therapy with most studies suggesting that one to two-thirds of individuals will eventually develop refractory pouchitis. A large study of over 1,000 individuals with IPAA surgery demonstrated pouchitis rates of 61 % at 5 years and 79 % at 10 years for individuals with PSC which was roughly double the rates seen in individuals with only ulcerative colitis [11]. In addition to increased risks of pouchitis, individuals with PSC and coexisting IBD do suffer with high rates of colorectal neoplasia that is predicted to be 25 % lifetime risk. The current guidelines for surveillance in these individuals requires an annual colonoscopy with four quadrant biopsies every 10 cm to detect mucosal dysplasia. This may be improved with the use of high definition colonoscopy or dye spray techniques to highlight flat neoplastic lesions or dysplastic glands for targeted biopsies. A further technique which is promising is the use of confocal laser endomicroscopy which allows a microscopic assessment of the colonic mucosa to detect very early changes in gland pattern as occurs with dysplasia (Fig. 4.5). The risk of colorectal cancer remains after liver transplantation and hence surveillance is indicated post successful liver transplantation. Some studies have suggested that ursodeoxycholic acid or 5-aminosalicylate preparations can lower the risk of PSC associated colorectal cancer [23]. However, in a recent study of high dose ursodeoxycholic acid, there were suggestions that this drug might increase the development of neoplasia [24].

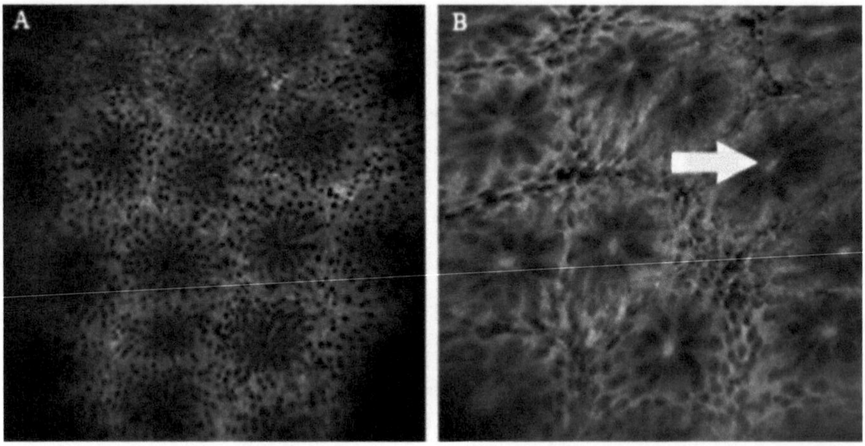

Fig. 4.5 Confocal microscopy images of normal colon (**a**) and active colitis (**b**). During active colitis crypts are irregular, dilated and the central crypt opening bright in appearance due to fluorescein leakage (*arrow*)

For many individuals who suffer with either refractory IBD or dysplasia, a panproctocolectomy would be indicated and given the high rates of pouchitis a standard end ileostomy would be the preferred surgery. This is however not entirely without complications as peristomal varices can occur in individuals with advancing liver disease and increasing portal hypertension.

Cholangiocarcinoma and Other Biliary Tract Cancers

Patients with PSC are at risk of cholangiocarcinoma, gallbladder polyps or subsequent transformation to gallbladder cancer and when they have become cirrhotic, there is a risk of hepatic cellular carcinoma [25]. Cholangiocarcinoma represents the most devastating complication of PSC with up to a third of cholangiocarcinomas being diagnosed within the first year of making the diagnosis of PSC. The presentation is highly variable ranging from minimal abnormalities at cholangiogram to mass lesions with obstructive jaundice. The normal risk of cholangiocarcinoma ranges from between 0.5 and 2 % with a predicted lifetime risk of nearly 15 %. Cholangiocarcinoma is classified based on its position within the biliary tree which also helps to guide the appropriate treatment [26]. Cholangiocarcinoma that affects predominantly the extrahepatic biliary tree or the intrapancreatic segment of the common bile duct can be treated by surgical resection of the extrahepatic bile ducts with or without a Whipple procedure. This procedure though has a roughly 30–40 % survival at 5 years. The vast majority of individuals will present with early lymph node involvement and local spread at diagnosis and would not be suitable for liver transplantation or resection as this is associated with variable prognosis and the survival of less than 2 % at 2 years. Cholangiocarcinoma as a whole is a tumour that is relatively sensitive to standard chemo and radio therapeutic agents with the median survival following diagnosis being 9 months. A small proportion of individuals with a cholangiocarcinoma involving the mid common bile duct extending up to the hilum without local spread may be suitable for the Mayo liver transplantation protocol for cholangiocarcinoma [27]. This involves neo adjuvant chemotherapy followed by intraductal brachytherapy and liver transplantation. In these cases, survival rates of 85 % have been reported at 1 year which persists at 5 years with greater than 80 % survival. Unfortunately, this is only available to highly selected patients with early disease. Because of this increased risk of cholangiocarcinoma, current recommendation is for cross sectional imaging of the liver which may be done by ultrasound scanning, CT scanning or MRI scanning on an annual basis with six monthly CA 19-9 levels. The diagnosis is made on positive histology with suggestive imaging findings. Brushings obtained from ERCP or PTC typically have a low yield which can be improved by a combination of CA19-9 levels or by in situ hybridisation to detect chromosomal abnormalities. Most promising is the use of direct visualisation of the bile duct system by technology such as Spyglass which allows direct light microscopy views of the affected area and targeted biopsies. Similarly, confocal endomicroscopy probes may be placed into the biliary tree to detect mucosal changes as well as submucosal alterations in blood flow suggestive of neoplasia. Staging of cholangiocarcinoma is done through cross sectional imaging to determine distant spread and lymph node involvement. Lymph node sampling is mandatory which can be achieved either percutaneously or through endoscopic ultrasound and fine needle aspiration. Further detection of tumour spread can be obtained by CT-PET scanning. Patients with PSC are also at risk of gallbladder dysfunction, the development of gallbladder polyps and gallbladder cancer.

Gallbladder diseases such as cholelithiasis, gallbladder polyps and gallbladder cancers are increased among patients with PSC. Gallbladder cancer develops in 2 % of individuals with PSC. However, in those who develop gallbladder polyps, the risk of a carcinoma is in excess of 50 % with the remainder of the individuals demonstrating epithelial dysplasia. Most guidelines advocate in favour of cholecystectomy when gallbladder polyps are found regardless of size; however, some caution should exist as one study did not find neoplasia in polyps less than 0.8 cm but reported a 40 % morbidity associated with cholecystectomy in PSC patients with advanced liver disease. Current AASLD guidelines suggest an annual ultrasound scan to detect gallbladder polyps and a cholecystectomy regardless of polyp size if liver disease severity permits [1].

Complications of PSC

Whilst cholangiocarcinoma and gallbladder cancer are relatively unique complications of PSC, patients with PSC are at also at risk of common complications of liver cirrhosis such as portal hypertension with variceal haemorrhage and ascites, hepatic encephalopathy and the development of hepatocellular cancer and should receive screening and supportive therapy as per general cirrhosis guidelines [1].

Chronic cholestasis of all causes leads to additional complications such as pruritus and fat soluble vitamin deficiencies with associated metabolic bone disease [28]. All patients with PSC should receive a baseline bone density scan and at 2–3 yearly intervals. Supplementation of vitamin A, D (at least 1,000 IU/day), E, K and calcium (1–1.5 g/day) may be necessary. In some instances of severe metabolic bone disease the use of bisphosphonates and calcitonin might be indicated. Pruritus in some instances may respond to restoring adequate biliary drainage such as the dilatation of a biliary stricture or PTC. However, in the majority of patients, there will be extensive intrahepatic cholestasis as a driver of pruritus that may respond to oral bile salt binders such as cholestyramine, bile salt detoxification with UDCA, the use of enzyme inducers such as rifampicin, opioid antagonists such as naltrexone or the serotonin reuptake inhibitor sertraline.

Recurrent bacterial sepsis of the biliary tree is common in advanced PSC and ranges in severity from requiring the occasional short course of oral antibiotic therapy to rotating oral antibiotic therapy (often consisting sequential use of a cephalosporin, metronidazole and a quinolone each for 4 weeks on a rolling basis) to extreme cases of continuous intravenous antibiotic dependence. In addition to the development of portal hypertension and progression to end stage liver disease, the presence of deteriorating extrahepatic bile duct disease with recurrent cholangitis and/or intractable pruritus are established indications for liver transplantation.

Medical Therapy

The Use of Ursodeoxycholic Acid

Ursodeoxycholic acid (UDCA) is a naturally occurring hydrophobic bile acid that is widely used in the treatment of a range of cholestatic liver diseases. It has multiple biologic effects, ranging from a choloretic agent to the ability to dissolve small gallstones. The effect that UCDA has on the biliary epithelium is one of cytoprotection and the ability to influence the inflammatory signals in this microenvironment. Another mechanism of action is that UDCA is able to alter the composition of the total bile acid pool to lessen the harmful effects of the more toxic endogenous bile acids during cholestasis [29].

Because of these potential beneficial effects, UDCA has gained a prominent role as an effective treatment in Primary Biliary Cirrhosis (PBC). In PBC, it has been known for a number of years that it improves liver biochemistry, by improving cholestasis and subsequently pruritus. UDCA has been shown to provide a survival benefit in PBC. Until relatively recently, it was widely accepted that UDCA was a safe treatment without significant adverse effects.

For the last 20 years, it has been proposed that UDCA might have a similar role in PSC. Pilot studies performed during the period 1990–1997, using predominantly low dose UDCA at the range of 10–15 mg/kg per day or total daily doses of 750–1,250 mg/day, suggested potential benefit. The majority of these studies found improvements in PSC as measured by liver biochemistry tests. In some instances, UDCA was evaluated along with other treatments such as methotrexate or therapeutic ERCP and demonstrated a trend towards a beneficial effect with UDCA at a low dose, but ultimately these studies were all insufficiently powered to demonstrate a clear survival benefit. This culminated into the most prominent trial for low dose UDCA that was performed by Lindor et al. in 1997 using 13–15 mg/kg of UDCA per day in a randomised double blind placebo controlled trial. The primary outcomes of this trial were defined as death, liver transplantation, histological progression, the development of varices, ascites or encephalopathy, worsening of liver biochemistry or symptoms such as fatigue or pruritus. One hundred and five patients were recruited and randomised. Fifty-one patients in each group were followed up for at least 3 months with a medium follow-up of 2.2 years. The conclusion from this study using low dose UDCA was that at this dose, UDCA did not have any benefits above placebo in patients with PSC.

Because of these disappointing findings with low dose UDCA in the progression of PSC, two pilot studies were performed to assess the benefits of UDCA at higher doses. Mitchell et al. performed a randomised placebo control trial using 26 patients with PSC to receive either 20 mg/kg daily of UDCA or placebo. Cholangiography and liver biopsy were performed at entry and at 2 years. Symptoms, clinical signs and liver biochemistry tests were recorded at three monthly intervals. At the end of the study, they concluded that high-dose UDCA did not influence symptoms but they noted significant improvements in the liver biochemistry ($p=0.03$), delayed progression of cholangiographic appearances ($p=0.015$) and improved liver fibrosis staging ($p=0.05$). In this study, there were no significant adverse effects reported. They concluded that high dose UDCA may be of benefit in PSC but that larger studies were needed to determine whether this translated to improved long-term survival.

This study was followed by a larger multi-centre randomised control study from Sweden where a total of 219 patients with PSC were randomised to 17–23 mg/kg of UDCA per day or placebo for 5 years. They reported that the combined endpoint of death or liver transplantation occurred in 7.2 % of PSC patients in the UDCA treatment group versus 10.9 % of patients in the placebo controlled group ($p=0.368$). They saw a similar trend when using liver transplantation as a single endpoint. Importantly, there were no differences between the two groups in symptoms or quality of life measures. This study hinted at a potential survival benefit using high dose UDCA in PSC but concluded that larger study with greater power was required to test this hypothesis further. It is important to note that no significant adverse effects were reported in this study. During this period, another study was done by Cullen, et al. where they randomised 31 patients with PSC to either 10 mg/kg of

UDCA or 20 or 30 mg/kg for 2 years. Consistent with the other two studies, there was a trend in the 30 mg/kg group towards histological improvement and the reduction in their Mayo Risk score. No adverse effects were noticed in any of the three treatment groups.

Given the potential benefit of high dose UDCA, Lindor et al. conducted a large long-term randomised double-blind controlled high dose UDCA versus placebo study. Patients received UDCA at a range of 28–30 mg/kg per day with 150 patients with PSC enrolled into this study. Liver biopsy and cholangiography were performed before randomisation and at 5 years and the primary outcome measures were the development of cirrhosis, varices, cholangiocarcinoma, liver transplantation or death. Seventy-six patients were recruited to UDCA arm and 74 to placebo. Both groups were similar with respect to sex, age, duration of disease, serum AST and alkaline phosphatase levels as well as liver histology and Mayo Risk score. The study was terminated after 6 years due to futility as 39 % of the UDCA group versus 26 % of the placebo group reached the pre-established clinical endpoints. The risk of reaching any of these primary endpoints was 2.3 times greater for the patients on UDCA than for those on placebo ($p<0.1$). Most importantly, serious adverse events were more common in the UDCA group than placebo (63 % vs. 37 %, $p<0.01$). Closer examination of these endpoints revealed that high doses of UDCA were associated with an increased rate of portal hypertension and the development of bleeding oesophageal varices [30]. There was in increase in patients requiring liver transplantation as well as reaching minimal listing criteria for liver transplantation. The risk for cholangiocarcinoma remained stable between both groups. An interesting finding in this study was that it was the patients with relatively early PSC that were most at risk of progressing to these endpoints. Because of this data, it is now recommended by the American Association for the Study of Liver Diseases that high dose UDCA has no place in the management of PSC (randomised controlled trial data showing harm).

Some have questioned whether UDCA might have a beneficial effect in the associated condition of IBD and the increased risks of colorectal cancer that exist in patients who suffer with PSC. This is supported by historical data by Tung et al. who performed a cross sectional retrospective study in 2001 evaluating the risk in 59 patients with ulcerative colitis and PSC who were undergoing colonoscopic surveillance for colonic dysplasia. After adjusting for sex, age, onset of colitis, duration of colitis, duration of PSC and severity of liver disease, they concluded that the use of UDCA was strongly associated with a decreased prevalence of colonic dysplasia with an odds ratio of 0.18 and $p=0.005$. This study was followed by another study by Pardi et al. where they interrogated the data from their original low dose randomised placebo controlled trial of UDCA in PSC at the Mayo clinic. In this study, they had 52 patients that were followed up for a total of 355 person years and demonstrated a relative risk of 0.26 for developing colorectal dysplasia or cancer whilst on UDCA ($p=0.034$). They concluded that UDCA significantly decreases the risk of developing colorectal cancer or dysplasia in patients with UC and PSC [23]. The majority of patients in this study received open label UDCA at a relatively low dose to 10–15 mg/kg per day. A further study by Wolf et al. in 2005 examined a historical cohort of PSC patients with ulcerative colitis consisting of 28 cases on a wide range of UDCA doses. In their study, they were unable to show a protective effect from UDCA in reducing the risk of developing cancer or dysplasia but interestingly saw a trend towards a reduced mortality.

At this stage, most clinicians were comfortable with using low dose UDCA as a chemo-preventive agent to reduce colorectal cancer in IBD associated with PSC despite the disappointment of high dose UDCA as PSC treatment. However, this enthusiasm was short lived as Eaton et al. published in 2011 data from the original high dose UDCA trial that was prematurely stopped because of worse outcomes in the UDCA group. They reanalysed their data from this study and evaluated the patients' risk for the development of colorectal neoplasia. They reported that patients who had received high dose UDCA compared to placebo had a significantly increased risk of developing colorectal cancer with a hazard ratio of 4.44 and a confidence interval of 1.30–20.10 ($p=0.02$). Thus concluding, that high dose UDCA has no place as a chemo-preventive agent in PSC [24].

A big question in clinical practice when managing PSC patients is whether there is any rationale at present to use UDCA as a treatment. Certainly based on our current evidence, high dose UDCA is harmful and accelerates not only the liver disease but also the development of colorectal cancer. Low dose UDCA certainly has no beneficial effects on the liver but based on small historical studies that might be some benefit in lessening the risk of colorectal cancer. Overall, the field is split on whether UDCA has any role in future and this is borne out by the fact that the American Association for Liver Disease is advocating against the use of UDCA at any dose in PSC whilst the European Association for the Study of Liver Disease has commented that low dose UDCA might be of use [1].

It is unlikely that further studies will be done using UDCA in its current form but some hope exists that a novel bile acid, 24-norursodeoxycholic acid might hold promise where UDCA has failed. It may be that there is a sub-population of PSC that derive benefit from UDCA to account for some of the positive trends that were seen with the earlier studies and these might have been identified by more rigorous phenotypical stratification into subtypes such as small duct PSC, large duct PSC or IgG4 associated autoimmune cholangiopathy. As genome-wide association scans and personalised medicine develop, it might well be that we will be able in future to determine a patient subgroup that will benefit from UDCA. As it stands at present, there is certainly no place for high dose UDCA and until we can demonstrate a beneficial role for low dose UDCA, the use of this drug in PSC will be limited.

Antibiotic Therapy in PSC

The role of the gut microbiota is increasingly being recognised as critically important in IBD disease pathogenesis through both direct interactions with the enteric immune system and indirectly via activation of pathogen recognition receptors such as the

Toll-like receptors (TLRs) and NOD-like receptors by bacterial motifs such as LPS. This represents a modifiable therapeutic target that has seen significant successes such as the use antibiotic or probiotic treatments for pouchitis or stool transplants in selected cases with difficult to treat colitis. Given the close relationship between PSC and IBD, similar interactions with the microbiome have been proposed and explored in case series and prospective trials. Tetracycline, metronidazole, vancomycin and azithromycin (often in combination with UDCA) have all been shown in case reports to significantly reduce hepatic inflammation as measured by AST, ALT and/or alkaline phosphatase.

This has led to three prospective studies. Eighty patients with PSC were randomised to 36 months of UDCA (15 mg/kg/day) plus metronidazole or UDCA alone by Farkkila et al. They reported superiority of metronidazole and UDCA over UDCA alone with significant improvements in alkaline phosphatase, Mayo PSC risk score, and histologic stage and grade. Similarly, 16 patients with PSC treated with minocycline for 1 year had significant decreases in alkaline phosphatase. Unfortunately 25 % of the patients withdrew from the study due to intolerance to minocycline. The most notable study to date has been a double blind, randomised pilot study of 35 PSC cases randomised to: low-dose vancomycin (125 mg qid), high-dose vancomycin (250 mg qid), low-dose metronidazole (250 mg tid) or high-dose metronidazole (500 mg tid). Low- and high-dose vancomycin groups were superior to metronidazole and achieved significant decreases in serum alkaline phosphatase levels at 12 weeks [31]. The beneficial effects of oral vancomycin are particularly encouraging in paediatric patients. A prospective series of 14 paediatric cases have reported significant decreases in alkaline phosphatase and disease symptoms in almost all cases. Prospective validation of these results in large randomised trials are required to fully establish the utility of antibiotics in PSC and correct patient selection.

Immunosuppressive Therapy

The use of immunosuppressive drugs in PSC has been largely disappointing. Despite evidence of altered autoimmunity in PSC, the use of immunosuppressive drugs in PSC has had little impact with no evidence of long-term efficacy or delay in progression to end stage PSC or complications. The majority of studies using immunosuppressive drugs were performed as uncontrolled pilot studies and have included the use of azathioprine, cyclosporine, tacrolimus, methotrexate and corticosteroids. Tacrolimus, azathioprine and corticosteroids did show modest improvements in liver biochemistry but these effects were either not sustained or the outcomes assessed over prolonged periods to assess progression to cirrhosis [32]. A criticism is that the majority of these studies included advanced PSC with significant fibrosis with potentially minimal active inflammation to target.

Endoscopic or Surgical Interventions

Management of Dominant Biliary Strictures

Dominant strictures of the extra-hepatic biliary system are reported to occur in 50 % of cases and are associated with increased colonisation of bile by bacteria, sudden deterioration in liver function and increased symptoms such as jaundice, cholangitis and itching. These instances should always raise the suspicion of cholangiocarcinoma and be actively investigated by cross sectional imaging, biliary imaging and/or direct biliary sampling by ERCP, PTC or Spyglass technology. The majority of dominant strictures will be benign and are amenable to intervention to improve or restore liver function or symptoms. Some case reports have suggested that aggressive biliary dilatation regimes delay the need for liver transplantation; however, the exact benefit in altering disease course is yet to be established in prospective randomised studies.

Endoscopic or percutaneous treatment of dominant strictures by dilatation alone or dilation and stent placement can restore biliary drainage but at a cost of potentially introducing bacteria into a sterile system with aggravation of cholangitis. There are no randomised studies to guide selection between dilatation alone or dilation and stent placement; however, retrospective data would suggest that the combination of stenting and dilation leads to increased morbidity and complications. Single treatments appear to have limited benefit with most cases requiring interventions every 6–8 weeks for up to a year to resolve strictures. The risk of procedure-related cholangitis is substantial with most guidelines recommending 5–10 days of oral antibiotics. Predictors of adverse outcomes to biliary intervention include the presence of cirrhosis, active IBD, endoscopist experience, a sphincterotomy or the placement of a biliary stent.

Prognostic Models and the Timing for Liver Transplantation

Traditionally large duct PSC is associated with a 13 year median time from presentation to requiring liver transplantation. This is however not the case for the small duct variant of IBD where the majority of these individuals will not develop end stage liver disease. Approximately 15–25 % of these individuals will over time convert to large duct disease and subsequently require liver transplantation. Recent work has suggested that individuals with persistently raised alkaline phosphatase levels are at a high risk of progression whilst those with intermittent normalisation of this parameter carried a low risk of progression to end stage liver disease. Similar work is emerging to suggest that the absolute IgG4 level in these cases may also be used as a prognostic marker with those higher than twice the upper limit of normal more frequently progressing to end stage liver disease. The biggest difficulty at present is that there is no robust clinical score or biomarker that may be used to predict the outcome of PSC in its early stages. Once the disease progresses to more advanced stages of liver fibrosis and dysfunction, the most common scoring system used is the MELD score. Unfortunately the score was not developed for PSC and frequently underscores the severity of their liver disease, particularly in those with advanced large duct disease that require rotating antibiotics because of continuous sepsis. Subsequently the Mayo PSC risk score was developed which relies on the presence of raised bilirubin, albumin levels, age, the presence or absence of variceal haemorrhage and AST levels. This provides a more robust prediction of survival for individuals with late PSC [33]. However, this has not been adopted into models to prioritise for liver transplantation where a scoring system such as MELD, Na-MELD and UKELD still predominate.

Liver Transplantation for PSC

Liver transplantation for PSC is currently the only viable treatment option for individuals who have developed either refractory biliary disease requiring rotating antibiotics or have progression to classical features of liver failure such as portal hypertension and hepatic encephalopathy. Traditional duct to duct anastomosis has become a less favoured surgical procedure in these individuals given the high risk of anastomotic strictures and the risk of cholangiocarcinoma in the remaining biliary remnant. This has led to the majority of centres currently performing a resection of the extrahepatic biliary tree at the same time as transplantation and the formation of a Roux-en-Y biliary anastomosis with the allograft. The outcomes from liver transplantation in this group have been excellent with 5 year survivals in excess of 85 % (Fig. 4.6).

Twenty percentage of individuals with PSC will develop recurrent disease at 5 years. Recurrent PSC may be difficult to distinguish from chronic allograft rejection as both could lead to ductopaenia. PSC along with other autoimmune liver diseases such as PBC and autoimmune hepatitis are at higher risk of developing rejection and hence requires relatively higher levels of immunosuppression. There is some suggestion that cyclosporine might be beneficial over tacrolimus in as far as preventing recurrent disease with similar data for azathioprine being superior to mycophenolate. Rapamycin has also been proposed as a compound that leads to less recurrent PSC but requires formal validation in prospective studies as the majority of this data is obtained from historical cohorts and retrospective analysis.

Recurrent PSC Post-liver Transplant

Liver transplantation is not a cure for PSC as it recurs in 20–25 % of recipients over a 5–10 year period after liver transplantation with cadaveric organs and possibly at even higher rates using living related organs. As an example, a cohort of 230 PSC

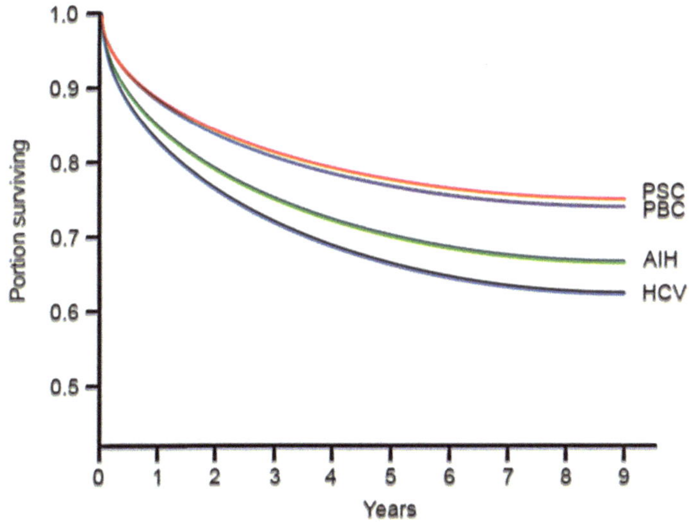

Fig. 4.6 Disease specific survival post-transplant. Modified from Roberts et al. Liver Transplantation 2004;10(7)

recipients with a median follow-up time of 82.5 months found a rate of recurrent PSC (rPSC) of 23.5 %, with a time to developing rPSC of 4.1 years. A study in 2004 analysed 3,309 patients transplanted for PSC from the UNOS database and found a higher retransplantation rate and a lower survival when compared to PBC recipients from the same study population at 7 years post-transplant. Recent studies suggest that PSC is only second to hepatitis C as a leading cause for recurrent disease and subsequent graft loss (Fig. 4.7) [34].

The diagnosis of recurrent disease can be difficult and relies on the exclusion of secondary causes of sclerosing cholangitis such as ischemia of the biliary tree, hepatic artery thrombosis, acute or chronic ductopenic rejection, ABO mismatch and infection (bacterial or viral) and usually occurs more than 90 days post-transplant. Graziadei proposed the Mayo Clinic criteria which require a confirmed diagnosis of PSC prior to transplant; cholangiograms showing non-anastomotic biliary strictures of the biliary tree with beading and irregularity occurring more than 90 days post-transplantation or liver histology revealing fibrous cholangitis and/or fibro-obliterative lesions of large bile ducts, with or without ductopaenia or biliary cirrhosis whilst excluding secondary causes.

The majority of these individuals will not develop graft failure. However, as the majority of PSC patients are of a relatively young age group, a few individuals will require second or third liver transplants. The risk of recurrent disease appears to be closely linked to their IBD with some studies suggesting that a high IBD activity peritransplant is associated with recurrent disease [35]. A further study has demonstrated that a curative colectomy for IBD before transplant was associated with very low rates of recurrent PSC suggesting an important interaction between the gut and the liver in this disease (Fig. 4.8) [36]. As these individuals will continue to have a

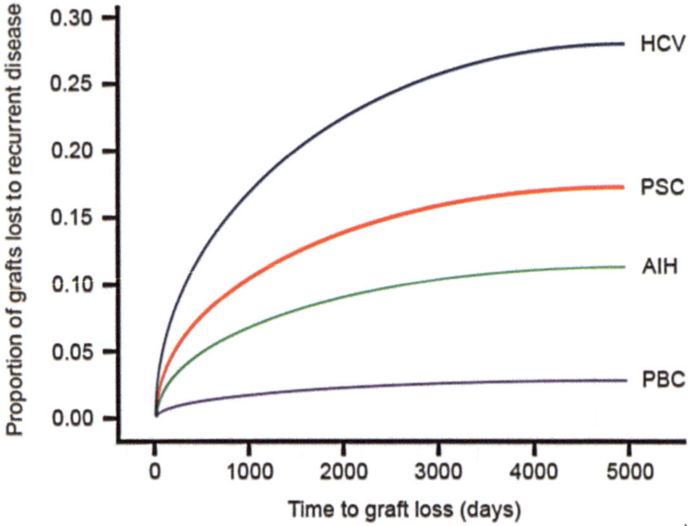

Fig. 4.7 Impact of disease recurrence on graft survival. Modified from Rowe et al. Transplant International 2008;21 and reanalysis of original data set

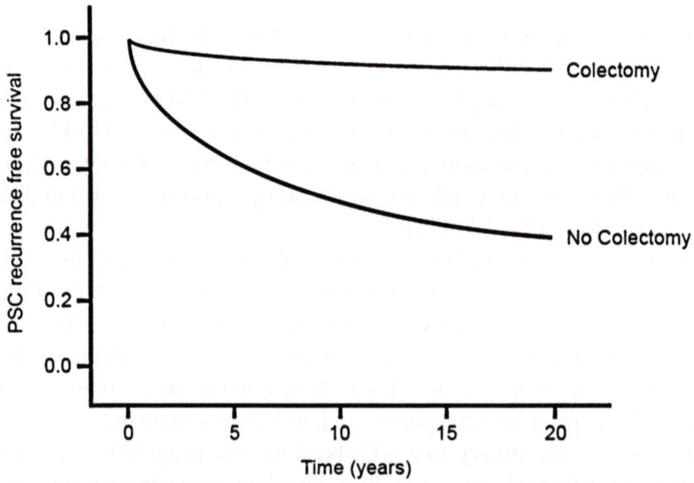

Fig. 4.8 PSC recurrence post-transplant. Patients who undergo colectomy pre-liver transplant or at the time of liver transplant are significantly less likely to develop recurrent PSC. Modified from Alabraba et al. Liver Transplantation 2009;15 and reanalysis of extended data set

high risk of colorectal cancer, it might not be unreasonable in some individuals with difficult to control IBD to consider a colonic resection pre-transplant as this would place them at low risk of recurrent PSC and also obviate the need for frequent endoscopic screening thereafter. Recurrent PSC again has the risk of cholangiocarcinoma.

With the relative scarcity of the cadaveric organs, attention has shifted to the use of living related liver donation as a mechanism to provide allografts for these individuals. This has been associated with excellent results. However, there is some suggestion that these individuals might be at higher risk of recurrent disease which may be indicative of shared PSC susceptibility genes between siblings and potential risks of PSC within their immediate family. Further risk factors for rPSC include male sex, a history of acute cellular rejection, the use of extended donor criteria cadaveric grafts human leukocyte antigen DRB1*08 (HLADRB1*08).

No medical therapy has been shown to prevent PSC recurrence or stop disease progression. The data that colectomy pre-transplant is associated with less rPSC suggests a critical role of the inflamed colon in recurrent disease pathogenesis with the hope that the widespread use of potent biological therapies for IBD might result in a "chemical colectomy" to reduce rPSC. Currently the only option for recurrent PSC is re-transplantation but is associated with increased mortality and complication than the initial transplant.

Summary

PSC represents a syndrome of polygenic susceptibility leading to altered immunity that ultimately leads to a common pathway of chronic immune-mediated bile duct destruction and liver cirrhosis. The emerging importance of antibiotics in the management of PSC suggests a unique relationship between host genetics, the immune system and the gut microbiome. Thus the next steps in deciphering PSC will be to link genotypes to altered biology and disease phenotypes to develop targeted therapies. As an example, those who carry the FUT2 risk alleles with altered biliary microbiota might respond best to antibiotic treatments such as Vancomycin. In contrast, those that carry IL-2/IL-2 receptor risk loci alleles which are associated with classical autoimmunity, might be the sub-population of PSC that does respond to standard immunomodulation. Cases reports have highlighted many compounds that are potentially of benefit in PSC but have failed in larger cohort studies. It may well be that these responders reflect relatively rare PSC risk allele carriers (subtypes) which are lost in larger studies but can now be captured based on genotyping. By incorporating genotyping to define subsets of PSC as part of future treatment studies, we have the ability to select those who benefit most from a therapy when perhaps it does not apply generically to all of PSC and thus personalise PSC care. Although we can use existing risk loci to sub-classify PSC, this does not exclude the need for further genetic discovery during these studies as other genes might dictate disease progression of the emergence of complications such as the MMP2 gene loci which is not a risk loci for PSC but does determine its progression. Metagenomic studies in PSC are in its infancy and represent the next big frontier in unravelling the causes of PSC.

References

1. Chapman R, Fevery J, Kalloo A, et al. Diagnosis and management of primary sclerosing cholangitis. Hepatology. 2010;51:660–78.
2. Eaton JE, Talwalkar JA. Lazaridis KN, et al. Gastroenterology: Pathogenesis of Primary Sclerosing Cholangitis and Advances in Diagnosis and Management; 2013.
3. Molodecky NA, Myers RP, Barkema HW, et al. Validity of administrative data for the diagnosis of primary sclerosing cholangitis: a population-based study. Liver Int. 2011;31:712–20.
4. Molodecky NA, Kareemi H, Parab R, et al. Incidence of primary sclerosing cholangitis: a systematic review and meta-analysis. Hepatology. 2011;53:1590–9.
5. Molodecky NA, Soon IS, Rabi DM, et al. Increasing incidence and prevalence of the inflammatory bowel diseases with time, based on systematic review. Gastroenterology. 2012;142:46–54. e42; quiz e30.
6. Bjornsson E, Olsson R, Bergquist A, et al. The natural history of small-duct primary sclerosing cholangitis. Gastroenterology. 2008;134:975–80.
7. Boberg KM, Chapman RW, Hirschfield GM, et al. Overlap syndromes: the International Autoimmune Hepatitis Group (IAIHG) position statement on a controversial issue. J Hepatol. 2011;54:374–85.
8. Culver EL, Chapman RW. Systematic review: management options for primary sclerosing cholangitis and its variant forms – IgG4-associated cholangitis and overlap with autoimmune hepatitis. Aliment Pharmacol Ther. 2011;33(12):1273–91.
9. Hirschfield GM, Karlsen TH. Lindor KD, et al. Lancet: Primary sclerosing cholangitis; 2013.
10. Loftus Jr EV, Harewood GC, Loftus CG, et al. PSC-IBD: a unique form of inflammatory bowel disease associated with primary sclerosing cholangitis. Gut. 2005;54:91–6.
11. Rahman M, Desmond P, Mortensen N, et al. The clinical impact of primary sclerosing cholangitis in patients with an ileal pouch-anal anastomosis for ulcerative colitis. Int J Colorectal Dis. 2011;26:553–9.
12. Andersen IM, Tengesdal G. Lie BA, et al. Smoking, and Hormones on Risk for Primary Sclerosing Cholangitis. Clin Gastroenterol Hepatol: Effects of Coffee Consumption; 2013.
13. Hirschfield GM, Chapman RW, Karlsen TH, et al. The genetics of complex cholestatic disorders. Gastroenterology. 2013;144:1357–74.
14. Mells GF, Kaser A, Karlsen TH. Novel insights into autoimmune liver diseases provided by genome-wide association studies. J Autoimmun. 2013;46:41–54.
15. Liu JZ, Hov JR, Folseraas T, et al. Dense genotyping of immune-related disease regions identifies nine new risk loci for primary sclerosing cholangitis. Nat Genet. 2013;45:670–5.
16. Melum E, Franke A, Schramm C, et al. Genome-wide association analysis in primary sclerosing cholangitis identifies two non-HLA susceptibility loci. Nat Genet. 2011;43:17–9.
17. Wannhoff A, Hov JR, Folseraas T, et al. FUT2 and FUT3 genotype determines CA19-9 cut-off values for detection of cholangiocarcinoma in patients with primary sclerosing cholangitis. J Hepatol. 2013;59(6):1278–84.
18. Folseraas T, Melum E, Rausch P, et al. Extended analysis of a genome-wide association study in primary sclerosing cholangitis detects multiple novel risk loci. J Hepatol. 2012;57:366–75.
19. Karlsen TH, Franke A, Melum E, et al. Genome-wide association analysis in primary sclerosing cholangitis. Gastroenterology. 2010;138:1102–11.
20. Trivedi PJ, Adams DH. Mucosal immunity in liver autoimmunity: a comprehensive review. J Autoimmun. 2013;46:97–111.
21. Adams DH, Eksteen B. Aberrant homing of mucosal T cells and extra-intestinal manifestations of inflammatory bowel disease. Nat Rev Immunol. 2006;6:244–51.
22. Eksteen B, Grant AJ, Miles A, et al. Hepatic endothelial CCL25 mediates the recruitment of CCR9+ gut-homing lymphocytes to the liver in primary sclerosing cholangitis. J Exp Med. 2004;200:1511–7.
23. Pardi DS, Loftus Jr EV, Kremers WK, et al. Ursodeoxycholic acid as a chemopreventive agent in patients with ulcerative colitis and primary sclerosing cholangitis. Gastroenterology. 2003; 124:889–93.

24. Eaton JE, Silveira MG, Pardi DS, et al. High-dose ursodeoxycholic acid is associated with the development of colorectal neoplasia in patients with ulcerative colitis and primary sclerosing cholangitis. Am J Gastroenterol. 2011;106:1638–45.
25. Boberg KM, Bergquist A, Mitchell S, et al. Cholangiocarcinoma in primary sclerosing cholangitis: risk factors and clinical presentation. Scand J Gastroenterol. 2002;37:1205–11.
26. Rizvi S, Gores GJ. Pathogenesis, diagnosis, and management of cholangiocarcinoma. Gastroenterology. 2013;145:1215–29.
27. Darwish Murad S, Kim WR, Harnois DM, et al. Efficacy of neoadjuvant chemoradiation, followed by liver transplantation, for perihilar cholangiocarcinoma at 12 US centers. Gastroenterology. 2012;143:88–98. e3; quiz e14.
28. Angulo P, Therneau TM, Jorgensen A, et al. Bone disease in patients with primary sclerosing cholangitis: prevalence, severity and prediction of progression. J Hepatol. 1998;29:729–35.
29. Roma MG, Toledo FD, Boaglio AC, et al. Ursodeoxycholic acid in cholestasis: linking action mechanisms to therapeutic applications. Clin Sci (Lond). 2011;121:523–44.
30. Lindor KD, Kowdley KV, Luketic VA, et al. High-dose ursodeoxycholic acid for the treatment of primary sclerosing cholangitis. Hepatology. 2009;50:808–14.
31. Tabibian JH, Weeding E, Jorgensen RA, et al. Randomised clinical trial: vancomycin or metronidazole in patients with primary sclerosing cholangitis – a pilot study. Aliment Pharmacol Ther. 2013;37:604–12.
32. Talwalkar JA, Gossard AA, Keach JC, et al. Tacrolimus for the treatment of primary sclerosing cholangitis. Liver Int. 2007;27:451–3.
33. Kim WR, Poterucha JJ, Wiesner RH, et al. The relative role of the Child-Pugh classification and the Mayo natural history model in the assessment of survival in patients with primary sclerosing cholangitis. Hepatology. 1999;29:1643–8.
34. Rowe IA, Webb K, Gunson BK, et al. The impact of disease recurrence on graft survival following liver transplantation: a single centre experience. Transpl Int. 2008;21:459–65.
35. Joshi D, Bjarnason I, Belgaumkar A, et al. The impact of inflammatory bowel disease post-liver transplantation for primary sclerosing cholangitis. Liver Int. 2013;33:53–61.
36. Alabraba E, Nightingale P, Gunson B, et al. A re-evaluation of the risk factors for the recurrence of primary sclerosing cholangitis in liver allografts. Liver Transpl. 2009;15:330–40.

Chapter 5
IgG4 Related Cholangitis

Said Al Mamari, Emma L. Culver, and Roger W. Chapman

Introduction

IgG4 associated cholangitis (IAC) is a distinct form of chronic cholangitis that is responsive to corticosteroids and has characteristic histological manifestations including a dense infiltration of the affected bile duct walls with IgG4 positive plasma cells [1–4]. It is the biliary manifestation of the novel multisystem IgG4 related disease (IgG4-RD) that affects most commonly, among many other organs, the pancreas. Although isolated cases of IAC are reported, it occurs most frequently in association with autoimmune pancreatitis (AIP). The clinical significance of IAC originates from the similar clinical, biochemical, radiological and even histological features that it shares with primary sclerosing cholangitis (PSC) and cholangiocarcinoma (CCA).In contrast to these disorders, IAC patients respond dramatically to corticosteroid therapy when treated in its inflammatory phase. Distinguishing IAC from these disease mimics is important in order to institute appropriate therapy early enough to prevent fibrotic complications and unnecessary major surgical interventions. Nevertheless, this distinction is not straightforward and can be challenging. This is related to the lack of pathognomonic features of IAC even on histology. This chapter focuses on the current available knowledge on pathogenesis, prevalence, clinical features, radiology and histology findings, diagnosis, treatment and natural history of IAC.

S. Al Mamari, M.D. M.R.C.P. (UK) (✉)
Liver Unit, Sultan Qaboos Hospital, 23 July Street, Salalah, Dhofar 211/98, Oman
e-mail: saidalmammari@hotmail.com

E.L. Culver, B.Sc. (Hons.), M.B.Ch.B., M.R.C.P.
Translational Gastroenterology Unit, John Radcliffe Hospital, Oxford, UK

R.W. Chapman, M.D., F.R.C.P.
Translational Gastroenterology, Oxford University Hospital Trust, Oxford, UK

E.J. Carey and K.D. Lindor (eds.), *Cholestatic Liver Disease*, Clinical Gastroenterology,
DOI 10.1007/978-1-4939-1013-7_5, © Springer Science+Business Media New York 2014

The Concept of IgG4 Related Disease

IgG4-RD is a fibro-inflammatory multisystem disease characterised by unique histological manifestations including a dense lymphoplasmacytic infiltrate, obliterative phlebitis and storiform fibrosis with prominent IgG4-positive plasma cell infiltration in involved organs, that responds dramatically to corticosteroid treatment [5–8]. It often manifests with tumefactive lesions that can mimic malignancy and other inflammatory diseases. The disease was first described as a chronic inflammatory sclerosis of the pancreas in 1961. In [9], Yoshida et al. coined the term "autoimmune pancreatitis" in Japan. The association with increased serum IgG4 levels was described in 2001 by Hamano et al. [10]. A distinction was later made between type I AIP (classical AIP and the pancreatic manifestation of systemic IgG4-RD) and type II AIP (with distinct clinical and histological manifestations which are not IgG4-related). Type I AIP only will be discussed further in this chapter. The systemic nature of this disease was subsequently appreciated in 2003 with the sequential reporting of different organs with similar histological findings [8, 11].

The biliary manifestation of IgG4-RD were first described in 2004 [12], however, the first description may date back to 1963 when Bartholomew et al. from the Mayo Clinic reported the association of PSC and pancreatitis in two cases [13]. Since that time, several descriptive terms have been used to report cases with concomitant biliary strictures and pancreatitis [14]. In 2011, the organising committee of an international symposium on IgG4-RD proposed that bile duct involvement should be termed "IgG4-related sclerosing cholangitis" [15]. In this chapter the term "IgG4 associated cholangitis" will be used to refer to this condition, as agreed by the European Association for the Study of the Liver (EASL) clinical practice guidelines for cholestatic liver diseases [16] as there is seldom histological evidence concomitant with a sclerosing cholangitis.

Aetiopathogenesis

The pathogenesis of IgG4-RD has received increasing attention with new insights into the genetic and immunological aspects of the disease (Fig. 5.1). Several lines of evidence; including the frequent detection of non-specific autoantibodies, hypergammaglobulinemia (particularly increased IgG4), the dense infiltration of the affected tissues with immune cells (T cells, B cells and IgG4 positive plasma cells) and the dramatic response to steroid therapy, strongly support an immune-mediated phenomenon [1, 4, 17]. It remains unclear, however, whether the immune responses are secondary to chronic stimulation by an unknown antigen or allergen or autoimmune in nature.

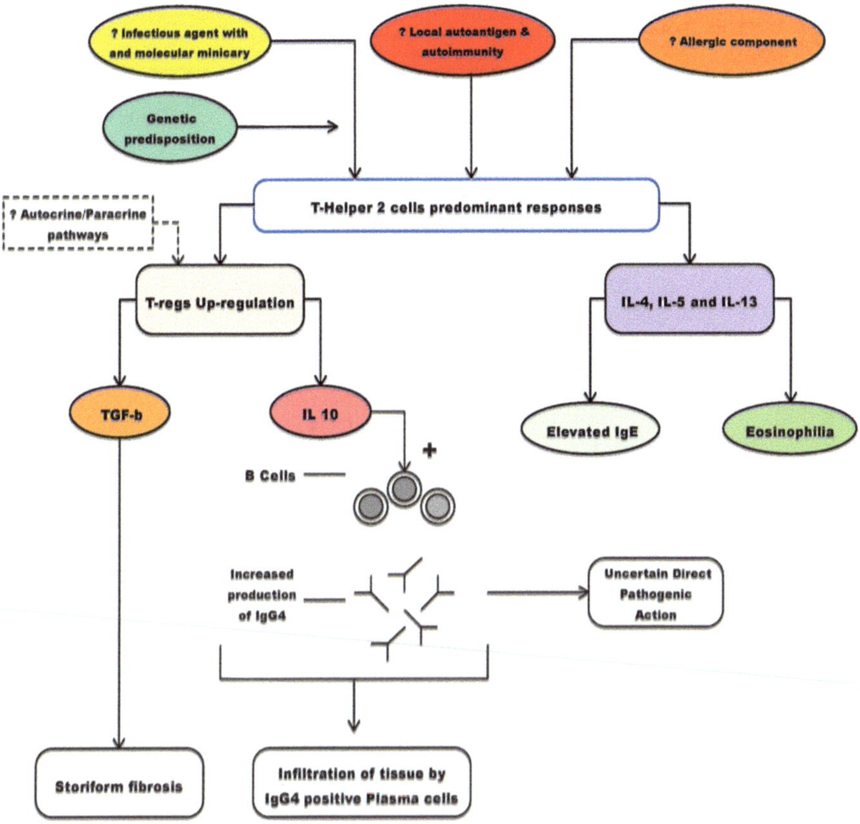

Fig. 5.1 Schematic representation of the current hypotheses on the aetiopathogenesis of IgG4-RD and IAC. (With thanks to WouterSmit (AMC, Amsterdam) for his contribution in illustrating this figure)

Role of Genetic Factors

HLA class II serotypes DRB1*0405 and DQB1*0401 have been associated with increased disease susceptibility in Japan [18]. In contrast, this was not demonstrated in Korea, where disease relapse was associated with aspartic acid substitution at DQβ1-57 [19]. Single nucleotide polymorphisms (SNP) involved in disease susceptibility or recurrence have been reported to be present within genes encoding cytotoxic T-lymphocyte-associated antigen 4 (CTLA-4), tumour necrosis factor-alpha (TNFα) and Fc receptor-like 3 (FcR-3) [20–23] (Table 5.1). However, most genetic studies have centred on AIP in Asian patients and the applicability of this to other ethnic groups remains uncertain.

Table 5.1 Single nucleotide polymorphisms associated with AIP

Proteins	SNP	Association	References
CTLA-4	49A haplotype	Higher in AIP in China	Chang et al. [20]
	−318C/+49A/CT60G	Increased susceptibility to AIP in China	Chang et al. [20]
	+6233 3′-untranslated region	Increased susceptibility to AIP in Japan	Umemura et al. [22]
	+6230G/G	AIP susceptibility	Umemura et al. [22]
	+6230A	AIP resistance	
	49A/A and +6230A/A genotypes	Increase AIP relapse in Japan	
TNF-α	863A haplotype	Extra-pancreatic involvement in China	Chang et al. [20]
FcR-3	−110A/A genotype	Increased susceptibility to AIP in Japan (serum IgG4 correlated to susceptible alleles)	Umemura et al. [21]

Loco-regional Factors

The involvement of the biliary tract, gallbladder and liver in many patients with AIP may suggest loco-regional factor(s) in pathogenesis. Peribiliary glands, which are physiologically distributed around the extrahepatic and intrahepatic large bile ducts [24] may be severely damaged in patients with IAC [25]. These glands are known to contain small amounts of exocrine pancreatic acini [26]. It has been postulated that a common antigen could be expressed in these glands, leading to the spectrum of manifestations observed in the hepato-biliary-pancreatic ductal system.

Helicobacter pylori and Molecular Mimicry

A role for gastric *Helicobacter pylori* in the pathogenesis of AIP was suggested in 2005 on the basis that *H. pylori* was associated with other autoimmune disorders and an increased detection of peptic ulcers in patients with AIP [27]. Significant homology between human carbonic anhydrase-II (CA-II) and α-carbonic anhydrase of *H. pylori* in segments containing the binding motif of the susceptibility HLA molecule DRB1_0405 was demonstrated [28], and the authors proposed that this pathogen may trigger AIP in genetically predisposed individuals by means of molecular mimicry. This hypothesis was supported by the detection of antibodies against plasminogen-binding protein of *H. pylori* in 94 % of patients in an Italian cohort with AIP [29]. In a recent study, no sequences of *H. pylori* DNA could be demonstrated in tissue or pancreatic juice from patients with AIP suggesting a direct infection was unlikely [30]. The role of this pathogen remains undetermined.

Autoimmunity and Autoantigens

Several autoantigens have been investigated based on the theory that IgG4-RD is an autoimmune disorder. Non-specific antinuclear antibodies are identified in more than half of patients. Autoantibodies against lactoferrin (LF) and carbonic anhydrase (CA)-II, expressed in exocrine organs including the pancreas, salivary gland, bile duct, and renal tubules, can be detected in 73 and 54 % AIP patients, respectively [31]. A strong positive correlation between increased serum IgG4 levels and anti-CA-II antibody levels has been reported [32]. Anti-CA-IV antibodies, expressed in the epithelial cells of several organs, have also been detected in 34 % of AIP patients [33]. The wide distribution of LF and CA was suggested to provide a unifying explanation for the multisystem involvement in IgG4-RD, but these antibodies are non-specific for the disease. Antibodies against pancreatic secretory trypsin inhibitor (PSTI) were detected in 30–40 % of AIP patients [34] and autoantibodies against pancreatic exocrine enzymes and anti-PSTI antibodies were demonstrated by RNA microarray of pancreatic tissue and immunoassays in AIP patients from Europe [35]. In a proteomics study from Japan, a 13.1-kDa protein was identified as a candidate autoantigen, although the sequence has not been determined [36].

Role of IgG4 Molecule

IgG4 is the least common IgG subclass representing less than 5 % of total IgG in the serum [37]. However, it can account for up to 80 % of total IgG after chronic exposure to certain antigens. IgG4 is a unique antibody with important amino acid differences to IgG1 in the CH2 domain resulting in an inability to activate complement via the classical pathway and reduced cellular immune responses due to decreased binding to the Fc-gamma receptors of effector cells [17, 38]. In the core hinge region, an amino acid switch allows IgG4 to undergo exchange of half-antibodies generating functionally monovalent antibodies which cannot cross-link antigens or form large immune complexes. IgG4 can bind the Fc portion of other IgG molecules at its constant domain, contributing to its anti-inflammatory function.

A direct role for IgG4 antibody in the pathogenesis of IgG4-RD has not been confirmed. IgG4 autoantibodies have not been detected in IgG4-RD although they have been shown to play an important role in unrelated immune-mediated disorders such as pemphigus vulgaris [39]. Interestingly, IgG4 in sera from patients with AIP can bind with normal human bile and pancreatic duct epithelia, a reaction that was abolished with steroid therapy [40]. The dense infiltration of the affected tissues with IgG4-positive plasma cells and the elevated levels of serum IgG4 seen in the majority of patients is still unexplained, but may be an epiphenomenon of the disease [10].

Role of Type 2 Helper (Th2) T-Cell Immune Responses

The immune-pathogenesis underlying the prominent lymphoplasmocytic infiltration with abundant IgG4 positive plasma cells in this disease is not fully understood. On immunohistochemistry, both CD20+ B cells and CD4+ T cells are present. In tissue and blood, a Th2 immune response predominates with increased expression of IL-4, IL-5 and IL-13 [41, 42], unlike other autoimmune disorders such as PSC and PBC where Th1 immune responses result in increased production of IFN-γ [43, 44]. These Th2 responses and related cytokine profile may explain some of the findings in IAC including the elevated serum IgE level, peripheral and tissue eosinophilia seen in some patients [45]. A role for Th2 cytokines in the bile of IAC patients in disrupting the biliary epithelial cell barrier function leading to chronic biliary inflammation in these patients has also been proposed [42]. There is a well-known association of Th2 responses with allergic disorders, and a history of allergy reported in over half of patients with AIP, although an allergic trigger has not been demonstrated so far.

Role of T Regulatory Cells (Tregs)

Inducible-memory T regulatory cells (Tregs) and their regulatory cytokines were found to be up-regulated in both peripheral blood [46] and the affected tissues [41] of AIP and IAC patients. The reasons for this are not completely understood. Tregs are well known to play an important role in prevention of autoimmune disorders [47] and the attenuation of immune reactions associated with allergic and infectious disorders [48] by producing the regulatory cytokines IL-10 and tumour growth factor-b (TGF-b). The up-regulation of Tregs in IAC and AIP, therefore, may represent a secondary reaction to the excessive Th2 responses. It has been demonstrated previously that IL-10 can induce B cells to isotype switch to produce IgG4 [49] and that TGF-b is an important cytokine involved in tissue fibrogenesis. Therefore, the up-regulation of these two regulatory cytokines may mediate the two major histological manifestations of IgG4-RDs, i.e. infiltration of IgG4-positive plasma cells in affected tissues and storiform fibrosis.

Epidemiology and Demographics

Epidemiological data on the prevalence of IAC is scarce due to the lack of population-based studies. Most studies come from Japan and focus mainly on AIP. The estimated prevalence of AIP was reported to be 0.8 cases per 100,000 persons in Japan and the incidence was estimated to be 0.28–1.08/100,000, with approximately 336–1300 new cases per year [6]. Around 74 % of AIP patients are reported to have a concomitant IAC whereas isolated IAC is seen only in 8 % of cases [50].

Therefore, the prevalence of IAC may be estimated to be around three quarters that of AIP. Approximately 10 % of patients originally diagnosed with "sclerosing cholangitis" will have steroid-responsive strictures of the biliary tract with lymphoplasmocyticinfiltrates and IgG4-positive plasma cells in their bile ducts histology—these patients most likely have IAC rather than PSC, although diagnostic criteria should be adhered to when making this diagnosis [51].

The prevalence of IAC among patients diagnosed as PSC was evaluated by some previous studies that reported that approximately 7–9 % of patients presenting as PSC have features of IAC [52, 53]. In the largest two series of patients reported from Mayo Clinic [50] and King's College in London [2], the majority of patients were adults, male and typically older than 50 years.

Clinical Features

Clinical Manifestations

The spectrum of clinical manifestations in IAC is highly variable. Compared to classical PSC [54], 75 % of IAC patients present abruptly with obstructive jaundice [14]. The pancreas is involved in more than 90 % of IAC patients, therefore manifestations of pancreatic insufficiency including anorexia, weight loss, steatorrhoea and new-onset diabetes mellitus are often present [1, 4, 14]. Other common symptoms may include abdominal pain, pruritus, pancreatitis, and cholestatic biochemistry [50]. IAC patients may also present with a pancreatic mass, common bile duct/hilar strictures or hepatic mass mimicking pancreatic cancer, CCA and hepatocellular carcinoma (HCC) respectively. Differentiating AIP and IAC from these malignancies is impossible based on symptoms alone and can result in inappropriate major surgical interventions unless considered early and excluded [2, 4].

Laboratory Findings

Around 90 % of patients with IAC have elevated serum alkaline phosphatase and gamma-glutamyltransferase levels at diagnosis. Serum bilirubin levels are usually higher compared to classical PSC patients, particularly in those presenting with obstructive jaundice [38, 55].

Hypergammaglobulinemia is common [55–58], however, it is usually caused by the significantly higher IgG4 levels compared to PSC patients where IgG1 is predominant [55]. Markedly raised IgG4 levels >2.8 g/L (twice the upper limit of normal) are more suggestive of IAC and >5.6 g/L (four times the upper limit of normal) are highly specific for IAC, whereas moderately raised levels >1.4–2.8 g/L can be seen in otherwise classical PSC [53], cholangiocarcinoma [59], pancreatic cancer [60] and other inflammatory and infective disorders. Furthermore, serum IgG4 levels >1.4 g/L can be seen in 5 % of healthy individuals. IgG4 levels can be normal in almost 20 % of patients at diagnosis [58] and can define a milder clinical phenotype with lower risk of relapse and fewer organs involved. Specificity and sensitivity of 97 and 50 % for IAC, respectively, were obtained using IgG4 levels >2.8 g/L [59]. Specificity and sensitivity of 100 and 26 %, respectively, using a cut-off of IgG4 >5.6 g/L was reported [59]. Therefore a very high serum IgG4 is highly specific for IAC but below a cut-off of 5.6 g/L there are limitations to differentiate from other disease mimics. The utility of biliary IgG4 levels for IAC was recently explored in a single small study which showed promise but needs further clarification [61]. The use of ratios such as the IgG4-positive plasma cell/mononuclear cell ratio was found to be significantly higher in IAC than PSC and needs extended studies [62].

ANAs and other disease non-specific autoantibodies, eosinophilia, and/or elevated IgE levels might be seen in around 20–40 % of IAC cases but are non-specific. Anti-neutrophil cytoplasmic antibodies (pANCA), which are frequently detected in PSC, are usually absent in IAC. Tumour markers are also not specific to distinguish IAC from malignancy, with high serum Ca19-9 observed in IAC (63 % in one study) [56, 58] and normal or minimally elevated CEA levels in most IAC patients [58].

Cholangiography and Imaging Features

The spectrum of radiological features in IAC is variable and nonspecific. As only a few cases present with isolated biliary disease, pancreatic disease is usually evident on imaging. Dynamic computed tomography (CT) and magnetic resonance cholangiopancreatography (MRCP) may show diffuse enlargement of the pancreas or a focal lesion that mimics pancreatic cancer [63] (Fig. 5.2). Other less commonly described findings include acute pancreatitis, pancreatic atrophy and diffuse enhancement [50] (Fig. 5.3). Although the ability of MRCP to delineate abnormalities of the main pancreatic duct is limited as compared to retrograde cholangiopancreatography (ERCP) in almost half of patients with diffuse type AIP [64], it continues to be a valuable non-invasive tool for the detection of pancreatic gland abnormalities as well as for follow-up of patients with IAC/AIP. Hilar space-occupying lesions or hepatic mass-like lesions mimicking CCA and HCC, respectively, are among other possible findings.

Strictures, wall thickening or both are the most frequently reported radiological abnormalities in patients with IAC. Circular and symmetrical thickening of the bile duct wall, smooth outer and inner margins, and a homogenous internal echo can be demonstrated on abdominal ultrasonography (US) [65], CT [66], MRCP, endoscopic ultrasound (EUS) and intraductal ultrasonography (IDUS). Interestingly, these features can be demonstrated in both stenotic and non-stenotic areas as well as in the gallbladder wall.

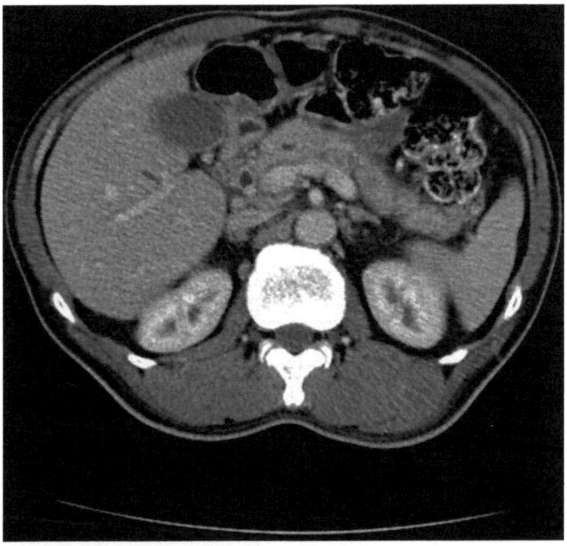

Fig. 5.2 CT abdomen and pelvis with contrast showing a mass at the head of the pancreas obstructing the distal common bile duct with proximal intra hepatic duct dilatation and mild pancreatic duct dilatation

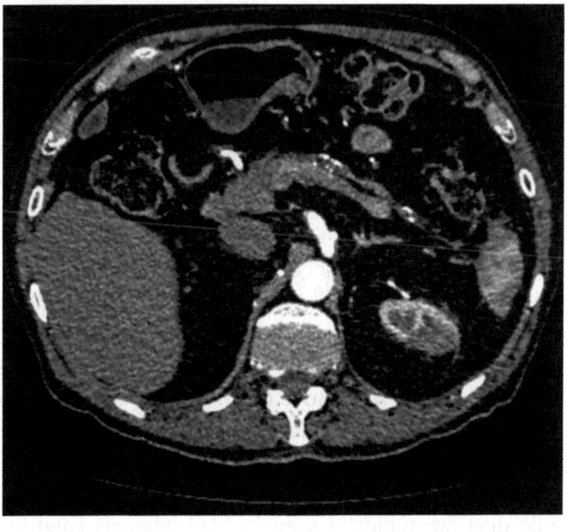

Fig. 5.3 CT abdomen and pelvis with contrast showing an atrophic pancreas in a patient with AIP and IAC. Bile duct resection with Roux en Y anastomosis for recurrent cholangitis originally diagnosed as PSC

The distribution of the radiological changes in IAC is variable. Although a distal common bile duct (CBD) stricture is classical (Fig. 5.4), the involvement of both intrahepatic and extrahepatic bile ducts is evident in approximately 50 % of patients [55, 67] (Fig. 5.5). Inflammation and/or edema of the pancreas may contribute to the stricture; however, thickening of the bile duct itself can usually be demonstrated [68]. MRCP is helpful for delineating the distribution and the extent of the strictures; nevertheless, direct assessment by ERCP or percutaneous transhepatic cholangiography is usually indicated. Advantages of ECRP in this regard relate to its better

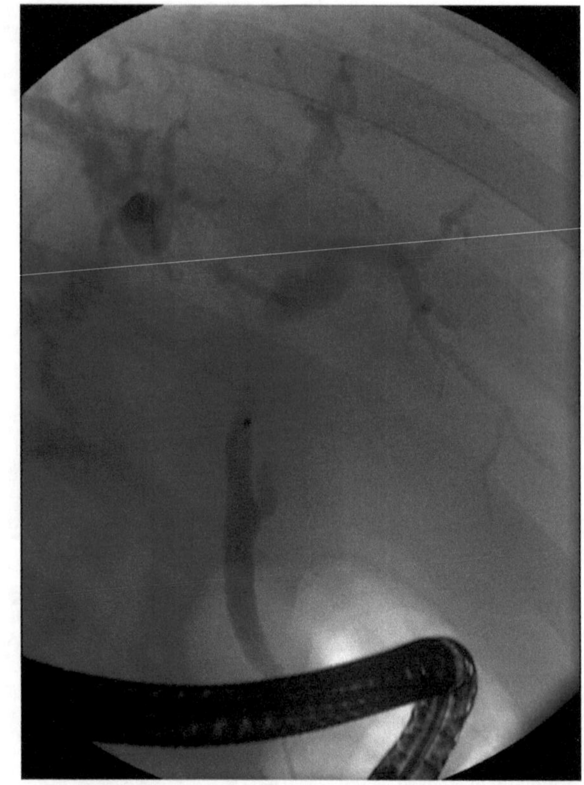

Fig. 5.4 ERCP showing a common hepatic duct stricture with distal right and left hepatic duct dilatation in a patient with isolated IAC. Stent was placed into the left hepatic duct system. This patient had a normal serum IgG4 and proceeded to hepatic resection for presumed cholangiocarcinoma. Resection confirmed classical changes of IAC

sensitivity for the detection of subtle changes in the biliary tree and the main pancreatic duct as well as its therapeutic implications including obtaining brushings and biopsies for histopathology assessment and temporary stent insertion to relieve obstructive jaundice or cholangitis [38, 64]. EUS has a role to obtain fine needle aspirates (FNA) to exclude dysplasia and biopsy of a mass where possible.

Due to "similar" cholangiography findings, IAC was thought once to represent a PSC variant. There are however subtle differences on imaging [69]. Segmental strictures, long strictures with pre-stenotic dilatation and strictures of the distal common bile duct are typically seen in IAC whereas band-like strictures, beading, pruned-tree appearance and diverticulum-like out-pouching are more typical of classical PSC. Recently, Japanese investigators proposed a cholangiography-based classification for IAC [70]. According to this IAC can be classified into four types. IAC Type 1 is characterised by an isolated distal CBD stricture with chronic pancreatitis—pancreatic cancer and CCA being the most relevant differential diagnosis, which can be distinguished by IDUS [71], EUS-FNA [72] and/or biopsy of the bile duct [7, 71]. In IAC type 2, both the intrahepatic and extrahepatic bile ducts are involved and it must be differentiated from PSC. Based on the presence or absence of pre-stenotic dilatation with the intrahepatic strictures, this type is further subdivided into Type 2a and 2b respectively. The significance of these subtypes is unclear; however, Type 2b is thought

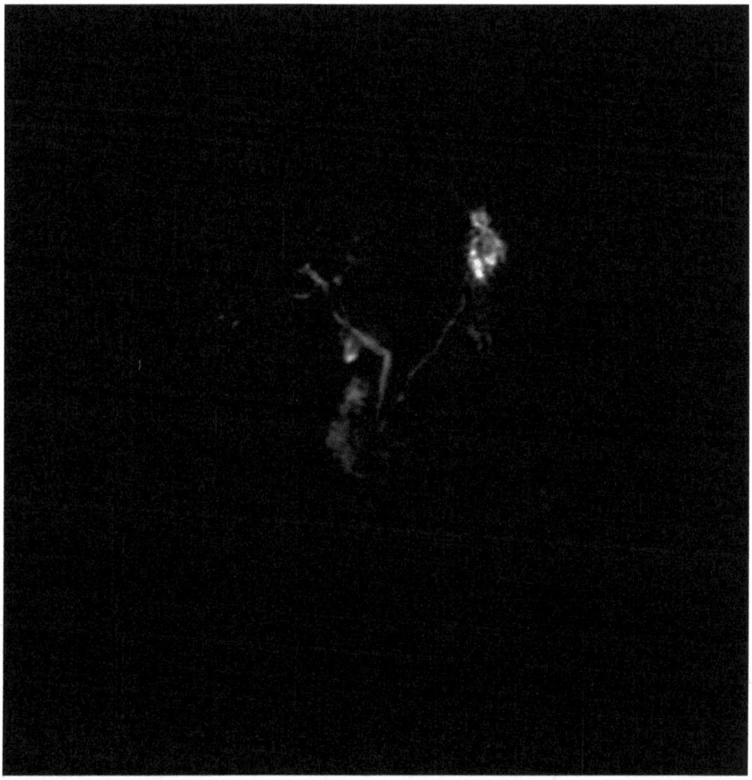

Fig. 5.5 MRCP showing diffuse intrahepatic duct irregularities of IAC with an extrahepatic duct stricture. This patient was originally diagnosed with PSC. Biopsy of the liver and bile duct confirmed IAC and response to corticosteroids was seen

to result from marked lymphoplasmocytic infiltration into the peripheral bile ducts. IAC Type 3 is characterised by hilar and distal CBD strictures whereas Type 4 shows only hilar strictures and both should be distinguished from CCA by means of EUS, IDUS, cytology and/or biopsy of the bile duct. It must be mentioned, however, that the cholangiography findings in some patients with IAC do not fit into any of these four types and the clinical utility of this approach has not been validated.

Histopathology Features

Although the microanatomy of the affected organs and probably the age of the lesions may cause some variability, the histological findings in IAC are generally similar to those seen in other organs involved in IgG4-RD. The large bile ducts are usually affected; however, changes in the small intrahepatic bile ducts can be occasionally demonstrated on liver biopsy.

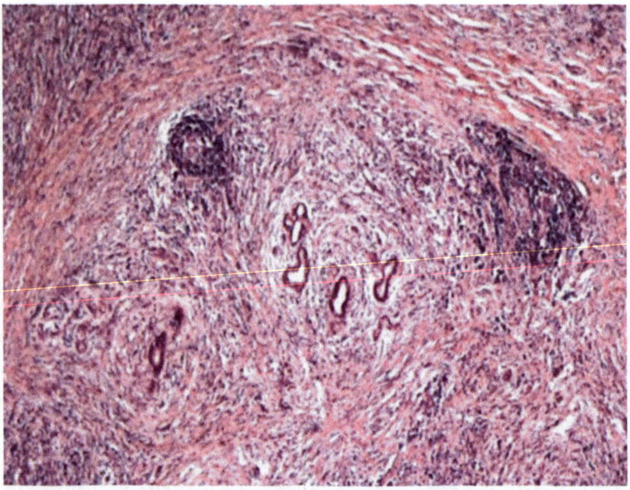

Fig. 5.6 Histology (H and E) from a bile duct resection demonstrating a lymphoplasmacytic cell infiltrate with peri-ductal distribution and a storiform fibrosis

Histopathological Characteristics of Large Duct Disease

Extrahepatic, hilar and perihilar bile ducts, and also frequently the gallbladder are involved in IAC [12, 14, 50]. Macroscopically, resected bile ducts appear diffusely thickened leading to a "pipe-stem" fibrosis like appearance. Mucosal surfaces are usually normal. Occasionally, periductal inflammatory mass lesions in the resected hilar and perihilar ducts can be seen [73]. The classical findings of IAC on histology include a dense lymphoplasmacytic infiltrate, storiform fibrosis and obliterative phlebitis. The combination of these findings coupled with the presence of a significant number of IgG4-positive plasma cells (>10 IgG4-positive plasma cells per mean of three high-power fields (hpf) on biopsy and >50 IgG4-positive plasma cells per mean of three hpf on surgical resection) and an IgG4/IgG ratio of over 40 % is strongly suggestive of IAC in the correct clinical context.

The lymphoplasmacytic infiltrates consist of evenly distributed lymphocytes that often organise into lymphoid aggregates with occasional germinal centres (Fig. 5.6). T-Cells usually predominate, with scattered aggregates of B-cells. Plasma cells are an essential component and may predominate the cellular infiltrates. These cells are polyclonal, in fact a clonal population of plasma cells is sufficient to exclude IgG4-RD. A few macrophages, histocytes and moderate tissue eosinophilia is not uncommon [2, 12, 74]. The inflammatory process is intermingled with a unique storiform pattern of fibrosis that resembles the spokes of a cartwheel with spindle cells radiating from a centre. Compared to PSC, the biliary epithelium appears normal, unless a biliary stent is present. The fibro-inflammatory process usually extends to the peribiliary adventitial veins, nerves and glands [12]. Obliterative phlebitis results from obliteration of adventitial venous channels within the dense lymphoplasmacytic infiltrates (Fig. 5.7). Lymphocytes and plasma cells can be seen

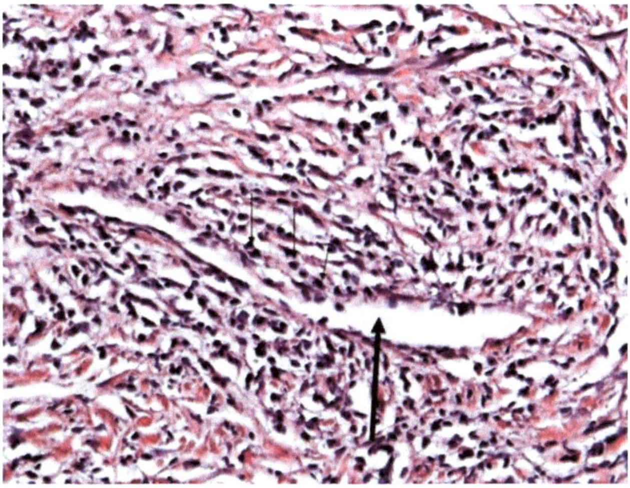

Fig. 5.7 Histology (H and E) showing obliterative phlebitis

within the wall and the lumen of the veins. Occasionally, the obliteration can be partial. Arteritis is not a usual finding, although its presence does not exclude the diagnosis. The inflammatory process involving the hilar/perihilar region is largely confined to the portal tracts, with only minimal extension into the adjacent liver parenchyma [2, 12, 74].

Although not entirely specific, demonstration of IgG4-positive plasma cells on immunohistochemistry is important for diagnosis. However, these cells have been also demonstrated in a number of other disorders [2, 74]. The number of IgG4-positive plasma cells in IAC and other IgG4-RDs, however, has been shown in multiple studies to be significantly higher than other disorders. The exact cutoff of IgG4-positive plasma cells with which the diagnosis can be made with high confidence is controversial. It varies between organs and depending on the presence of fibrosis. A recent consensus statement proposed that >50/HPF in surgical specimens and >10/HPF in biopsy samples are required for diagnosis of IAC [75]. It should be remembered, however, that these cutoffs are not essential for the diagnosis, as fewer cells can be seen in some patients with long standing fibrotic disease [75] (Fig. 5.8). IgG4/IgG cell counts ratio >40 % was found to be particularly helpful in discriminating IgG4-RD from other disorders with moderate number of IgG4-positive plasma cells [74, 75]. Nevertheless, this ratio itself is not sufficient to establish the diagnosis and should be interpreted in conjunction with other clinical, radiological, serology and histopathology findings [75].

Histopathology Findings of Small Duct Lesions

Although frequently variable and inconclusive, small bile duct involvement can be demonstrated on liver biopsy [76]. The spectrum of possible histological changes includes sclerotic changes with dense periportal fibrosis, marked portal inflammation

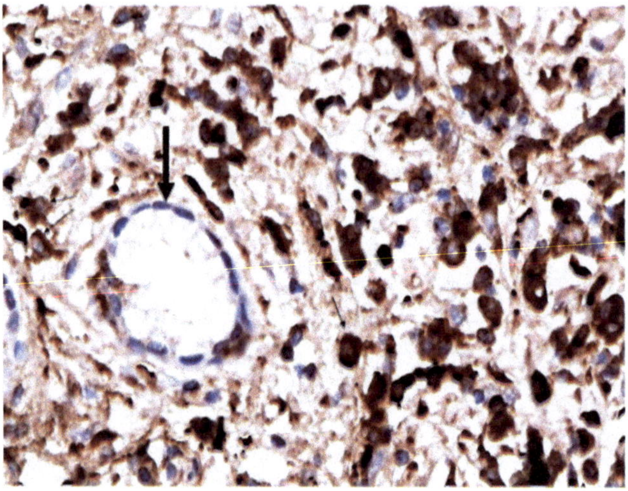

Fig. 5.8 Immunostaining of the bile duct showing IgG4-positive plasma cells >10/HPF (*dark brown*)

with many plasma cells, ductular reaction, lobular inflammation and canalicular cholestasis [76]. Characteristic features like obliterative phlebitis can be demonstrated when a medium-sized portal vein is present in the specimen obtained. More than 10/HPF IgG4-positive plasma cells (20 % of biopsy samples) [76–78] and small inflammatory nodules in peripheral portal tracts that are composed of spindle cells, lymphocytes, plasma cells, and eosinophils are specific findings for IAC [77, 78]. Ductopaenia and periductal fibrosis, typically seen in PSC, argues strongly against IAC [76–78].

Diagnosis

There is no pathognomonic feature of IAC. Common features seen in IAC such as pancreatic duct abnormalities (7–15 %), increased serum IgG4 (9–36 %) and IgG4-positive plasma cells (23 %) were reported to occur also in patients with PSC and other disorders [3]. Therefore, IAC diagnosis must be based on a combination of clinical, serologic, imaging, and histologic findings [4]. Multiple diagnostic criteria have been proposed in order to distinguish IAC from other conditions that may share similar features. The HISORt (histology, imaging, serology, other organ involvement and response to corticosteroid) criteria for AIP [63] and its IAC version [50] (Table 5.2), Asian consensus criteria [79] and most recently new Japanese criteria [80] (Table 5.3) are the most widely applied. Although these criteria share almost the same diagnostic items, the combination of criteria required to establish a definite diagnosis is variable. For example, a definite diagnosis can be established in the presence of either typical histology from a previous resection or biopsy or

Table 5.2 The HISORt criteria for IAC [50]

	Diagnostic criterion	Description
1	Histology of bile duct	Lymphoplasmacytic sclerosing cholangitis on resection specimens (lymphoplasmacytic infiltrate with >10 IgG4-positive cells/HPF within and around bile ducts with associated obliterative phlebitis and storiform fibrosis). Bile duct biopsy specimens often do not provide sufficient tissue for a definitive diagnosis; however, presence of >10 IgG4-positive cells/HPF is suggestive of IAC
2	Imaging of bile duct	One or more strictures involving intrahepatic, proximal extrahepatic, or intrapancreatic bile ducts Fleeting/migrating biliary strictures
3	Serology	Increased serum IgG4 level (normal, 8–140 mg/dL)
4	Other organ involvement	Pancreas: classic features of AIP on imaging or histology; suggestive pancreatic imaging findings: focal pancreatic mass/enlargement without pancreatic duct dilation, multiple pancreatic masses, focal pancreatic duct stricture without upstream dilatation, pancreatic atrophy Retroperitoneal fibrosis Renal lesions: single or multiple parenchymal low-attenuation lesions (round, wedge-shaped, or diffuse patchy) Salivary/lacrimal gland enlargement
5	Response to steroid therapy	Normalisation of liver enzyme increase or resolution of stricture (although complete resolution of stricture may not be seen early in the course of treatment or in patients with predominantly fibrotic strictures)

N.B: 1 or 2+3=definite diagnosis

Table 5.3 Japanese IgG-4 sclerosing cholangitis diagnostic criteria

Diagnostic item	1. Biliary tract imaging shows diffuse or segmental narrowing of the intrahepatic or extrahepatic bile duct associated with the thickening of bile duct wall 2. Increased serum IgG4 levels (>135 mg/dL) 3. Coexistence of AIP, IgG4-related dacryoadenitis/sialoadenitis, or IgG4-related retroperitoneal fibrosis 4. Histology shows: a. Marked lymphocytic and plasmacyte infiltration and fibrosis b. Infiltration of IgG4-positive cells (>10 cells/high-power field) c. Storiform fibrosis d. Obliterative phlebitis Option: effectiveness of steroid therapy (as determined at specialised facility)
Diagnosis (once PSC, malignant diseases and secondary sclerosing cholangitis have been excluded)	Definite: combinations of (1) and (3); (1), (2) and (4) a/b; (4) a/b/c; (4) a/b/d Probable: combination of (1), (2) and option Possible: combination of (1) and (2)

From Ohara H, Okazaki K, Tsubouchi H, et al. Clinical diagnostic criteria of IgG4-related sclerosing cholangitis 2012. J HepatobiliaryPancreatSci 2012;19:538. Reprinted with permission from Springer classic imaging of AIP/IAC with increased serum IgG4 levels according to the HISORtcriteria [50]. In patients who have do not meet these criteria and have a high index of suspicion, every effort should be made to rule out malignancy. This is followed by a re-evaluation after 4 weeks of corticosteroids therapy and if a response is observed the diagnosis of IAC can be confirmed. In contrast, response to steroids is considered as an optional criterion by the Asian and Japanese criteria and its presence cannot establish a definite diagnosis in the absence of other criteria that are considered crucial for definite diagnosis [79, 80].

Although these criteria are helpful in clinical practice for establishing the diagnosis, every effort must be done to exclude other disorders including malignancy. Pancreatic cancer, CCA, PSC and other causes of lymphoplasmacytic cholangitis are the most relevant differential in this situation and will often require biopsy to exclude (Table 5.3).

Treatment

Distinguishing IAC from other disorders is not of academic interest only. Given the dramatic response to corticosteroids in the inflammatory stage, establishing the correct diagnosis early in the course of the disease is important to prevent progressive fibrotic stricturing complications and unnecessary major surgical interventions for misdiagnosed disease.

Alleviation of jaundice, abdominal discomfort, improvement of radiological and biochemical abnormalities constitute the main objectives in the initial phase of treatment. This is usually achieved in most cases with a course of steroids for 4–8 weeks with gradual taper as response is seen. A trial of corticosteroids may be initiated in those patients in whom IAC is highly suspected but who do not fulfil the diagnostic criteria for definite IAC (after best possible exclusion of malignancy) with the objective of confirming the diagnosis if a response is observed [81]. Although spontaneous resolution has been described [50], steroids have consistently been shown to hasten clinical and radiological remission and reduce the risk of future relapse. The minority of strictures will fail to show response to the treatment due to irreversible fibrosis in long-standing biliary strictures. In these patients remission of pancreatic disease or other organ involvement may be seen.

There is no international consensus on an appropriate steroid regimen, duration of treatment or the management of relapse due to a lack of randomised clinical trials. Therefore, treatment recommendations are based mainly on the clinical experience of experts in the treatment of IAC. The most widely applied regimens come from the Mayo Clinic and Japan [82, 83]. The recommendations from the Mayo Clinic suggest prednisone 40 mg/day for 4 weeks as an initial dose, followed by repeat laboratory tests and imaging in 4–6 weeks' time. If clinical and radiological response is achieved, prednisone dose should be tapered by 5 mg every week to complete a treatment course of 11 weeks [82]. In contrast, a weight-based dose of prednisolone (0.6 mg/kg/day) that can be tapered gradually to 5 mg/day over 3–6 months in patients with clinical and radiological response is recommended by the Japanese. A maintenance dose of steroids (2.5–10 mg/day) for at least 6 months and possibly up to 3 years is instituted [83].

Due to the dramatic response to steroids, therapeutic intervention with ERCP and biliary stenting are not required after steroid initiation. Nevertheless, biliary stenting is usually performed in many patients before establishing the diagnosis with quick resolution of symptoms. Repeat stenting is not usually needed in patients who achieve remission. In patients with long standing strictures, who may not respond to therapy prolonged stenting might be required [50].

After initial response, approximately 30–50 % of IAC patients may experience disease recurrence either during the tapering phase or within the first 3 years [83, 84] after stopping corticosteroids. Several factors were proposed to predict early relapse in these patients. These include increasing levels of AlkPhos and IgG4 [85], persistently high serum IgG4 levels [83, 85] and the involvement of proximal bile duct [50, 83]. There is no consensus regarding the management of disease recurrence. However, European and US groups recommend resuming the original dose of steroids that can be subsequently replaced by a steroid sparing agent like azathioprine [50, 86, 87], 6-mercaptopurine or mycophenolate mofetil [50, 87, 88] for long-term immunosuppression. The Mayo group recently reported relapse free survival with prednisolone alone was similar to prednisolone plus an immunosuppressive [86].

In patients with refractory disease or frequent relapses treatment options are more challenging. Successful use of immunosuppressive drugs like budesonide and rituximab has been reported [89, 90]. Recently, investigators from the Mayo Clinic proposed a treatment algorithm for management of disease relapses in patients with definite IAC and AIP [87]. According to this algorithm a course of steroids should be repeated in all patients followed by re-evaluation of disease activity in 6–8 weeks' time. Patients with rapid response should proceed with steroid taper with or without maintenance treatment. Alternatively, an immunomodulator can be started in conjunction with steroids over an overlap tapering period of 8 weeks. Patients who do not achieve complete remission and those who are steroid dependent (requiring prednisone doses of 20 mg/day or higher to maintain remission) or intolerant to steroids or immunomodulator may benefit from treatment with rituximab [87].

Refinements of the current treatment strategies for IAC are certainly required. It remains unclear whether the high rate of disease recurrence is an intrinsic feature of this disease or the result of suboptimal treatment regimens. Randomised clinical trials are certainly required to clarify the optimal initial management as well as the management of the disease relapse. Current recommendations are summarised in Fig. 5.9.

Prognosis and Natural History

Due to the short follow-up in most case series, prognosis and natural history of IAC are not well characterised. Spontaneous remissions in IAC are reported. However, without treatment, cases of biliary cirrhosis have also been reported [50].

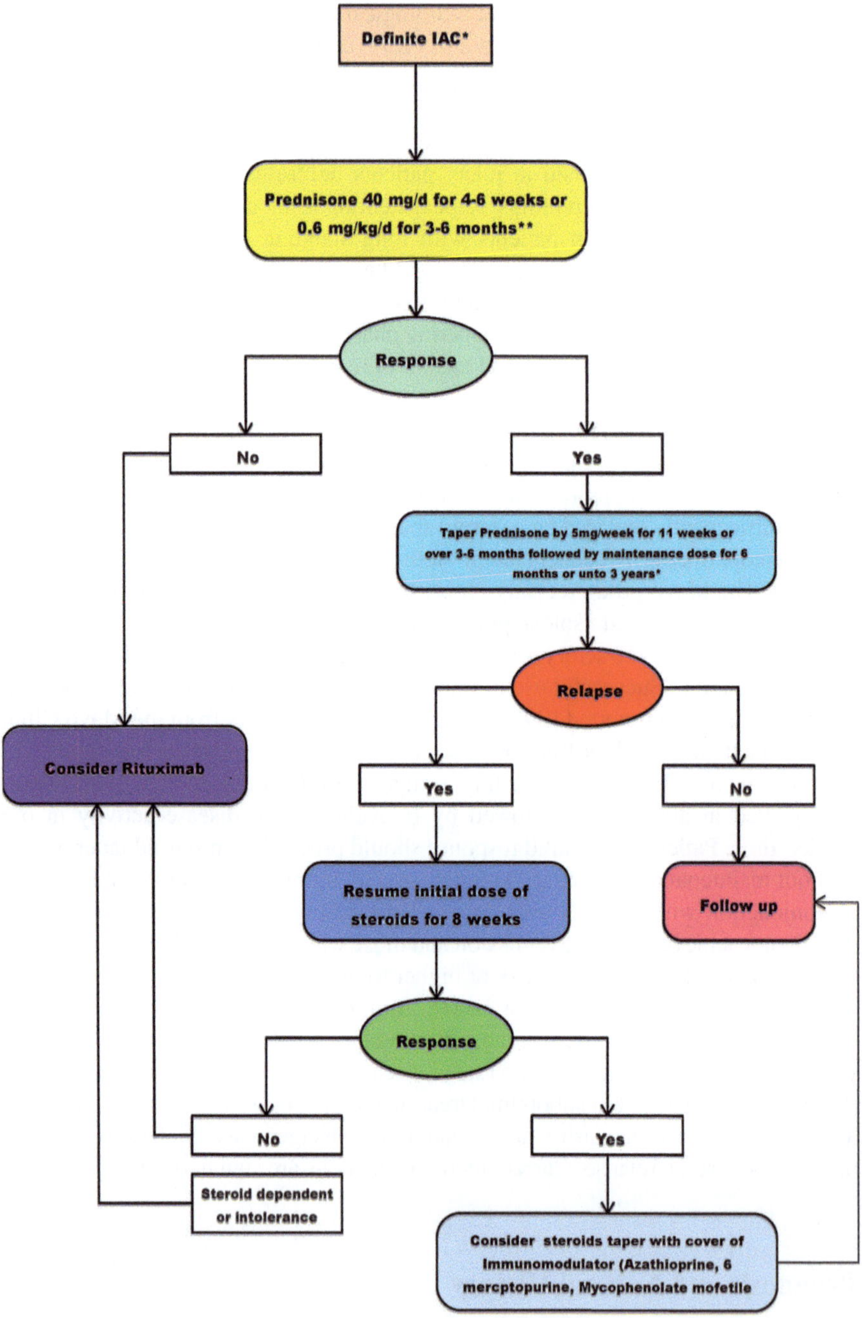

Fig. 5.9 Current recommendations for the initial treatment of definite IAC and management of relapse. (*Asterisk*) Every effort should be made to rule out malignancy. (*Double asterisks*) Japanese recommendations

The prevalence of cirrhosis in patients with IAC and the rate of progression to advanced fibrosis remains controversial. In this regard, four of 53 patients in one cohort developed portal hypertension and cirrhosis within 5 years of initial symptoms [50], whereas only one patient with untreated IAC developed early cirrhosis in another cohort [2].

In contrast to PSC, prognosis of patients with steroid responsive IAC is more favourable [52]. The need for liver transplantation seems to be exceedingly rare, as only one case of established IAC and another case with probable IAC has been reported so far [1]. Furthermore, cholangiocarcinoma in patients with IAC was not observed in the largest case series reported [52].

Summary

IAC is the biliary manifestation of IgG4-RD and occurs most frequently in older men in association with AIP type1. The immunopathogenesis of the disease including the role of IgG4, disease-specific antigens, Th2 immune response and genetics continues to be unravelled. The clinicopathological definition of IAC continues to evolve. Histology reveals a lymphoplasmacytic infiltrate, storiform fibrosis and obliterative phlebitis with a marked infiltration of IgG4-positive plasma cells. Overlap with similar diseases is becoming increasingly recognised and differentiation from disease mimics such as cancer and inflammatory disorders is important and challenging. Diagnostic algorithms have been developed to aid identification of this disease, and it is unlikely that any single criterion will be diagnostic in isolation. Treatment options continue to expand as 50 % of patients relapse and experience with B cell depletion therapies in refractory disease grows. Prospective studies of IAC patients are required to clarify the natural history and long-term outcome of patients, although it seems to have a favourable prognosis compared to PSC.

References

1. MD MGS. IgG4-associated cholangitis. Clin Liver Dis [Internet]. 2013;17:255–68.
2. Zen YY, Nakanuma YY, Portmann BB. Immunoglobulin G4-related sclerosing cholangitis: pathologic features and histologic mimics. Semin Diagn Pathol [Internet]. 2012;29:205–11.
3. Webster GJM, Pereira SP, Chapman RW. Autoimmune pancreatitis/IgG4-associated cholangitis and primary sclerosing cholangitis – overlapping or separate diseases? J Hepatol. 2009; 51:398–402.
4. Björnsson E. Immunoglobulin G4-associated cholangitis. Curr Opin Gastroenterol [Internet]. 2008;24:389–94.
5. Stone JH, Zen Y, Deshpande V. IgG4-related disease. N Engl J Med. 2013;366:539–51.
6. The Research Program for Intractable Disease by Ministry of Health, Labor and Welfare (MHLW) Japan G4 Team, Umehara H, Okazaki K, Masaki Y, Kawano M, Yamamoto M, et al. A novel clinical entity, IgG4-related disease (IgG4RD): general concept and details. Mod Rheumatol [Internet]. 2011;22:1–14.

7. Kamisawa T, Funata N, Hayashi Y, Eishi Y, Koike M, Tsuruta K, et al. A new clinicopathological entity of IgG4-related autoimmune disease. J Gastroenterol. 2003;38:982–4.
8. (null). IgG4-related disease: nomenclature, clinical features, and treatment. Semin Diagn Pathol [Internet]. 2012;29:177–90.
9. Yoshida K, Toki F, Takeuchi T, Watanabe S-I, Shiratori K, Hayashi N. Chronic pancreatitis caused by an autoimmune abnormality. Digest Dis Sci. 1995;40:1561–8.
10. Hamano H, Kawa S, Horiuchi A, Unno H, Furuya N, Akamatsu T, et al. High serum IgG4 concentrations in patients with sclerosing pancreatitis. N Engl J Med. 2001;344:732–8.
11. Kamisawa T, Okamoto A. Autoimmune pancreatitis: proposal of IgG4-related sclerosing disease. J Gastroenterol. 2006;41:613–25.
12. Zen YY, Harada KK, Sasaki MM, Sato YY, Tsuneyama KK, Haratake JJ, et al. IgG4-related sclerosing cholangitis with and without hepatic inflammatory pseudotumor, and sclerosing pancreatitis-associated sclerosing cholangitis: do they belong to a spectrum of sclerosing pancreatitis? AM J Surg Pathol [Internet]. 2004;28:1193–203.
13. Bartholomew LG, Cain JC, Woolner LB, Utz DC, Ferris DO. Sclerosing cholangitis. N Engl J Med. 1963;269:8–12.
14. Björnsson E, Chari ST, Smyrk TC, Lindor K. Immunoglobulin G4 associated cholangitis: description of an emerging clinical entity based on review of the literature. Hepatology. 2007; 45:1547–54.
15. Stone JH, Khosroshahi A, Deshpande V, Chan JKC, Heathcote JG, Aalberse R, et al. Recommendations for the nomenclature of IgG4-related disease and its individual organ system manifestations. Arthrit Rheumat. 2012;64:3061–7.
16. European Association for the Stud. EASL clinical practice guidelines: management of cholestatic liver diseases. J Hepatol. 2009;51:237–67.
17. Nakanuma Y, Zen Y. Pathology and immunopathology of immunoglobulin G4-related sclerosing cholangitis: the latest addition to the sclerosing cholangitis family. Hepatol Res. 2007; 37:S478–86.
18. Kawa S, Ota M, Yoshizawa K, Horiuchi A, Hamano H, Ochi Y, et al. HLA DRB10405-DQB10401 haplotype is associated with autoimmune pancreatitis in the Japanese population. Gastroenterology. 2002;122:1264–9.
19. Do Hyun do HP, Kim M-HM, Oh HBH, Kwon O-JO, Choi Y-JY, Lee S-SS, et al. Substitution of aspartic acid at position 57 of the DQ@b1 affects relapse of autoimmune pancreatitis. Gastroenterology. 2008;134:7–7.
20. Chang M-C, Chang Y-T, Tien Y-W, Liang P-C, Jan I-S, Wei S-C, et al. T-Cell regulatory gene CTLA-4 polymorphism/haplotype association with autoimmune pancreatitis. Clin Chem. 2007;53:1700–5.
21. Umemura T, Ota M, Hamano H, Katsuyama Y, Kiyosawa K, Kawa S. Genetic association of Fc receptor-like 3 polymorphisms with autoimmune pancreatitis in Japanese patients. Gut. 2006;55:1367–8.
22. Umemura T, Ota M, Hamano H, Katsuyama Y, Muraki T, Arakura N, et al. Association of autoimmune pancreatitis with cytotoxic T-lymphocyte antigen 4 gene polymorphisms in Japanese patients. Am J Gastroenterol. 2008;103:588–94.
23. Umemura T, Katsuyama Y, Hamano H, Kitahara K, Takayama M, Arakura N, et al. Association analysis of Toll-like receptor 4 polymorphisms with autoimmune pancreatitis. Hum Immunol. 2009;70:742–6.
24. Terada T, Nakanuma Y, Ohta G. Glandular elements around the intrahepatic bile ducts in man; their morphology and distribution in normal livers. Liver. 2008;7:1–8.
25. Lazaridis KN, Gores GJ. Primary sclerosing cholangitis and cholangiocarcinoma. Semin Liver Dis. 2006;26:042–51.
26. Terada T, Nakanuma Y. Pathological observations of intrahepatic peribiliary glands in 1,000 consecutive autopsy livers. III Survey of necroinflammation and cystic dilatation. Hepatology. 1990;12:1229–33.
27. Kountouras J, Zavos C, Chatzopoulos D. Autoimmune pancreatitis, *Helicobacter pylori* infection, and apoptosis: a proposed relationship. Pancreas. 2005;30:192.

28. Guarneri F, Guarneri C, Benvenga S. Helicobacter pylori and autoimmune pancreatitis: role of carbonic anhydrase via molecular mimicry? J Cell Mol Med. 2005;9:741–4.
29. Frulloni L, Lunardi C, Simone R, Dolcino M, Scattolini C, Falconi M, et al. Identification of a novel antibody associated with autoimmune pancreatitis. N Engl J Med. 2009;361:2135–42.
30. Jesnowski R, Isaksson B, Möhrckea C, Bertsch C, Bulajic M, Schneider-Brachert W, et al. Helicobacter pylori in autoimmune pancreatitis and pancreatic carcinoma. Pancreatology. 2010;10:462–6.
31. Okazaki K, Uchida K, Ohana M, Nakase H, Uose S, Inai M, et al. Autoimmune-related pancreatitis is associated with autoantibodies and a Th1/Th2-type cellular immune response. Gastroenterology. 2000;118:573–81.
32. Aparisi L, Farre A, Gomez-Cambronero L, Martinez J, De Las Heras G, Corts J, et al. Antibodies to carbonic anhydrase and IgG4 levels in idiopathic chronic pancreatitis: relevance for diagnosis of autoimmune pancreatitis. Gut. 2005;54:703–9.
33. Nishimori I. Serum antibodies to carbonic anhydrase IV in patients with autoimmune pancreatitis. Gut. 2005;54:274–81.
34. Asada M, Nishio A, Uchida K, Kido M, Ueno S, Uza N, et al. Identification of a novel autoantibody against pancreatic secretory trypsin inhibitor in patients with autoimmune pancreatitis. Pancreas. 2006;33:20–6.
35. Löhr JM, Faissner R, Koczan D, Bewerunge P, Bassi C, Brors B, et al. Autoantibodies against the exocrine pancreas in autoimmune pancreatitis: gene and protein expression profiling and immunoassays identify pancreatic enzymes as a major target of the inflammatory process. Am J Gastroenterol. 2010;105:2060–71.
36. Yamamoto M, Naishiro Y, Suzuki C, Kokai Y, Suzuki R, Honda S, et al. Proteomics analysis in 28 patients with systemic IgG4-related plasmacytic syndrome. Rheumatol Int. 2009;30:565–8.
37. Morell A, Skvaril F, Hitzig WH, Barandun S. IgG subclasses: development of the serum concentrations in "normal" infants and children. J Pediatr. 1972;80:960–4.
38. de Buy Wenniger LM, Rauws EA, Beuers U. What an endoscopist should know about immunoglobulin-G4-associated disease of the pancreas and biliary tree. Endoscopy. 2012;44:66–73.
39. Rock B, Martins CR, Theofilopoulos AN, Balderas RS, Anhalt GJ, Labib RS, et al. The pathogenic effect of IgG4 autoantibodies in endemic Pemphigus foliaceus (Fogo Selvagem). N Engl J Med. 1989;320:1463–9.
40. Aoki S, Nakazawa T, Ohara H, Sano H, Nakao H, Joh T, et al. Immunohistochemical study of autoimmune pancreatitis using anti-IgG4 antibody and patients' sera. Histopathology. 2005;47:147–58.
41. Zen Y, Fujii T, Harada K, Kawano M, Yamada K, Takahira M, et al. Th2 and regulatory immune reactions are increased in immunoglobin G4-related sclerosing pancreatitis and cholangitis. Hepatology. 2007;45:1538–46.
42. Müller T, Beutler C, Picó AH, Otten M, Dürr A, Abadi Al H, et al. Increased T-Helper 2 cytokines in bile from patients with IgG4-related cholangitis disrupt the tight junction-associated biliary epithelial cell barrier. Gastroenterology. 2013;144:1116–28.
43. Harada K, Van de Water J, Leung PS, Coppel RL, Ansari A, Nakanuma Y, et al. In situ nucleic acid hybridization of cytokines in primary biliary cirrhosis: predominance of the Th1 subset. Hepatology. 1997;25:791–6.
44. Lit LC-W, Wong C-K, Li EK-M, Tam L-S, Lam CW-K, Lo Y-MD. Elevated gene expression of Th1/Th2 associated transcription factors is correlated with disease activity in patients with systemic lupus erythematosus. J Rheumatol. 2007;34:89–96.
45. Guma M, Firestein GS. Best practice & research clinical rheumatology. Best Pract Res Clin Rheumatol. 2012;26:425–38.
46. Miyoshi H, Uchida K, Taniguchi T, Yazumi S, Matsushita M, Takaoka M, et al. Circulating naïve and CD4+CD25 high regulatory T cells in patients with autoimmune pancreatitis. Pancreas. 2008;36:133–40.

47. Maloy KJ, Salaun L, Cahill R, Dougan G, Saunders NJ, Powrie F. CD4+CD25+ TR cells suppress innate immune pathology through cytokine-dependent mechanisms. J Exp Med. 2002;197:111–9.
48. Vignali DAA, Collison LW, Workman CJ. How regulatory T cells work. Nat Rev Immunol. 2008;8:523–32.
49. Satoguina JS, Weyand E, Larbi J, Hoerauf A. T Regulatory-1 cells induce IgG4 production by B cells: role of IL-10. J Immunol. 2005;174:4718–26.
50. Ghazale A, Chari ST, Zhang L, Smyrk TC, Takahashi N, Levy MJ, et al. Immunoglobulin G4-associated cholangitis: clinical profile and response to therapy. Gastroenterology. 2008;134:10.
51. Kamisawa T. Sclerosing cholangitis associated with autoimmune pancreatitis differs from primary sclerosing cholangitis. WJG. 2009;15:2357.
52. Takikawa H, Takamori Y, Tanaka A, Kurihara H, Nakanuma Y. Analysis of 388 cases of primary sclerosing cholangitis in Japan presence of a subgroup without pancreatic involvement in older patients. Hepatol Res. 2004;29:153–9.
53. Mendes FD, Jorgensen R, Keach J, Katzmann JA, Smyrk T, Donlinger J, et al. Elevated serum IgG4 concentration in patients with primary sclerosing cholangitis. Am J Gastroenterol. 2006;101:2070–5.
54. Chapman RW, Arborgh BA, Rhodes JM, Summerfield JA, Dick R, Scheuer PJ, et al. Primary sclerosing cholangitis: a review of its clinical features, cholangiography, and hepatic histology. Gut. 1980;21:870–7.
55. Nakazawa T, Ohara H, Sano H, Ando T, Aoki S, Kobayashi S, et al. Clinical differences between primary sclerosing cholangitis and sclerosing cholangitis with autoimmune pancreatitis. Pancreas. 2005;30:20.
56. Kawaguchi K, Koike M, Tsuruta K, Okamoto A, Tabata I, Fujita N. Lymphoplasmacytic sclerosing pancreatitis with cholangitis: a variant of primary sclerosing cholangitis extensively involving pancreas. Hum Pathol. 1991;22:387–95.
57. Ichimura T, Kondo S, Ambo Y, Hirano S, Ohmi M, Okushiba S-I, et al. Primary sclerosing cholangitis associated with autoimmune pancreatitis. Hepatogastroenterology. 2002;49:1221–4.
58. Hirano K, Shiratori Y, Komatsu Y, Yamamoto N, Sasahira N, Toda N, et al. Involvement of the biliary system in autoimmune pancreatitis: a follow-up study. Clin Gastroenterol Hepatol. 2003;1:453–64.
59. Oseini AM, Chaiteerakij R, Shire AM, Ghazale A, Kaiya J, Moser CD, et al. Utility of serum immunoglobulin G4 in distinguishing immunoglobulin G4-associated cholangitis from cholangiocarcinoma. Hepatology. 2011;54:940–8.
60. Ghazale A, Chari ST, Smyrk TC, Levy MJ, Topazian MD, Takahashi N, et al. Value of serum IgG4 in the diagnosis of autoimmune pancreatitis and in distinguishing It from pancreatic cancer. Am J Gastroenterol. 2007;102:1646–53.
61. Vosskuhl K, Negm A, Framke T, Weismüller T, Manns M, Wedemeyer H, et al. Measurement of IgG4 in bile: a new approach for the diagnosis of IgG4-associated cholangiopathy. Endoscopy. 2011;44:48–52.
62. Uehara T, Hamano H, Kawa S, Sano K, Honda T, Ota H. Distinct clinicopathological entity "autoimmune pancreatitis-associated sclerosing cholangitis". Pathol Int. 2005;55:405–11.
63. Chari ST, Smyrk TC, Levy MJ, Topazian MD, Takahashi N, Zhang L, et al. Diagnosis of autoimmune pancreatitis: the Mayo Clinic experience. Clin Gastroenterol Hepatol. 2006;4:1010–6.
64. Kamisawa T, Tu Y, Egawa N, Tsuruta K, Okamoto A, Kodama M, et al. Can MRCP replace ERCP for the diagnosis of autoimmune pancreatitis? Abdom Imaging. 2008;34:381–4.
65. Koyama R, Imamura T, Okuda C, Sakamoto N, Honjo H, Takeuchi K. Ultrasonographic imaging of bile duct lesions in autoimmune pancreatitis. Pancreas. 2008;37:259–64.
66. Itoh S, Nagasaka T, Suzuki K, Satake H, Ota T, Naganawa S. Lymphoplasmacytic sclerosing cholangitis: assessment of clinical, CT, and pathological findings. Clin Radiol. 2009;64:1104–14.

67. Nishino T, Toki F, Oyama H, Oi I, Kobayashi M, Takasaki K, et al. Biliary tract involvement in autoimmune pancreatitis. Pancreas. 2005;30:76.
68. Hirano K, Tada M, Isayama H, Yamamoto K, Mizuno S, Yagioka H, et al. Endoscopic evaluation of factors contributing to intrapancreatic biliary stricture in autoimmune pancreatitis. Gastrointest Endosc. 2010;71:85–90.
69. Nakazawa T, Ohara H, Sano H, Aoki S, Kobayashi S, Okamoto T, et al. Cholangiography can discriminate sclerosing cholangitis with autoimmune pancreatitis from primary sclerosing cholangitis. Gastrointest Endosc. 2004;60:937–44.
70. Nakazawa T, Ohara H, Sano H, Ando T, Joh T. Schematic classification of sclerosing cholangitis with autoimmune pancreatitis by cholangiography. Pancreas. 2006;32:229.
71. Naitoh I, Nakazawa T, Ohara H, Ando T, Hayashi K, Tanaka H, et al. Endoscopic transpapillary intraductal ultrasonography and biopsy in the diagnosis of IgG4-related sclerosing cholangitis. J Gastroenterol. 2009;44:1147–55.
72. Mizuno N, Bhatia V, Hosoda W, Sawaki A, Hoki N, Hara K, et al. Histological diagnosis of autoimmune pancreatitis using EUS-guided trucut biopsy: a comparison study with EUS-FNA. J Gastroenterol. 2009;44:742–50.
73. Zen Y, Fujii T, Sato Y, Masuda S, Nakanuma Y. Pathological classification of hepatic inflammatory pseudotumor with respect to IgG4-related disease. Mod Pathol. 2007;20:884–94.
74. Deshpande V. The pathology of IgG4-related disease: critical issues and challenges. Semin Diagn Pathol. 2012;29:191–6.
75. Deshpande V, Zen Y, Chan JK, Yi EE, Sato Y, Yoshino T, et al. Consensus statement on the pathology of IgG4-related disease. Mod Pathol. 2012;25:1181–92.
76. Umemura T, Zen Y, Hamano H, Kawa S, Nakanuma Y, Kiyosawa K. Immunoglobin G4-hepatopathy: association of immunoglobin G4-bearing plasma cells in liver with autoimmune pancreatitis. Hepatology. 2007;46:463–71.
77. Naitoh I, Zen Y, Nakazawa T, Ando T, Hayashi K, Okumura F, et al. Small bile duct involvement in IgG4-related sclerosing cholangitis: liver biopsy and cholangiography correlation. J Gastroenterol. 2010;46:269–76.
78. Deshpande V, Sainani NI, Chung RT, Pratt DS, Mentha G, Rubbia-Brandt L, et al. IgG4-associated cholangitis: a comparative histological and immunophenotypic study with primary sclerosing cholangitis on liver biopsy material. Mod Pathol. 2009;22:1287–95.
79. Otsuki M, Chung JB, Okazaki K, Kim M-H, Kamisawa T, Kawa S, et al. Asian diagnostic criteria for autoimmune pancreatitis: consensus of the Japan-Korea symposium on autoimmune pancreatitis. J Gastroenterol. 2008;43:403–8.
80. Ohara H, Okazaki K, Tsubouchi H, Inui K, Kawa S, Kamisawa T, et al. Clinical diagnostic criteria of IgG4-related sclerosing cholangitis 2012. J Hepatobiliary Pancreat Sci. 2012;19:536–42.
81. Pannala R, Chari ST. Corticosteroid treatment for autoimmune pancreatitis. Gut. 2009;58:1438–9.
82. Ghazale A, Chari ST. Optimising corticosteroid treatment for autoimmune pancreatitis. Gut. 2007;56:1650–2.
83. Kamisawa T, Shimosegawa T, Okazaki K, Nishino T, Watanabe H, Kanno A, et al. Standard steroid treatment for autoimmune pancreatitis. Gut. 2009;58:1504–7.
84. Sah RP, Chari ST, Pannala R, Sugumar A, Clain JE, Levy MJ, et al. Differences in clinical profile and relapse rate of type 1 versus type 2 autoimmune pancreatitis. Gastroenterology. 2010;139:140–8.
85. Tabata T, Kamisawa T, Takuma K, Egawa N, Setoguchi K, Tsuruta K, et al. Serial changes of elevated serum IgG4 levels in IgG4-related systemic disease. Intern Med. 2011;50:69–75.
86. Church NI, Pereira SP, Deheragoda MG, Sandanayake N, Amin Z, Lees WR, et al. Autoimmune pancreatitis: clinical and radiological features and objective response to steroid therapy in a UK series. Am J Gastroenterol. 2007;102:2417–25.
87. Hart PA, Topazian MD, Witzig TE, Clain JE, Gleeson FC, Klebig RR, et al. Treatment of relapsing autoimmune pancreatitis with immunomodulators and rituximab: the Mayo Clinic experience. Gut. 2012;62(11):1607–15.

88. Sodikoff JB. Mycophenolate mofetil for maintenance of remission in steroid-dependent autoimmune pancreatitis. WJG. 2012;18:2287.
89. Khosroshahi A, Carruthers MN, Deshpande V, Unizony S, Bloch DB, Stone JH. Rituximab for the treatment of IgG4-related disease. Medicine. 2012;91:57–66.
90. Topazian M, Witzig TE, Smyrk TC, Pulido JS, Levy MJ, Kamath PS, et al. Rituximab therapy for refractory biliary strictures in immunoglobulin G4-associated cholangitis. Clin Gastroenterol Hepatol. 2008;6:364–6.

Chapter 6
Rare Causes of Cholestasis

Tamir Miloh and Ozlem Pinar Bulut

Introduction

Cholestasis is an important manifestation of a variety of liver diseases. Intrahepatic cholestasis can result from a variety of genetic defects of hepatocytes that may be associated with multisystem manifestation. Extrahepatic cholestasis can result from a spectrum of obstructive processes. Cholestatic syndromes have different phenotypic expression, diagnosis method, natural course, prognosis and therapy. Molecular studies in humans have provided insight into rare cholestatic syndromes and may be the target of new interventions.

The term cholestasis means stagnation of bile in the liver, resulting in failure of normal amounts of bile to reach the duodenum. Cholestasis can be classified into either extrahepatic or intrahepatic. Extrahepatic cholestasis is marked by a mechanical obstruction of the bile ducts. In contrast, intrahepatic cholestasis occurs when there is an inherited or acquired defect of bile formation/transport within the liver epithelia (i.e., hepatocytes or biliary epithelia). Genetic and molecular studies have identified several genes associated with intrahepatic cholestatic disorders. These disorders include Alagille syndrome (AGS), various forms of progressive familial intrahepatic cholestasis (PFIC), benign recurrent intrahepatic cholestasis, Aagenaes syndrome (AS): Northern American Indian cirrhosis (NAIC), and arthrogryposis, renal dysfunction, and cholestasis (ARC) syndrome among others.

T. Miloh, M.D. (✉)
Pediatrics Department, Phoenix Children's Hospital,
1919 E. Thomas Road, Phoenix, AZ 85016, USA
e-mail: tmiloh@phoenixchildrens.com

O.P. Bulut, M.D.
Pediatric Gastroenterology, Hepatology & Nutrition, Phoenix Children's Hospital,
1919 E. Thomas Road, Phoenix, AZ 85016, USA
e-mail: obulut@phoenixchildrens.com

E.J. Carey and K.D. Lindor (eds.), *Cholestatic Liver Disease*, Clinical Gastroenterology,
DOI 10.1007/978-1-4939-1013-7_6, © Springer Science+Business Media New York 2014

The hepatocytes produce primary bile, which is delivered into the intrahepatic followed by the extrahepatic bile ducts before it arrives at the small intestine to serve its physiological functions. The intrahepatic bile ducts are lined by biliary epithelial cells, termed cholangiocytes that modify the composition of hepatic bile. Primary bile is originated at the apical or canalicular domain of the hepatocyte with the contribution of transmembrane transporters. The majority of these molecules are ATP-binding cassette (ABC) transporters. Genetic defects of these hepatic transporters can cause rare inherited cholestatic diseases. However, other genes not directly interfering with the canalicular transport of bile are likely contribute to the development of rare cholestatic syndromes.

Biliary Atresia

Biliary atresia (BA) is a progressive idiopathic inflammatory process that results in obliteration and fibrosis of the extrahepatic biliary tract and presents in the first few weeks of infancy with jaundice leading to cirrhosis before 2 years of age [1]. The overall incidence is 1:10,000. The most common form is BA without any other anomalies or malformations, also named perinatal BA. These patients are born anicteric and develop progressive jaundice and acholic stools within the first weeks of life. In approximately 15 % of cases, BA is associated with other malformations such as asplenia, polysplenia, situs inversus, malrotation, interrupted inferior vena cava, and cardiac anomalies and is also named BASM (biliary atresia splenic malformation) or embryonic BA [2]. In a smaller percentage BA may be associated with other congenital malformations, such as intestinal atresia, imperforate anus, kidney anomalies, and/or heart malformations [3].

The etiology remains idiopathic and is likely multifactorial: genetic, immunologic, viral and toxic [4]. Most infants are born full term and develop progressive jaundice and pale/acholic stools over the first weeks of life. Laboratory studies reveal elevated direct bilirubin and GGT with moderate increase in transaminases. Coagulopathy is likely the consequence of vitamin K deficiency [5]. Alpha 1 antitrypsin deficiency and Alagille may mimic BA. Ultrasonography may reveal absent or irregular gallbladder, absent common bile duct and occasionally the triangular cord sign (echogenicity of the portal hepatis remnant of the common bile duct) [6]. Hepatobiliary scintigraphy, usually primed with phenobarbital, does not reveal intestinal secretion. Liver biopsy is important to exclude other causes of cholestasis and is significant for expanded portal tracts with edema, inflammation and fibrosis with ductular proliferation, canalicular and bile duct biliary plugs. An intraoperative cholangiogram is considered the gold standard and reveals biliary obstruction. Alternatively, ERCP or percutaneous cholangiography may be performed [7].

Hepatoportoenterostomy (HPE, also known as the Kasai procedure) is resection of the fibrotic biliary remnant in the hilum with reconstruction of a Roux-en-Y loop of intestine to the liver hilum. HPE performed before 60 days of life have a better prognosis [8]. Postoperative management of patients after Kasai may include administration of ursodeoxycholic acid, nutritional support (calories and fat-soluble vitamins) [9], and prevention of cholangitis with prophylactic antibiotics [10]. There is controversy around the utility of corticosteroids with some studies showing efficacy short term without reducing the need for liver transplantation [11]. If jaundice persists beyond 3 months after the Kasai, the patient should be referred for liver transplant evaluation. Long-term complications include recurrent cholangitis, portal hypertension and liver tumors [12, 13]. Despite successful HPE and restoration of bile flow, 70–80 % of children require liver transplantation before adulthood and biliary atresia continues to be the most common indication for liver transplantation in children. However, with improvement in surgical technique and postoperative care, a percentage of patients are now reaching adulthood before transplantation.

Alagille Syndrome

AGS is an autosomal dominant inherited, highly variable, multi-systemic condition with an estimated prevalence of approximately 1 per 70,000 live births [14] with both genders being equally affected. The majority of cases are due to mutation in JAG1 in the Notch signaling pathway, and a small portion of cases are due to mutation in NOTCH2 [15, 16]. Reduced penetrance and variable expression are common in this disorder, and somatic/germ line mosaicism may also be relatively frequent. Main clinical and pathological features are intrahepatic bile duct paucity which results in chronic cholestasis, peripheral pulmonary artery stenosis, vertebral anomalies, characteristic facies, posterior embryotoxon, pigmentary retinopathy, dysplastic kidneys, and vascular abnormalities [17–19].

The multiple manifestations of AGS in humans suggest that JAG1 and Notch interactions are critical for normal embryogenesis of the heart, kidney, eye, face, skeleton, and other organs affected in this syndrome [20, 21]. Multiple mutations within the coding region of JAG1 have been documented in patients with AGS. The majority of JAGI mutations in patients are new and not found in either parent [22, 23]. Nonetheless, mutations can be present in 70 % of patients who meet clinical criteria for AGS [24]. Nearly half of these mutations are frameshift or nonsense mutations leading to premature truncation of the protein. The remaining mutations include gene deletions and missense mutations [25].

It is unclear as to whether missense mutations may cause milder variants of AGS or perhaps even single-organ abnormalities, though phenotypic differences between whole gene deletions and isolated point mutations have not been reported. Both copies of JAG1 are necessary for normal embryogenesis in humans [20, 21, 26]. However, the mechanism by which mutated JAG1 results in AGS remains unclear.

The clinical presentation of AGS is variable. Even within families, there is extreme variability in the severity of the disease, likely to be a result of other genetic and environmental modifying factors. Given the clinical variability and incomplete penetrance of the disorder, AGS often goes undiagnosed. Patients may present with progressive pruritus, cirrhosis, or liver failure. Still other individuals may lack or have few symptoms. Importantly, AGS is one of the more common etiologies of cholestasis in the neonatal period and must be differentiated from biliary atresia, which requires prompt surgical intervention. This is important, because the Kasai portoenterostomy is not beneficial in AGS [27].

Conjugated hyperbilirubinemia within the first 3 months of life is often the first presenting symptoms in the majority of patients with AGS. Progressive liver disease, eventually causing cirrhosis and failure, and requiring liver transplantation, occurs in approximately 15 % of cases [19]. Characteristic liver histology shows bile duct paucity in addition to major extrahepatic findings including characteristic facies, cardiac murmur, vertebral anomalies, and posterior embryotoxon. Cardiovascular anomalies can occur in close to 90 % of individuals with AGS [28]. Involvement of the pulmonary outflow tract is the most common type of congenital heart disease, with peripheral pulmonary stenosis (PPS) affecting at least two-thirds of cases. Tetralogy of Fallot (TOF) is the most common complex structural anomaly, occurring in up to 16 % of cases [19, 28]. Posterior embryotoxon has been reported in up to 90 % of ALG patients [29], however can also be found in up to 15 % of the normal population. Vascular accidents have been reported to occur in up to 15 % of cases, and were a cause of death in 34 % in one series [19, 30]. Intracranial bleeding may occur as a consequence of relatively minor head trauma.

There are currently no effective medical therapies for AGS. Supportive measures can be offered for nonspecific complications including pruritus. Medical therapies to improve pruritus include ursodeoxycholic acid, rifampin, cholestyramine, naltrexone, alimemazine, non-sedating antihistamine agents, and phenobarbitone or antihistamines; if these fail, biliary diversion may be required [31, 32]. The management of cholestatic pruritus in AGS is difficult and often suboptimal. Pruritus may remain intractable even with combination medical treatment, and at this stage, surgery or liver transplantation is indicated [32]. The survival post-liver transplantation for AGS patients is reduced compared to biliary atresia patients; the 1-year patient survival in patients with AGS is approx. 87 % compared to 96 % for biliary atresia patients. Deaths in AGS patients mostly occur within the first month post transplantation. Biliary, vascular, central nervous system, and renal complications after liver transplantation are associated with death in AGS patients; and renal insufficiency in the AGS patients usually worsens after liver transplantation [33].

Progressive Familial Intrahepatic Cholestasis

PFIC represents a heterogeneous group of autosomal recessive disorders of bile formation disruption. PFIC is the cause of cholestasis in approximately 10–15 % of children with an estimated incidence of 1/50,000–1/100,000 births [34]. PFIC is noted by the onset of cholestasis in infancy or early childhood that persists throughout life and often leads to liver cirrhosis within the first decade unless treated. There are three types of PFIC related to mutations in genes controlling the hepatocellular formation and transport of bile. Patients with PFIC-1 and PFIC-2 present with low serum GGT; patients with PFIC-3 have high serum GGT.

PFIC-1, also known as Byler's disease, was first described in Amish descendants of Jacob Byler [35], in the Inuit population in Greenland and Canada and other populations [36]. PFIC-1 is autosomal recessive caused by mutation for PFIC-1 to mutation of the FIC1 gene, on chromosome 18q21-22 [37, 38]. FIC1 encodes a P-type ATPase (ATP8Bl) involved in aminophospholipid flippase from the outer to the inner leaflet of plasma membranes, which is important in protection against the high bile salt concentration in the canalicular lumen and maintaining canalicular membrane integrity [38]. Expression of FIC1 has been found in a number of tissues including the intestine (highly expressed), liver, biliary tract, pancreas, and kidney [34]. The mechanism by which ATP8Bl defects lead to PFIC-1 remains unknown. Impaired ATP8Bl function results in downregulation of farnesoid X receptor (FXR) and subsequent Bile Salt Export Pump (BSEP) down regulation which leads to upregulation of the ASBP Apical Sodium Bile salt Transporter (ASBP) in the intestine [39]. Cystic Fibrosis Transmembrane Conductance Regulator (CFTR) downregulation has been reported in PFIC-1 that may explain some of the extrahepatic features [34].

Patients with PFIC- 1 usually present in the first weeks of life with severe pruritus disproportionate to the degree of jaundice [40]. Cholestasis can be initially episodic but becomes progressive. Progression to cirrhosis and end-stage liver disease occurs at a variable rate. Extrahepatic manifestation includes chronic diarrhea, short stature, failure to thrive, deafness, pancreatitis, biliary stones, and respiratory symptoms [40]. PFIC-1 is characterized by low serum GGT, high primary serum bile salts (chenodeoxycholic acid and cholic acid) and direct bilirubin, moderately elevated transaminase activities, normal serum cholesterol, and low biliary chenodeoxycholic concentrations. Liver imaging is normal [34, 40]. Liver histology reveals a "bland" picture of cholestasis and electron microscopy may show coarse granular bile [41, 42]. Mutational analysis of the ATP8B1 gene is the cornerstone of the diagnosis [43]; however, many patients are compound heterozygous.

Medical management is mostly supportive, assuring adequate nutrition and preventing fat soluble vitamins deficiency. Treatment with UDCA may be effective in some patients [34]. Treating pruritus is very challenging and children with PFIC-1 and PFIC-2 may benefit from surgical partial biliary diversion: external or internal before progression to cirrhosis [44, 45]. In partial external biliary diversion (PEBD) the gallbladder is connected to a cutaneous stoma by a loop of small bowel leading to reduction of the bile salt pool and inducing a shift to less toxic hydrophilic bile salts [46]. Internal biliary diversions are intestinal conduits between the gallbladder and the cecum, bypassing the terminal ileum, without external stoma [47]. However, recurrence of cholestasis has been reported in a few cases [48]. In ileal bypass (IB) the terminal ileum is skipped by an ileocolonic anastomosis [45]. Nasobiliary drainage may help selecting potential responders to biliary diversion [34]. Liver transplantation is performed in cirrhosis, portal hypertension and refractory pruritus [49]. Patients with PFIC-1 may experience worsening watery diarrhea (responsive to bile salt sequestrants) and liver graft steatosis which may progress to steatohepatitis [34, 40, 50].

PFIC-2 is an autosomal recessive disease caused by a mutation ABCB11 gene on chromosome 2q24 encoding the bile salt export pump (BSEP). Inhibition of BSEP leads to reduced bile salt secretion, reduced bile flow, and cholestasis. The spectrum of PFIC-2 is associated with the BSEP mutation. Jaundice, pruritus, failure to thrive, hepatomegaly, and splenomegaly present within the first months of life and cirrhosis has been noted as early as in the neonatal period [34, 40]. PFIC-2 patients manifest with a more severe hepatobiliary disease in comparison to PFIC-1 [51]. Significant coagulopathy with bleeding and hypocalcaemia due to vitamin D deficiency may be the presenting symptoms. Patients are a high risk of developing hepatocellular carcinoma at a young age and surveillance is warranted [52]. Hepatoblastoma and cholangiocarcinoma were also described at a young age [40]. There are no extrahepatic manifestations in PFIC-2 [51].

Laboratory findings include direct hyperbilirubinemia, elevated aminotransferase and Alpha fetoprotein (higher than PFIC-1), normal GGT, elevated serum bile acids, and decreased biliary bile salts [51]. Imaging studies show a normal biliary tree. Liver biopsy reveals giant cell transformation with canalicular cholestasis. Immunostaining for BSEP protein is negative. Electron microscopy reveals amorphous or finely filamentous bile [34]. Medical management is mostly supportive and often unsatisfactory. Surgical diversions may be effective, especially in those with functionally milder mutations [34]. Diversion should be offered early in the course of PFIC-2 as they it may slow progression of disease [53]. Treatment of a child with PFIC-2 with a mutation specific chaperone with 4-phenylbutyrate resulted in improved cholestasis and liver function [54]. Liver transplantation is indicated in cirrhosis, failed medical and surgical approaches, intractable pruritus, or HCC. Alloimmune mediated BSEP dysfunction may occur after liver transplantation in PFIC-2 patients leading to a PFIC-2 like phenotype recurrence [55].

PFIC-3 disease is caused by mutation of the multidrug-resistance-3, MDR3 glycoprotein, which is coded by the ABCB4 gene on chromosome 7q21 [34, 56]. MDR3 protein is an ATP dependent phosphatidylcholine flippase and expressed primarily within hepatocytes, though detected in other tissues. Consequently, PFIC-3 patients lack MDR-3 on the canalicular domain of the hepatocyte and have a significant decrease (<15 % of normal) in biliary phospholipid concentrations despite normal canalicular excretion of bile salts, promoting lithogenic hydrophobic bile with crystallized cholesterol. Disease-causing mutations on both alleles were found to be associated with reduced liver expression of ABCB4 protein, lack of response to ursodeoxycholic acid therapy, and progression to cirrhosis and end-stage liver disease, whereas mild genotypes, including single heterozygous mutations, were generally associated with less severe disease and, often, absence of symptoms [57]. MDR3 deficiency has been documented in several disease phenotypes, including intrahepatic and gallbladder cholesterol lithiasis, intrahepatic cholestasis of pregnancy, and progressive familial intrahepatic cholestasis type 3 (PFIC3).

PFIC-3 may present in infancy in half of the cases or later in life with jaundice, pale stools, pruritus, hepatomegaly, and splenomegaly (as a manifestation of portal hypertension) [58]. Children with PFIC3 are also at risk to develop intrahepatic and gallbladder cholesterol cholelithiasis and drug-induced cholestasis (DIC) [59]. Liver function tests showed elevated aminotransferases, AlkPhos, GGT, total serum bile acid and conjugated hyperbilirubinemia and absent serum lipoprotein X. Bile analysis revealed low concentrations of phospholipids and elevated ratios of bile salt to phospholipid and cholesterol to phospholipid. Liver imaging is typically normal, but may show a large gallbladder or biliary stones. Liver biopsy reveals ductular proliferation, biliary fibrosis, and immunohistochemical staining for MDR3 shows complete absence of canalicular staining. UDCA has variable results depending on the severity of the mutation: complete normalization of liver function test in 41 %, negative response in 37 %, and partial improvement in 20 % the rest [58]. UDCA benefit may be related to the modulation of biliary bile acid composition in favor of hydrophilic bile acids. Refractory progressive cases may require a liver transplantation [59].

Benign Recurrent Intrahepatic Cholestasis

BRIC is characterized by intermittent attacks of jaundice and pruritus separated by symptom-free intervals usually manifesting at adolescence [60] and was first described in 1959 [61]. There are two types of BRIC, affecting the ATP8B1 (BRIC 1) or ABCB11 (BRIC 2) gene, respectively [34]. It is postulated that in BRIC the protein is only partially impaired. Unlike PFIC, there is no permanent liver damage, no progression to cirrhosis, and no long-term complications of chronic liver disease [34]. Attacks consist of 2- to 4-weeks pre-icteric phase of malaise, anorexia, and pruritus, and an icteric phase lasting from usually 2–3 months. The number of discrete cholestatic episodes varies from a few episodes per year to one episode per decade and later in life, the cholestatic episodes become less frequent. Flares may have seasonal variation and exacerbation with infection, pregnancy, or contraception [62]. Patients with BRIC-1 may have significant weight loss, pancreatitis, and steatorrhea [62]. Patients with BRIC-2 have a higher incidence of cholelithiasis [63]. Attacks result in a characteristic cholestatic liver enzyme panel except that serum GGT remains low. Liver biopsy shows no pathologic characteristics even during episodes. Clinical, laboratory, and histologic features of BRIC remain normal during the asymptomatic phase [34]. Some patients present in childhood with recurrent attacks of cholestasis (BRIC) and cholestasis may gradually become permanent [64].

Medical therapies during the BRIC pruritic flare include UDCA and bile salt sequestrates with conflicting results [34]. Nasobiliary drain [65], extracorporeal albumin dialysis (MARS) [66], and the extracorporeal artificial liver support (Prometheus) have been shown to alleviate pruritus in refractory cases [67]. There is no proven effective therapy to avoid prevent or to shorten the cholestatic episodes in BRIC.

Dubin–Johnson Syndrome

Dubin–Johnson syndrome (DJS) is a rare autosomal recessive liver disorder characterized by elevation of both conjugated and unconjugated bilirubin, with more than 50 % of the total bilirubin being conjugated [68]. Hepatomegaly can sometimes be seen but transaminases, GGT and bile acids are within normal limits [69].

Total urine excretion of coproporphyrin isomer I is >80 % (normal 25 %) excretion and excretion of coproporphyrin isomer III is concomitantly decreased [70, 71]. Jaundice can worsen with use of oral contraceptives and pregnancy [72, 73].

Liver biopsy shows characteristic brown to black discoloration of the liver with otherwise normal histology. DJS is linked to a deficient hepatic excretion of non-bile salt organic anions at the apical canalicular membrane, by the ABC transport system known as canalicular multispecific organic anion transporter (cMOAT) encoded by the human gene MRP2 (ABCC2) located on chromosome 10q24 [74, 75].

This protein mediates ATPdependent transport of a broad range of endogenous and xenobiotic compounds across the canalicular membrane of the hepatocyte. Defects in cMOAT may account for the impaired hepatobiliary transport of non-bile salt organic anions seen in patients with DJS. Although jaundice is a lifelong finding in patients with DJS, no specific therapy is required. It is not associated with morbidity or mortality [76].

Rotor Syndrome

Rotor syndrome (RS) is an autosomal recessive inherited disorder with chronic elevation of conjugated and unconjugated serum bilirubin and can present in early childhood [77]. Liver functions tests and liver histology are normal. In RS there is a marked increase in urinary coproporphyrins with <80 % being coproporphyrin isomer I.

The SLCO1B1 and SLCO1B3 genes are involved in Rotor syndrome. Mutations in both genes are required for the condition to occur. The SLCO1B1 and SLCO1B3 genes provide instructions for making similar proteins, called organic anion transporting polypeptide 1B1 (OATP1B1) and organic anion transporting polypeptide 1B3 (OATP1B3), respectively. Both proteins are found in liver cells; they transport bilirubin and other compounds from the blood into the liver so that they can be cleared from the body. In the liver, bilirubin is dissolved in digestive fluid called bile and then excreted from the body.

The SLCO1B1 and SLCO1B3 gene mutations that cause Rotor syndrome lead to abnormally short, nonfunctional OATP1B1 and OATP1B3 proteins or an absence of these proteins. Without the function of either transport protein, bilirubin is less efficiently taken up by the liver and removed from the body. The buildup of this substance leads to jaundice in people with Rotor syndrome.

Crigler–Najjar Syndrome

Crigler–Najjar syndrome (CNS) is another rare genetic disorder resulting in chronic hyperbilirubinemia. Two types of CNS have been identified and recognized to be clinically distinct. Both are caused by an autosomal recessive defect in the UGTJA1 gene complex [78]. This gene encodes for the enzyme uridine diphosphate (UDP) glycosyltransferase 1 family, polypeptide AI, known to conjugate bilirubin.

In CNS type I, there is complete absence of functional UGTIAI. The unconjugated hyperbilirubinemia is severe and can lead to significant neurologic impairment due to bilirubin encephalopathy and permanent sequelae (kernicterus). The syndrome occurs in all races and has been associated with consanguinity in some patients. CNS 1 presents in the first days of life with elevated unconjugated bilirubin in the range of 20–25 mg/dL but can be as high as 50 mg/dL, normal transaminases, serum bile acids and no evidence of hemolysis. Stool is pigmented with low fecal urobilinogen excretion. The liver histology is normal.

In contrast, some functional UGT1Al activity is preserved in CNS type 2 (also known as Arias syndrome). Serum bilirubin is usually lower and jaundice may develop later in life and neurologic sequelae are less common. Jaundice may increase during fasting or intercurrent illness. CNS type 1 and type 2 are further differentiated by their response to phenobarbitol. (60–120 mg for 14 days) can significantly decrease serum bilirubin levels in CNS type 2 but have no effect on type I. Chromatographic analysis of bile collected from the duodenum reveals absence of conjugated bilirubin in CNS 1 and significant amount in CNS 2. DNA testing and prenatal diagnosis is available.

Treatment includes phototherapy (8–16 h per day) acting by converting a portion of bilirubin into a structural isomer that can be excreted in the bile without conjugation. This becomes less effective at puberty due to skin thickening and pigmentation, and decreased surface area in relation to body mass [79]. Late onset kernicterus may develop with treatment failure. Plasmapheresis is used to reduce bilirubin rapidly during a crisis to remove albumin bound bilirubin. Calcium carbonate and orlistat [80] can result in a modest reduction in bilirubin in patients with CNS1 on phototherapy by trapping intestinal bilirubin. Tin-protoporphyrin or tin-mesoporphyrin results in reduced bilirubin production [81]. Liver transplantation is considered the only definitive treatment for CNS 1 to prevent the risk of kernicterus [79]. Hepatocyte transplantation in a patient with CNS1 resulted in reduction of serum bilirubin levels that may be transient [82]. Gene therapy is being studied. Patients with CNS 2 affecting quality of life can be treated with phenobarbital or clofibrate [83].

Aagenaes Syndrome/Lymphedema-Cholestasis Syndrome

Aagenaes Syndrome (AS) is a form of familial intrahepatic cholestasis associated with lymphedema of the lower extremities and was first described in Norwegian patients in 1968 by the Norwegian pediatrician Aagenaes [84].

In the majority of cases, the disease follows autosomal recessive inheritance but de novo autosomal dominant mutation has been described as well [85]. The genetic locus, LCSJ, has been mapped to chromosome 15q in Norwegian kindred [86]. A second genetic locus, suggesting genetic heterogeneity of AS, may exist in other ethnic groups [87].

In affected individuals, jaundice manifests soon after birth and can reoccur episodically throughout life. Lymphedema in the lower extremities, is due to hypoplasia of lymphatic vessels, usually begins around school age and progresses, with its severity ranging from moderate to severe [88]. It has been postulated that the pathogenesis of this condition is due to abnormal development of hepatic lymphatics, though the underlying mechanism is not established. Initial cholestasis seems to resolve in early childhood, though recurrent bouts of cholestasis and lymphedema have been reported in adulthood [89]. Liver biopsies in infants show giant cell transformation and can show fibrosis or cirrhosis in older children [88].

Analysis of AS patients over a 10 year period who did not have signs of cholestasis showed significant elevation in serum transaminases compared to controls, and albumin was decreased in older patients with AS. Manifestation of lymphedema varied from moderate to massive. Patients with remission of liver disease by age 2–2.5 years showed a better prognosis. With proper nutritional and vitamin supplementation, more than 50 % of patients with AS can expect a normal life span. Most patients with AS have a relatively good prognosis compared to patients with other types of hereditary neonatal cholestasis syndromes [90].

Northern American Indian Childhood Cirrhosis

North American Indian Childhood Cirrhosis (NAIC) is an autosomal recessive, severe non-syndromic form of intrahepatic cholestasis first described in 30 North American Indian Children from Ojibway-Cree descent in the Abitibi region of northwestern Quebec, Canada [91].

Retrospective studies suggest a carrier frequency of 10 % in the indigenous children of northwestern Quebec [92]. Approximately 70 % of patients with NAIC present with conjugated hyperbilirubinemia and jaundice in the neonatal period. Despite clinical disappearance of jaundice, conjugated bilirubin, aminotransferases, GGT, and bile acids remain elevated beyond 1 year of age. Normal or moderately elevated cholesterol levels are found in most patients. The disorder is progressive and worsens with age, leading to biliary cirrhosis and portal hypertension in up to 90 % of patients [92]. The only effective therapy for NAIC is liver transplantation.

Early histology is characterized by giant cell hepatitis, biliary stasis, and neoductular proliferation which can rapidly progress to portal fibrosis and biliary cirrhosis. Electron microscopy demonstrates marked widening of pericanalicular ectoplasm with abundant pericanalicular microfilaments similar to changes seen in phalloidin intoxication [91]. Whether this marked accumulation of actin-containing microfilaments is because of dysfunctional contractile proteins or secondary to cholestatic injury is not known.

NAIC results from at least one known mutation in the CIRH1A gene on chromosome 16q22. The product of this gene is cirhin, a protein of unknown function. The encoded protein is preferentially expressed in embryonic liver, predicted to localize to mitochondria, and contains structural motifs frequently associated with molecular scaffolds. However, the function of cirhin and its role in NAIC pathogenesis remains unknown [93].

Arthrogryposis Multiplex Congenita, Renal Dysfunction, and Cholestasis Syndrome

ARC syndrome is an autosomal recessive multisystem disorder caused by mutations in the VPS33B gene characterized by neurogenic arthrogryposis (multiple joint contractures), renal tubular dysfunction with nephrocalcinosis, and low GGT neonatal cholestasis [94, 95]. The neurogenic muscular atrophy is related to rare damange of the anterior horn cells of the spinal cord. Affected infants generally die within the first year of life. Patients may have severe developmental delay, hypotonia, nerve deafness, poor feeding and failure to thrive, ichthyosis, microcephaly, defects of the corpus callosum, bleeding tendency and may have recurrent infections and diarrhea. Orthopedic sequelae include vertical talus, pes calcaneovalgus, hip dislocation, pathologic fractures, and rigid kyphosis [96]. Liver biopsy may be complicated by hemorrhage and reveals paucity of intrahepatic bile ducts and giant cell transformation of hepatocytes reported on liver biopsy [95–97].

Conclusion

Owing to the advancement of genetic methodologies and molecular biology techniques we now have better understanding of the causes of rare cholestatic syndromes. These discoveries could form the foundation to elucidate the mechanisms of and devise novel therapies for less infrequent diseases of intrahepatic cholestasis.

References

1. Haber BA, Russo P. Biliary atresia. Gastroenterol Clin North Am. 2003;32(3):891–911.
2. Shneider BL et al. A multicenter study of the outcome of biliary atresia in the United States, 1997 to 2000. J Pediatr. 2006;148(4):467–74.
3. Schwarz KB et al. Extrahepatic anomalies in infants with biliary atresia: results of a large prospective north american multicenter study. Hepatology. 2013;58(5):1724–31.
4. Mack CL, Feldman AG, Sokol RJ. Clues to the etiology of bile duct injury in biliary atresia. Semin Liver Dis. 2012;32(4):307–16.
5. Hartley JL, Davenport M, Kelly DA. Biliary atresia. Lancet. 2009;374(9702):1704–13.
6. Park WH et al. A new diagnostic approach to biliary atresia with emphasis on the ultrasonographic triangular cord sign: comparison of ultrasonography, hepatobiliary scintigraphy, and liver needle biopsy in the evaluation of infantile cholestasis. J Pediatr Surg. 1997;32(11): 1555–9.
7. Moyer V et al. Guideline for the evaluation of cholestatic jaundice in infants: recommendations of the North American Society for Pediatric Gastroenterology, Hepatology and Nutrition. J Pediatr Gastroenterol Nutr. 2004;39(2):115–28.
8. Schreiber RA et al. Biliary atresia: the Canadian experience. J Pediatr. 2007;151(6):659–65.
9. Shneider BL et al. Efficacy of fat-soluble vitamin supplementation in infants with biliary atresia. Pediatrics. 2012;130(3):e607–14.

10. Bu LN et al. Prophylactic oral antibiotics in prevention of recurrent cholangitis after the Kasai portoenterostomy. J Pediatr Surg. 2003;38(4):590–3.
11. Davenport M et al. Randomized, double-blind, placebo-controlled trial of corticosteroids after Kasai portoenterostomy for biliary atresia. Hepatology. 2007;46(6):1821–7.
12. Lykavieris P et al. Outcome in adulthood of biliary atresia: a study of 63 patients who survived for over 20 years with their native liver. Hepatology. 2005;41(2):366–71.
13. Shneider BL et al. Portal hypertension in children and young adults with biliary atresia. J Pediatr Gastroenterol Nutr. 2012;55(5):567–73.
14. Danks DM et al. Studies of the aetiology of neonatal hepatitis and biliary atresia. Arch Dis Child. 1977;52(5):360–7.
15. Li L et al. Alagille syndrome is caused by mutations in human Jagged1, which encodes a ligand for Notch1. Nat Genet. 1997;16(3):243–51.
16. Oda T et al. Mutations in the human Jagged1 gene are responsible for Alagille syndrome. Nat Genet. 1997;16(3):235–42.
17. Alagille D et al. Hepatic ductular hypoplasia associated with characteristic facies, vertebral malformations, retarded physical, mental, and sexual development, and cardiac murmur. J Pediatr. 1975;86(1):63–71.
18. Deprettere A, Portmann B, Mowat AP. Syndromic paucity of the intrahepatic bile ducts: diagnostic difficulty; severe morbidity throughout early childhood. J Pediatr Gastroenterol Nutr. 1987;6(6):865–71.
19. Emerick KM et al. Features of Alagille syndrome in 92 patients: frequency and relation to prognosis. Hepatology. 1999;29(3):822–9.
20. Crosnier C et al. JAGGED1 gene expression during human embryogenesis elucidates the wide phenotypic spectrum of Alagille syndrome. Hepatology. 2000;32(3):574–81.
21. Jones EA, Clement-Jones M, Wilson DI. JAGGED1 expression in human embryos: correlation with the Alagille syndrome phenotype. J Med Genet. 2000;37(9):658–62.
22. Krantz ID et al. Spectrum and frequency of jagged1 (JAG1) mutations in Alagille syndrome patients and their families. Am J Hum Genet. 1998;62(6):1361–9.
23. Crosnier C et al. Mutations in JAGGED1 gene are predominantly sporadic in Alagille syndrome. Gastroenterology. 1999;116(5):1141–8.
24. Piccoli DA, Spinner NB. Alagille syndrome and the Jagged1 gene. Semin Liver Dis. 2001;21(4):525–34.
25. Krantz ID, Piccoli DA, Spinner NB. Clinical and molecular genetics of Alagille syndrome. Curr Opin Pediatr. 1999;11(6):558–64.
26. Loomes KM et al. The expression of Jagged1 in the developing mammalian heart correlates with cardiovascular disease in Alagille syndrome. Hum Mol Genet. 1999;8(13):2443–9.
27. Kaye AJ et al. Effect of Kasai procedure on hepatic outcome in Alagille syndrome. J Pediatr Gastroenterol Nutr. 2010;51(3):319–21.
28. McElhinney DB et al. Analysis of cardiovascular phenotype and genotype-phenotype correlation in individuals with a JAG1 mutation and/or Alagille syndrome. Circulation. 2002;106(20):2567–74.
29. Hingorani M et al. Ocular abnormalities in Alagille syndrome. Ophthalmology. 1999;106(2):330–7.
30. Kamath BM et al. Vascular anomalies in Alagille syndrome: a significant cause of morbidity and mortality. Circulation. 2004;109(11):1354–8.
31. Emerick KM, Whitington PF. Partial external biliary diversion for intractable pruritus and xanthomas in Alagille syndrome. Hepatology. 2002;35(6):1501–6.
32. Kronsten V, Fitzpatrick E, Baker A. Management of cholestatic pruritus in paediatric patients with alagille syndrome: the King's college hospital experience. J Pediatr Gastroenterol Nutr. 2013;57(2):149–54.
33. Kamath BM et al. Outcomes of liver transplantation for patients with Alagille syndrome: the studies of pediatric liver transplantation experience. Liver Transpl. 2012;18(8):940–8.
34. Jacquemin E. Progressive familial intrahepatic cholestasis. Clin Res Hepatol Gastroenterol. 2012;36 Suppl 1:S26–35.

35. Clayton RJ et al. Byler disease. Fatal familial intrahepatic cholestasis in an Amish kindred. Am J Dis Child. 1969;117(1):112–24.
36. Klomp LW et al. A missense mutation in FIC1 is associated with Greenland familial cholestasis. Hepatology. 2000;32(6):1337–41.
37. Klomp LW et al. Characterization of mutations in ATP8B1 associated with hereditary cholestasis. Hepatology. 2004;40(1):27–38.
38. Bull LN et al. A gene encoding a P-type ATPase mutated in two forms of hereditary cholestasis. Nat Genet. 1998;18(3):219–24.
39. Chen F et al. Progressive familial intrahepatic cholestasis, type 1, is associated with decreased farnesoid X receptor activity. Gastroenterology. 2004;126(3):756–64.
40. Alissa FT, Jaffe R, Shneider BL. Update on progressive familial intrahepatic cholestasis. J Pediatr Gastroenterol Nutr. 2008;46(3):241–52.
41. Morotti RA, Suchy FJ, Magid MS. Progressive familial intrahepatic cholestasis (PFIC) type 1, 2, and 3: a review of the liver pathology findings. Semin Liver Dis. 2011;31(1):3–10.
42. Knisely AS. Progressive familial intrahepatic cholestasis: an update. Pediatr Dev Pathol. 2004;7(4):309–14.
43. Gonzales E, Spraul A, Jacquemin E. Clinical utility gene card for: progressive familial intrahepatic cholestasis type 1. Eur J Hum Genet. 2013.
44. Schukfeh N et al. Normalization of serum bile acids after partial external biliary diversion indicates an excellent long-term outcome in children with progressive familial intrahepatic cholestasis. J Pediatr Surg. 2012;47(3):501–5.
45. Davis AR, Rosenthal P, Newman TB. Nontransplant surgical interventions in progressive familial intrahepatic cholestasis. J Pediatr Surg. 2009;44(4):821–7.
46. Emond JC, Whitington PF. Selective surgical management of progressive familial intrahepatic cholestasis (Byler's disease). J Pediatr Surg. 1995;30(12):1635–41.
47. Mochizuki K et al. Partial internal biliary diversion for patients with progressive familial intrahepatic cholestasis type 1. Pediatr Surg Int. 2012;28(1):51–4.
48. Kalicinski PJ et al. Surgical treatment of progressive familial intrahepatic cholestasis: comparison of partial external biliary diversion and ileal bypass. Eur J Pediatr Surg. 2003;13(5):307–11.
49. Davit-Spraul A et al. Progressive familial intrahepatic cholestasis. Orphanet J Rare Dis. 2009;4:1.
50. Egawa H et al. Intractable diarrhea after liver transplantation for Byler's disease: successful treatment with bile adsorptive resin. Liver Transpl. 2002;8(8):714–6.
51. Pawlikowska L et al. Differences in presentation and progression between severe FIC1 and BSEP deficiencies. J Hepatol. 2010;53(1):170–8.
52. Knisely AS et al. Hepatocellular carcinoma in ten children under five years of age with bile salt export pump deficiency. Hepatology. 2006;44(2):478–86.
53. Stapelbroek JM et al. Liver disease associated with canalicular transport defects: current and future therapies. J Hepatol. 2010;52(2):258–71.
54. Gonzales E et al. Successful mutation-specific chaperone therapy with 4-phenylbutyrate in a child with progressive familial intrahepatic cholestasis type 2. J Hepatol. 2012;57(3):695–8.
55. Maggiore G et al. Relapsing features of bile salt export pump deficiency after liver transplantation in two patients with progressive familial intrahepatic cholestasis type 2. J Hepatol. 2010;53(5):981–6.
56. Deleuze JF et al. Defect of multidrug-resistance 3 gene expression in a subtype of progressive familial intrahepatic cholestasis. Hepatology. 1996;23(4):904–8.
57. Colombo C et al. Clinical features and genotype-phenotype correlations in children with progressive familial intrahepatic cholestasis type 3 related to ABCB4 mutations. J Pediatr Gastroenterol Nutr. 2011;52(1):73–83.
58. Jacquemin E et al. The wide spectrum of multidrug resistance 3 deficiency: from neonatal cholestasis to cirrhosis of adulthood. Gastroenterology. 2001;120(6):1448–58.
59. Davit-Spraul A et al. The spectrum of liver diseases related to ABCB4 gene mutations: pathophysiology and clinical aspects. Semin Liver Dis. 2010;30(2):134–46.
60. Paulusma CC, Elferink RP, Jansen PL. Progressive familial intrahepatic cholestasis type 1. Semin Liver Dis. 2010;30(2):117–24.

61. Summerskill WH, Walshe JM. Benign recurrent intrahepatic "obstructive" jaundice. Lancet. 1959;2(7105):686–90.
62. Brenard R, Geubel AP, Benhamou JP. Benign recurrent intrahepatic cholestasis. A report of 26 cases. J Clin Gastroenterol. 1989;11(5):546–51.
63. van Mil SW et al. Benign recurrent intrahepatic cholestasis type 2 is caused by mutations in ABCB11. Gastroenterology. 2004;127(2):379–84.
64. van Ooteghem NA et al. Benign recurrent intrahepatic cholestasis progressing to progressive familial intrahepatic cholestasis: low GGT cholestasis is a clinical continuum. J Hepatol. 2002;36(3):439–43.
65. Stapelbroek JM et al. Nasobiliary drainage induces long-lasting remission in benign recurrent intrahepatic cholestasis. Hepatology. 2006;43(1):51–3.
66. Sturm E et al. Extracorporal albumin dialysis (MARS) improves cholestasis and normalizes low apo A-I levels in a patient with benign recurrent intrahepatic cholestasis (BRIC). Liver. 2002;22 Suppl 2:72–5.
67. Oldakowska-Jedynak U. et al. Treatment of pruritus with Prometheus dialysis and absorption system in a patient with benign recurrent intrahepatic cholestasis. Hepatol Res. 2013.
68. Dubin IN. Chronic idiopathic jaundice; a review of fifty cases. Am J Med. 1958;24(2):268–92.
69. Javitt NB, Kondo T, Kuchiba K. Bile acid excretion in Dubin-Johnson syndrome. Gastroenterology. 1978;75(5):931–2.
70. Frank M, Doss M, de Carvalho DG. Diagnostic and pathogenetic implications of urinary coproporphyrin excretion in the Dubin-Johnson syndrome. Hepatogastroenterology. 1990;37(1): 147–51.
71. Kondo T, Kuchiba K, Shimizu Y. Coproporphyrin isomers in Dubin-Johnson syndrome. Gastroenterology. 1976;70(6):1117–20.
72. Cohen L, Lewis C, Arias IM. Pregnancy, oral contraceptives, and chronic familial jaundice with predominantly conjugated hyperbilirubinemia (Dubin-Johnson syndrome). Gastroenterology. 1972;62(6):1182–90.
73. Lindberg MC. Hepatobiliary complications of oral contraceptives. J Gen Intern Med. 1992;7(2):199–209.
74. Kartenbeck J et al. Absence of the canalicular isoform of the MRP gene-encoded conjugate export pump from the hepatocytes in Dubin-Johnson syndrome. Hepatology. 1996;23(5): 1061–6.
75. Paulusma CC et al. A mutation in the human canalicular multispecific organic anion transporter gene causes the Dubin-Johnson syndrome. Hepatology. 1997;25(6):1539–42.
76. Machida I et al. Mutational analysis of the MRP2 gene and long-term follow-up of Dubin-Johnson syndrome in Japan. J Gastroenterol. 2005;40(4):366–70.
77. Vest MF, Kaufmann HJ, Fritz E. Chronic non-haemolytic jaundice with conjugated bilirubin in the serum and normal liver histology: a case study. Arch Dis Child. 1960;35:600–4.
78. Kadakol A et al. Genetic lesions of bilirubin uridine-diphosphoglucuronate glucuronosyltransferase (UGT1A1) causing Crigler-Najjar and Gilbert syndromes: correlation of genotype to phenotype. Hum Mutat. 2000;16(4):297–306.
79. van der Veere CN et al. Current therapy for Crigler-Najjar syndrome type 1: report of a world registry. Hepatology. 1996;24(2):311–5.
80. Hafkamp AM et al. Orlistat treatment of unconjugated hyperbilirubinemia in Crigler-Najjar disease: a randomized controlled trial. Pediatr Res. 2007;62(6):725–30.
81. Kappas A et al. Direct comparison of Sn-mesoporphyrin, an inhibitor of bilirubin production, and phototherapy in controlling hyperbilirubinemia in term and near-term newborns. Pediatrics. 1995;95(4):468–74.
82. Ambrosino G et al. Isolated hepatocyte transplantation for Crigler-Najjar syndrome type 1. Cell Transplant. 2005;14(2–3):151–7.
83. Gabilan JC, Benattar C, Lindenbaum A. Clofibrate treatment of neonatal jaundice. Pediatrics. 1990;86(4):647–8.

84. Aagenaes O, van der Hagen CB, Refsum S. Hereditary recurrent intrahepatic cholestasis from birth. Arch Dis Child. 1968;43(232):646–57.
85. Morris AA et al. Parent-child transmission of infantile cholestasis with lymphoedema (Aagenaes syndrome). J Med Genet. 1997;34(10):852–3.
86. Bull LN et al. Mapping of the locus for cholestasis-lymphedema syndrome (Aagenaes syndrome) to a 6.6-cM interval on chromosome 15q. Am J Hum Genet. 2000;67(4):994–9.
87. Fruhwirth M et al. Evidence for genetic heterogeneity in lymphedema-cholestasis syndrome. J Pediatr. 2003;142(4):441–7.
88. Aagenaes O. Hereditary cholestasis with lymphoedema (Aagenaes syndrome, cholestasis-lymphoedema syndrome). New cases and follow-up from infancy to adult age. Scand J Gastroenterol. 1998;33(4):335–45.
89. Aagenaes O, Sigstad H, Bjorn-Hansen R. Lymphoedema in hereditary recurrent cholestasis from birth. Arch Dis Child. 1970;45(243):690–5.
90. Drivdal M et al. Prognosis, with evaluation of general biochemistry, of liver disease in lymphoedema cholestasis syndrome 1 (LCS1/Aagenaes syndrome). Scand J Gastroenterol. 2006;41(4):465–71.
91. Weber AM et al. Severe familial cholestasis in North American Indian children: a clinical model of microfilament dysfunction? Gastroenterology. 1981;81(4):653–62.
92. Drouin E et al. North American Indian cirrhosis in children: a review of 30 cases. J Pediatr Gastroenterol Nutr. 2000;31(4):395–404.
93. Yu B, Mitchell GA, Richter A. Nucleolar localization of cirhin, the protein mutated in North American Indian childhood cirrhosis. Exp Cell Res. 2005;311(2):218–28.
94. Gissen P et al. Clinical and molecular genetic features of ARC syndrome. Hum Genet. 2006;120(3):396–409.
95. Smith H et al. Associations among genotype, clinical phenotype, and intracellular localization of trafficking proteins in ARC syndrome. Hum Mutat. 2012;33(12):1656–64.
96. Jang JY et al. Clinical characteristics and VPS33B mutations in patients with ARC syndrome. J Pediatr Gastroenterol Nutr. 2009;48(3):348–54.
97. Horslen SP, Quarrell OW, Tanner MS. Liver histology in the arthrogryposis multiplex congenita, renal dysfunction, and cholestasis (ARC) syndrome: report of three new cases and review. J Med Genet. 1994;31(1):62–4.

Chapter 7
Cholestatic Variants of Viral Disease and Alcohol

Mary A. Atia and Bashar Aqel

Introduction

Viral or alcoholic hepatitis is classically characterized by elevations in the transaminases. However, cholestasis may occur with either of these disease states [1]. Recognizing this variant is imperative to making a prompt diagnosis and instituting the correct therapy.

Cholestasis can result from any defect in bilirubin metabolism. This includes decreased uptake of bilirubin, impaired conjugation in hepatocytes, disorders of bile excretion into the biliary system, or extrahepatic obstruction of the bile ducts. Clinical manifestations are primarily jaundice and pruritus with an associated elevation in bilirubin and alkaline phosphatase and GGT.

Cholestatic viral hepatitis was first reported by Eppinger in 1937 [2]. He described a "cholangitic" form of hepatitis marked by prolonged jaundice and cholestasis.

Cholestatic viral hepatitis can be caused by both hepatotropic and non-hepatotropic viruses. Non-hepatotropic viruses account for up to 10 % of viral hepatitis including cytomegalovirus (CMV), Epstein–Barr virus (EBV), herpes simplex virus, enterovirus, adenovirus, rubella, and parvovirus [3]. Among these, both CMV and EBV can present as cholestatic liver disease.

M.A. Atia, M.D. (✉) • B. Aqel, M.D.
Division of Gastroenterology & Hepatology, Mayo Clinic Arizona,
13400 East Shea Boulevard, Scottsdale, AZ 85259, USA
e-mail: Atia.Mary@mayo.edu; Aqel.bashar@mayo.edu

E.J. Carey and K.D. Lindor (eds.), *Cholestatic Liver Disease*, Clinical Gastroenterology, 127
DOI 10.1007/978-1-4939-1013-7_7, © Springer Science+Business Media New York 2014

Hepatitis A

Hepatitis A virus (HAV) was first identified in 1973; it is a positive strand RNA virus that is transmitted by the fecal-oral route. It is the most common acute viral hepatitis worldwide. After ingestion, virions reach the liver via the portal system. In hepatocytes, the virus replicates, assembles, and secretes into the biliary canalculus, from which it passes into the bile duct and small intestine. Clinical manifestations of acute infection depend on the host: less than 30 % of children display symptoms, whereas 80 % of adults develop a severe hepatitis with remarkably elevated aminotransferases [4]. Patients typically present with flu-like and gastrointestinal symptoms followed by jaundice. Chronic disease, cirrhosis, and/or hepatocellular carcinoma are not associated with HAV.

Atypical manifestations of hepatitis A have been reported. These include relapsing hepatitis, prolonged cholestasis, and autoimmune hepatitis. The prevalence of cholestatic HAV is between 2 and 4.7 % [5, 6]. Symptoms of pruritus, fever, fatigue, loose stools, and weight loss distinguish cholestatic hepatitis A. The duration of jaundice can exceed 12 weeks. On laboratory markers, patients have a bilirubin >10 mg/dl and alkaline phosphatase is more than 2–3 times the upper limit of normal with mild elevations in ALT and AST. Non-cholestatic HAV rather has a bilirubin <10 mg/dl and jaundice is present on average for 4 weeks [2]. IgM anti-HAV antibodies persist during the period of cholestasis. Associated risk factors of prolonged cholestasis are the following: advanced age, chronic hepatitis B, and low albumin [6]. Rare associations with cholestatic HAV include pancreatitis [7], acute kidney injury, cutaneous vasculitides and cryoglobulinemia [8], and toxic epidermal necrolysis [9].

Severe cholestasis related to HAV is illustrated on liver biopsy as well. The most common abnormality is centrilobular cholestasis. Other findings include dystrophy of the bile ducts, bile thrombi, cholestatic liver rosettes, and ductular transformation of hepatocytes. Periportal (zone 1) patchy necrosis is also present; this may cause an interruption in bile flow from the lobular parenchyma to the portal tract [10] (Fig. 7.1).

The precise mechanism of HAV cholestasis is unknown. Cholestasis by viral infection may be induced by inhibition of bile salt transporter function by proinflammatory cytokines, specifically tumor necrosis factor-alpha (TNF-a) and interleukin-1 (IL-1). Multidrug resistance-associated protein 2 (mrp2) is a transporter protein that is involved in the excretion of bilirubin; this protein is inhibited by TNF-a and IL-1 [11]. It has not been elucidated if virologic or host attributes are the primary factor. Jung et al. postulate that features of the host have a more significant role [6]. A study by Krawczyk et al. investigated genetic polymorphisms of different protein transporters responsible for bile secretion with certain genotypes associated with cholestasis—ABCB4 and ABCB11 [12]. The prevalence of the ABCB11 variant reaches 20–50 % in Europe; this potentially at-risk group may benefit from HAV vaccination. In contrast, Coppola et al. state that certain genotypes of HAV (Ia and Ib) may account for cholestasis and subsequently a more severe course of illness [13]. Further studies are required to better define the etiology of this disease process.

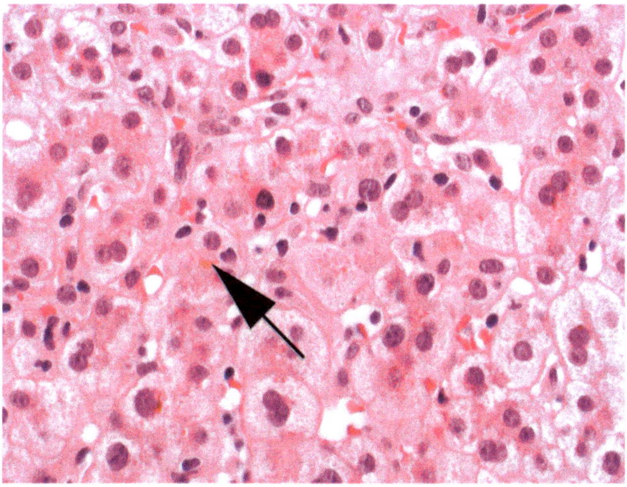

Fig. 7.1 Mild hepatocanalicular cholestasis (*arrow*) in a patient with acute Hepatitis A virus infection. Note the background lobular disarray and inflammation. H and E, 600×. (*Courtesy of Maxwell L. Smith, MD*)

Cholestasis will spontaneously resolve and the prognosis is good, though the majority of patients have a protracted course. This may result in extended length of hospital stay with associated increase in medical expenses. The use of corticosteroids has been discussed in the literature. It will hasten resolution of pruritus and result an improvement in bilirubin in two-thirds of patients [14]. However, there is a concern that steroids may predispose patients to relapse [15]. If pursued, the standard regimen is prednisone 40 mg po daily, then gradually tapered over 4 weeks. Other investigational treatments include ursodeoxycholic acid [16], rifampin and plasmapheresis [12].

Hepatitis B

Cholestatic viral hepatitis was first described in patients with hepatitis B by Davies et al. [17]. The most severe and ominous form is a distinct clinical and histologic entity known as fibrosing cholestatic hepatitis (FCH). The clinical course is characterized by progressive jaundice, mildly elevated aminotransferase levels, high levels of viremia, prolongation of prothrombin time, and rapid progression to liver failure evidenced by encephalopathy. It is primarily seen in recipients of liver allografts. However, it has also been identified overall in the setting of immunosuppression such as patients following renal transplantation [18–21], bone marrow transplantation [22], patients with HIV [23], and autoimmune diseases requiring high dose immunosuppression [24].

Histologically, there is ballooning degeneration of hepatocytes with ground-glass cytoplasm, and extensive periportal fibrosis. There is also severe canalicular and intracellular cholestasis. Interestingly, there are only mild inflammatory infiltrates. Notably, hepatitis B surface antigen and hepatitis B core antigen expression are prominent in the hepatocytes. As a result, the pathogenesis does not appear to be mediated by a host immune response, as typically seen in the immunocompetent patient. Instead, in the setting of immunosuppression the replication of the hepatitis B virus appears to have a direct cytopathic effect. Accumulation of hepatitis B surface antigen and hepatitis B core antigen in hepatocytes in the endoplasmic reticulum damages vital cell functions, leading to cell death [25].

Prior to the initiation of hepatitis B immunoglobulin (HBIG) and effective oral antiviral agents, recurrence of hepatitis B post-transplant was a frequent occurrence with the risk of development of FCH increased among those with the pre-core variant [26]. Pre-core mutant strains are able to undergo unrelenting viral replication because the lack of the hepatitis B e antigen enables the virus to avoid immune recognition. The prognosis of FCH is poor, with graft loss, liver failure, and death within weeks to months of onset. As a result, in the early 1990s, many transplant centers elected to deny transplantation to patients with chronic HBV. Initially, antiviral agents were used for the treatment of FCH including acyclovir, zidovudine, and ganciclovir. However, the advent of nucleoside and nucleotide analogues resulted in significant improvement in the outcomes of post-transplant HBV [27]. Due to the fact that liver injury in FCH is secondary to direct toxicity of high levels of HBV DNA, the majority of the literature has evaluated the role of lamivudine for treatment [28, 29]. The mechanism of action of a nucleoside analogue is inhibition of DNA synthesis by terminating the nascent proviral DNA chain through interference with the reverse transcriptase activity of HBV [29]. The standard dose of lamivudine is 100 mg administered daily, with suppression of HBV DNA to undetectable levels in 96 % of patients with chronic hepatitis B [30]. It can be given either alone or with HBIG. It has been shown to rapidly reduce the levels of HBV DNA, with subsequent improvement in liver function in a few months. However, the emergence of lamivudine resistance with prolonged use leading to the development of viral mutants is a notable concern. This has been observed in up to 14 % of patients after 1 year of therapy. Two mutations at codon 552 with substitution of methionine by isoleucine (M552I) or valine (M552V) have been identified [31]. As a result, newer agents such as tenofovir and entecavir have been used with promising results as they have in vitro as well as in vivo activities against lamivudine-resistant mutants [32]. For those patients who are still viremic at time of transplant, treatment with tenofovir or entecavir should be pursued to minimize the risk of developing FCH. Immunosuppression with tacrolimus rather than cyclosporine is favored [34]. A steroid sparing regimen is preferred, but if prednisone is required, it should be tapered quickly as it may potentiate HBV replication via the glucocorticoid-responsive element on the HBV genome [33]. If the above measures are ineffective, retransplantation may be required, with the caveat that FCH may recur [17, 23, 34].

Hepatitis C

Cholestatic hepatitis C primarily follows liver transplantation. Recurrent hepatitis C in the transplanted liver is nearly inevitable; with 70–90 % having histologic evidence of recurrence and up to 20 % of recipients developing cirrhosis within 5 years of transplantation. An infrequent but aggressive form of recurrence is cholestatic hepatitis C. It primarily affects patients who are immunosuppressed due to cytotoxic therapy, human immunodeficiency virus, bone marrow transplantation, or solid organ transplantation of the kidney, heart, or liver. Jaundice, high alkaline phosphatase and gamma-glutamyl transpeptidase levels, and very high serum HCV RNA levels characterize it. Cholestatic HCV has been reported to affect between 2 and 15 % of hepatitis C infected liver transplant recipients [35, 36]. The International Liver Transplant Society defined this entity in 2003 by the following criteria: occurs more than 1 month post-transplantation, patient is significantly immunosuppressed, serum bilirubin is great that 6 mg/dl, serum alkaline phosphatase and GTT are greater than five times the upper limit of normal, hepatitis C viral load is very high, histologic features of hepatocyte ballooning in the perivenular zone, absence of hepatic artery thrombosis and biliary strictures [37].

The pathogenesis of cholestatic HCV is hypothesized to be a consequence of direct viral cytotoxicity in the setting of immunosuppression (Fig. 7.2). The medications required to prevent rejection (i.e., corticosteroids, tacrolimus, mycophenolate mofetil) lead to increased HCV entry into hepatocytes via upregulation of the entry receptors occludin and scavenger receptor B1 (SRB1). However, the virus does not follow the same kinetics in all patients, and hence the variable clinical outcome of recurrent hepatitis C. In cholestatic HCV, there is a predominately Th2 cytokine response (IL-4/Il-10) at the messenger RNA and protein level. Conversely, in non-cholestatic recurrent HCV, the response is primarily Th1 with expression of IL-2 and IFN-gamma. Other data have investigated genetic diversification and quasispecies. A quasispecies is a population of closely related yet unique genomic RNA viral sequences; in cholestatic HCV the quasispecies become more homogenous [35]. The combination of these factors leads to high viral replication. Within the hepatocyte nucleus, the virus activates cell death, induces Il-8, and expresses high levels of interferon-stimulated genes. Histologic changes then become evident with hepatic inflammation, hepatocyte ballooning, and cholestasis, ultimately leading to allograft failure [38].

Early recognition is imperative as the disease has a rapid progression to liver failure and death independent of cirrhosis or fibrosis. A recent study by Verna et al. identified clinical and histologic features among patients with cholestatic HCV. Higher MELD scores at transplantation, older donor age, higher incidence of biopsy-proven acute cellular rejection (Banff grade >5), and total bilirubin >2 mg/dl were all predictive of cholestatic HCV. Interestingly, HCV viral load was not predictive of cholestatic HCV in this study [36]. Hanoumeh et al. found that donor IL28B genotype TT was associated with a higher incidence of cholestatic HCV. There was no association with the recipient IL28 receptor polymorphism [39].

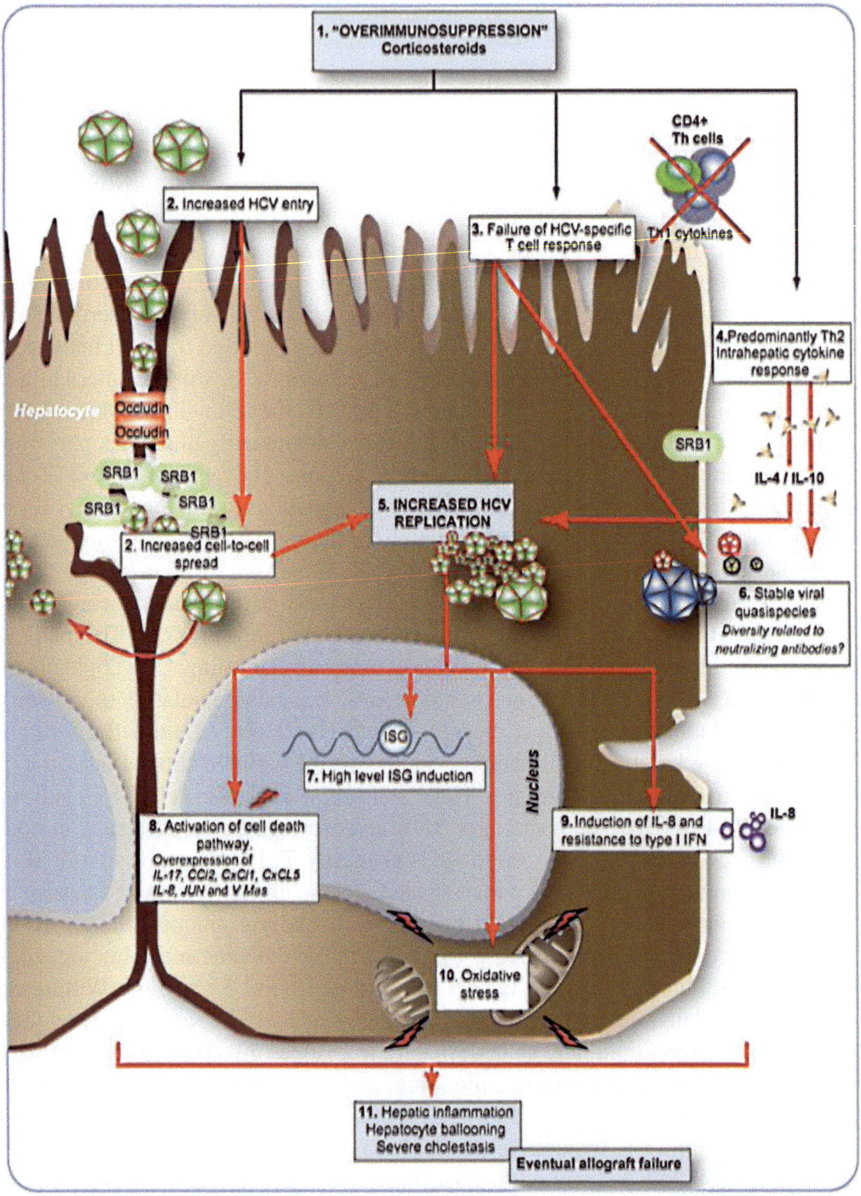

Fig. 7.2 Pathogenesis of cholestatic hepatitis C post liver transplantation. From McCaughan GW, Bowen DG. Pathogenesis of cholestatic hepatitis C. J Hepatol;54(2):392–4. Reprinted with permission from Elsevier Limited

On liver biopsy, patients with three out of the four following features had an increased risk of cholestatic HCV: prominent ductular reaction resembling a biliary obstruction, canalicular bile plugging and/or intracellular bile pigment, prominent

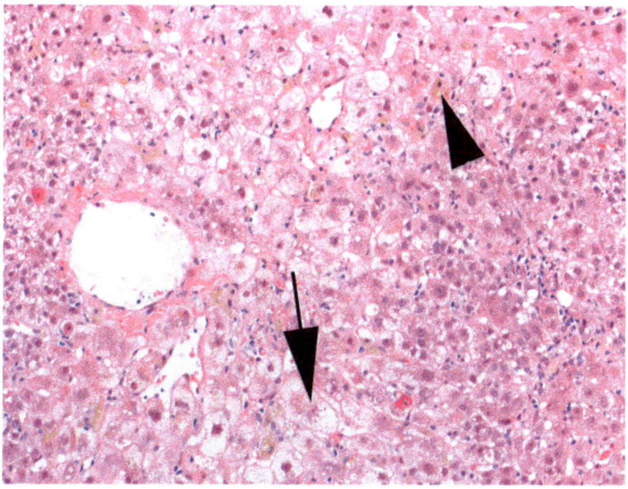

Fig. 7.3 Marked cholestasis (*arrow head*) with ballooning degeneration (*arrow*) in a centrilobular distribution in a patient with post-liver transplant fibrosing cholestatic Hepatitis C virus infection. H&E, 200×. (*Courtesy of Maxwell L. Smith, MD*)

hepatocyte ballooning with lobular disarray, and any degree of fibrosis (especially sinusoidal) (Fig. 7.3).

Distinguishing cholestatic HCV from other forms of chronic hepatitis in liver allografts is usually difficult and requires correlation with clinical, biochemical, and serologic profiles. Clinical risk factors include genotype (specifically 1b), immunosuppression, and high HCV viral load. Unfortunately, the available literature does not regularly report these details to confirm their relevance. In cholestatic HCV, the earliest histologic features are generally lobular without significant portal changes. This is distinct from acute cellular rejection, which typically displays endothelialitis, cholangitis, and mixed inflammatory cellular infiltrates. Clinically, patients exhibiting acute cellular rejection usually have an adjustment in the immune suppression protocol as the inciting event. Non-cholestatic recurrent hepatitis C shows chronic portal and lobular inflammation and acidophil bodies with or without fibrosis.

Graft loss has been reported to occur within 1–2 years after transplantation among patients with cholestatic HCV. Treatment of those patients is complex and should be initiated promptly to help salvage the liver transplant and prevent graft failure. The immunosuppression regimen should be modified and minimized. This will include a rapid steroid taper, elimination of mycophenolate mofetil, and in some patients conversion from tacrolimus to cyclosporine, as cyclosporine may have antiviral properties and inhibit HCV replication. Antiviral therapy should be initiated as well if patient clinical status will allow. Most published data is in the form of case series, evaluating the efficacy of pegylated interferon and ribavirin. In one of the largest case series, Aqel et al. described the experience of 17 patients with FCH. Fourteen patients qualified for treatment and viral clearance was only achieved in three patients—18 % of the entire cohort [40]. In another case series by Gopal and Rosen, seven patients with cholestasis were treated with interferon alfa-2b with ribavirin. Four had a response evidenced by an undetectable viral load and normalization of bilirubin. Two patients discontinued therapy with a rebound in cholestasis. The only two patients who survived required therapy indefinitely [41]. To date, there has yet to be any published data on the use or efficacy of the newer agents for HCV (protease and/or polymerase inhibitors) for the treatment of post-transplant cholestatic HCV. Several ongoing trials with interferon-free regimens are showing promising results for recurrent HCV post-transplant including patients with cholestatic HCV.

The prognosis of cholestatic HCV remains poor with nearly 50 % mortality even after treatment with antivirals. In a systematic review by Narang et al., 47 of 94 patients died between 2 months to 312 days after transplantation. Cholestatic HCV is considered a contraindication for retransplantation in most transplant centers given poor outcomes observed.

Hepatitis E

Hepatitis E (HEV) is a small spherical virus belonging to the genus *Hepevirus*. It is a linear, single-stranded, positive sense RNA virus. Hepatitis E is an enterically transmitted or food-borne disease with reservoirs in humans, swine, boar, and deer [42]. This distinct hepatotropic virus was first recognized in 1980 as an epidemic in Kashmir, India [43]. Other endemic areas include Pakistan and China [42]. It is uncommon in the USA or other developed countries.

HEV accounts for more than 50 % of acute viral hepatitis in young adults in developing nations. Clinically, HEV causes a self-limited illness with moderate jaundice and normalization of aminotransferases within 1–6 weeks [44]. Risk factors for hepatitis E infection include older age (median age 53 years) and recent travel history. Hyperbilirubinemia, coagulopathy, and hypoalbuminemia are more severe compared to hepatitis A [42]. There are cases of fatality (0.5–3 %); this is particularly among pregnant women with mortality up to 25 % [45]. No chronic sequelae have been identified.

Approximately 25 % of patients develop cholestatic features with acute HEV, evidenced by prolonged jaundice, pruritus, and acholic stools [46]. Compared to hepatitis A, protracted cholestasis is more prevalent with hepatitis E infection. Histopathology shows cholestasis with bile plugs in the canaliculi, feathery degeneration of hepatocytes and liver cell rosettes. In addition, lobular inflammation and fatty changes of the hepatocytes may be seen [45]. Treatment is supportive care.

Cytomegalovirus

Cytomegalovirus (CMV) is a herpes non-hepatotropic virus. Primary infection by CMV generally occurs subclinically as a mild flu-like syndrome with subsequent life-long latency within the host. Infection closely resembles EBV infectious mononucleosis with fever, atypical lymphocytosis, and splenomegaly. Liver involvement is manifested as subtle elevations in the transaminases. It is primarily seen among transplant recipients or in patients with other states of immunosuppression [47], though it can occasionally infect the immunocompetent patient as well [48].

The cholestatic variant is quite rare and only mentioned in a few case reports in the literature [49–53]. Diagnosis may be supported by an elevation in CMV PCR; however a liver biopsy is often necessary. Histopathology illustrates cholestasis in the form of canalicular biliary thrombi and an irregularly distributed lymphocytic infiltrate. With immunohistochemistry, CMV intranuclear inclusions are present. Extrahepatic biliary obstruction and/or dilation is also associated with CMV, and therefore an MRCP and/or ERCP may be pursued [47].

CMV cholestatic liver disease will spontaneously resolve with supportive care. However, there are cases of fatality and severe disease can be treated with ganciclovir [50].

Epstein-Barr Virus

EBV is a non-hepatotropic virus; it belongs to the human herpesvirus family [54]. More than 90 % of healthy subjects chronically carry EBV in B-lymphocytes. It is transmitted through close personal contact (via saliva, genital secretions) among children and adolescents. Infection classically causes a syndrome of fever, an exudative pharyngitis, fatigue, splenomegaly, and lymphadenopathy, known as infectious mononucleosis. Atypical lymphocytosis is a common biochemical feature. Liver involvement is frequent, affecting 90 % of patients. It is usually manifested by a mild and transitory elevation in transaminases.

This disease can present primarily with cholestasis, with one study reporting 65 % among all patients infected with EBV [55]. Jaundice occurs in only 6.6 % of patients [56]. Diagnosis is made by a positive EBV IgM antibody. Abdominal ultrasound usually illustrates hepatosplenomegaly, however there is occasional gallbladder wall thickening [56, 57]. Although not necessary, if a liver biopsy is pursued, inflammatory changes are noted with apoptotic hepatocytes, a mononuclear lymphocytic infiltration, granulomas, and centrilobular cholestasis.

Treatment is largely supportive. Steroids and antivirals (i.e., acyclovir, ganciclovir) have been used to treat severe cases; however randomized control trials have never been pursued. Some studies suggest use of ursodeoxycholic acid or cholestyramine to treat pruritic symptoms related to cholestasis. Molecular absorbent recycling system (MARS) has also been employed for severe cholestasis with subsequent decrease in hepatic encephalopathy [56]. Prognosis is favorable with natural recovery in weeks without concern for chronic liver disease.

The mechanism of EBV-induced cholestasis is not known. Theories have postulated that the virus inhibits MRP2, the main bilirubin transporter [56]. Other studies suggest that cytokines interfere with the sinusoidal and canalicular transporting systems that may lead to cholestasis [55] (Table 7.1).

Table 7.1 Cholestasis in viral disease

	Unique laboratory abnormalities	Histology	Course	Treatment
Hepatotropic viruses				
Hepatitis A	• IgM HAV	• Centrilobular cholestasis • Portal inflammation	Self-limiting	• Supportive • Steroids if severe and prolonged disease • UDCA
Hepatitis B	• Elevated HBV DNA	• Perisinusoidal fibrosis • Cholestasis • Ground-glass transformation • Hepatocyte ballooning • *Mild* inflammatory reaction	Rapidly progressive graft failure	• Lamivudine +/– HBIG • Adefovir • Reduce immunosuppression • Retransplanta-tion
Hepatitis C	• Elevated HCV RNA • Genotype 1b	• Perisinusoidal fibrosis • Cholestasis • Ground-glass transformation • Hepatocyte ballooning in zone 3 • *Mild* inflammatory infiltrate • Prominent ductular reaction	Rapidly progressive graft failure	• IFN and ribavirin • Reduce immunosuppression • Switch from tacrolimus to cyclosporine • New oral regimens once FDA approved
Hepatitis E		• Bile plugs in the canaliculi • Feathery degeneration of hepatocytes • Liver cell rosettes • Lobular inflammation	• Self-limiting • Rarely liver failure in pregnancy	• Supportive
Systemic viruses				
CMV	• Elevated CMV PCR	• Perisinusoidal fibrosis • Cholestasis • Hepatocyte ballooning • Mild mixed inflammatory reaction • CMV inclusions by immunohistochemistry	• Self-limiting	• Supportive • Gangciclovir if severe disease
EBV	• EBV IgM antibody	• Lymphocyte infiltration • Granulomas • Centrilobular cholestasis • Minimal hepatocyte involvement	• Self-limiting • One case of liver failure	• Supportive • Steroids and/or antivirals for severe cases

Alcoholic Liver Disease

Patients with alcoholic liver disease frequently manifest characteristics of cholestasis. Mallory first described this in 1911 [58]. The mechanism by which ethanol interacts with bile secretion is not well defined. Steatosis alone can cause cholestasis; early studies proposed that alcohol-associated cholestasis might be caused by hepatocyte necrosis resulting in edema and subsequent compression of intrahepatic biliary ductules. Other studies propose that ethanol interferes with the Na+,K+-ATPase pump on the basolateral membrane. There is also disruption in plasma membrane assembly, which disturbs the gradients. The combination of these factors inhibits Na+-dependent bile salt uptake, which is necessary for normal biliary secretion. There has also been research on the effect of alcohol on the microtubules, an essential component for intracellular vesicle trafficking. Acetaldehyde, the oxidative metabolite of ethanol, is hypothesized to interfere with microtubule formation [59].

Histologic cholestasis and clinical jaundice may be seen in all stages of alcohol liver disease. Steatosis is the most common histologic feature of alcoholic liver disease. Clinically, these patients exhibit an elevation of AST and ALT, typically in a 2:1 ratio. Rarely, patients with alcoholic steatosis have severe cholestasis as well. The presence of histologic cholestasis did not appear to be of prognostic significance in determining the risk of progression to cirrhosis [59]. In rare instances, isolated cholestasis without significant steatosis, hepatitis, or cirrhosis is ascribed to excess alcohol consumption. A study by Glover et al. [60] discussed three patients with alcohol related jaundice and severe cholestasis on liver biopsy but without histologic findings of steatosis or hepatitis.

Alcoholic hepatitis clinically is a more severe and acute condition than steatosis. Indicators of poor prognosis include malnutrition, encephalopathy, hyperbilirubinemia, and a prolonged prothrombin time. The Maddrey's discriminant function score (DF = 4.6 × [prothrombin time − control prothrombin time] + total bilirubin) utilizes the latter two variables for prognostication and therapeutic purposes, with a recommendation for treatment with corticosteroids for four weeks if the score is greater than 32 [61].

The association between cholestasis and alcoholic hepatitis was first described by Phillips and Davidson, who noted the accumulation of bile pigment in chronic alcoholics with acute decompensation [62]. The prevalence of histologic cholestasis is highly variable with studies ranging from 21 to 83 % [59]. However, the presence of histologic cholestasis does have a notable effect on prognosis. Patients with cholestatic hepatitis clinically had more severe disease, evidenced by ascites, encephalopathy, and higher discriminant function scores. On survival analysis, histologic cholestasis was associated with increased mortality; after 5 years 22 % of patients survived, whereas 54 % of patients without cholestasis were alive [63]. Histologically, tissue cholestasis correlated with increased fibrosis, parenchymal necrosis, bile duct proliferation, and portal inflammation (Fig. 7.4).

The role of liver biopsy in the patient with alcohol-related disease is debatable. It may be useful to exclude other contributing etiologies, assess the severity of liver disease, and establish prognosis. A study by Spahr et al. found that the presence of marked intraparenchymal cholestasis was an independent predictor of survival, along with age, and Maddrey score [64]. Other histologic lesions such as steatosis, polynuclear neutrophils, hepatocellular damage, ductular reaction, and iron deposition did not affect clinical outcome. Furthermore, while the majority of patients in the study had an elevated bilirubin, not all exhibited histologic cholestasis, suggesting that liver biopsy does provide additional prognostic information. However, given the

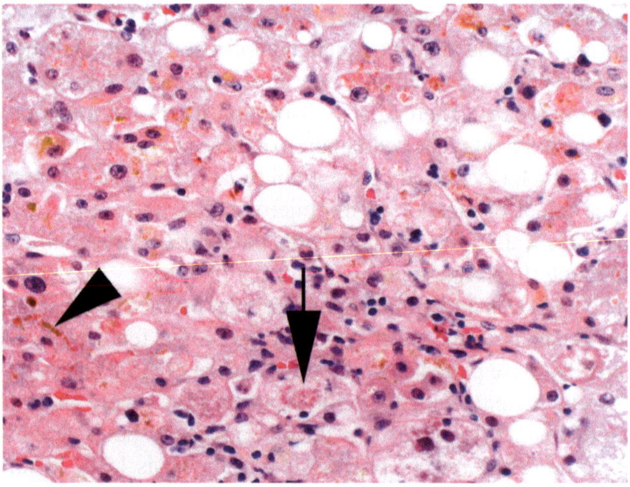

Fig. 7.4 Marked hepatocanalicular cholestasis (*arrow head*) in a patient with alcoholic hepatitis. Typical features of alcoholic steatohepatitis include ballooning degeneration with Mallory–Denk bodies (*arrow*), steatosis, and inflammation. H&E, 400×. (*Courtesy of Maxwell L. Smith, MD*)

Table 7.2 Evaluation of jaundice in the alcoholic patient

• Acetaminophen toxicity
• Acute alcoholic cholestasis
• Alcoholic steatosis
• Alcoholic hepatitis
• Alcoholic cirrhosis
• Acute viral hepatitis
• Drug reaction
• Hemolysis
• Biliary obstruction
• Acute pancreatitis
• Pancreatic carcinoma
• Pancreatic pseudocyst
• Choledocolithiasis
• Acute cholecystitis

Adapted from Tung BY, Carithers RL, Jr. Cholestasis and alcoholic liver disease. Clin Liver Dis 1999;3(3):585–601

fact that therapeutic options are largely limited to supportive care regardless of the etiology, some physicians are less inclined to pursue liver biopsy given the associated risks with this procedure. Finally, a jaundiced alcoholic patient with a cholestatic profile often presents a diagnostic challenge, especially in the setting of right upper quadrant pain, fever, and leukocytosis, as they both can be ascribed to alcoholic hepatitis or cholangitis. To differentiate between intrahepatic from extrahepatic disease, endoscopic retrograde cholangiopancreatography (ERCP) may be necessary to evaluate for biliary obstruction. One study reported biliary obstruction in 20 % of alcoholics with elevated bilirubin and/or alkaline phosphatase (Table 7.2).

Summary

Cholestatic variants of viral and alcohol-related hepatitis are more frequent than classically described. Prolonged cholestasis is associated with hepatotropic and non-hepatotropic viral hepatitides, specifically hepatitis A, hepatitis B, and CMV. Cholestatic hepatitis is a serious consequence after liver transplantation among recipients with chronic hepatitis B or C, with rapid progression to graft failure and mortality. For alcoholic hepatitis, cholestasis may be the presenting feature. As a result, it is important to maintain these disease entities in the differential diagnosis for cholestatic liver disease.

References

1. Burgart LJ. Cholangitis in viral disease. Mayo Clin Proc. 1998;73(5):479–82.
2. Gordon SC et al. Prolonged intrahepatic cholestasis secondary to acute hepatitis A. Ann Intern Med. 1984;101(5):635–7.
3. Tezer H et al. Cytomegalovirus hepatitis and ganciclovir treatment in immunocompetent children. Turk J Pediatr. 2008;50(3):228–34.
4. Jeong S-H, Lee H-S. Hepatitis A: clinical manifestations and management. Intervirology. 2010;53(1):15–9.
5. Petrov AI, Vatev NT, Atanasova MV. Cholestatic syndrome in viral hepatitis A. Folia Med (Plovdiv). 2012;54(1):30–5.
6. Jung YM et al. Atypical manifestations of hepatitis A infection: a prospective, multicenter study in Korea. J Med Virol. 2010;82(8):1318–26.
7. Agarwal KS, Puliyel J, Mathew A, Lahoti D, Gupta R. Acute pancreatitis with cholestatic hepatitis: an unusual manifestation of hepatitis A. Ann Trop Paediatr. 1999;19:391–4.
8. Ilan Y et al. Vasculitis and cryoglobulinemia associated with persisting cholestatic hepatitis A virus infection. Am J Gastroenterol. 1990;85(5):586–7.
9. Werblowsky-Constantini N et al. Toxic epidermal necrolysis associated with acute cholestatic viral hepatitis A. J Clin Gastroenterol. 1989;11(6):691–3.
10. Sciot R, Van Damme B, Desmet VJ. Cholestatic features in hepatitis A. J Hepatol. 1986;3(2):172–81.
11. Wolkoff AW. The hyperbilirubinemias, in Harrison's principles of internal medicine. New York, NY: McGraw Hill; 2008.
12. Krawczyk M et al. Prolonged cholestasis triggered by hepatitis A virus infection and variants of the hepatocanalicular phospholipid and bile salt transporters. Ann Hepatol. 2012;11(5): 710–4.
13. Coppola N et al. Acute hepatitis with severe cholestasis and prolonged clinical course due to hepatitis A virus Ia and Ib coinfection. Clin Infect Dis. 2007;44(9):e73–7.
14. Yoon EL et al. Clinical courses after administration of oral corticosteroids in patients with severely cholestatic acute hepatitis A; three cases. Korean J Hepatol. 2010;16(3):329–33.
15. Schiff ER. Atypical clinical manifestations of hepatitis A. Vaccine. 1992;10 Suppl 1:S18–20.
16. Fabris P et al. Effect of ursodeoxycholic acid administration in patients with acute viral hepatitis: a pilot study. Aliment Pharmacol Ther. 1999;13(9):1187–93.
17. Davies SE et al. Hepatic histological findings after transplantation for chronic hepatitis B virus infection, including a unique pattern of fibrosing cholestatic hepatitis. Hepatology. 1991;13(1): 150–7.
18. Lam PW et al. Fibrosing cholestatic hepatitis in renal transplant recipients. Transplantation. 1996;61(3):378–81.

19. Waguri N et al. Fibrosing cholestatic hepatitis after living related-donor renal transplantation. J Gastroenterol Hepatol. 1998;13(11):1133–7.
20. Longerich T et al. Acute liver failure in a renal transplant patient caused by adenoviral hepatitis superimposed on a fibrosing cholestatic hepatitis B. Hum Pathol. 2004;35(7):894–7.
21. Kairaitis LK, Gottlieb T, George CR. Fatal hepatitis B virus infection with fibrosing cholestatic hepatitis following renal transplantation. Nephrol Dial Transplant. 1998;13(6):1571–3.
22. Cooksley WG, McIvor CA. Fibrosing cholestatic hepatitis and HBV after bone marrow transplantation. Biomed Pharmacother. 1995;49(3):117–24.
23. Fang JW, Wright TL, Lau JY. Fibrosing cholestatic hepatitis in patient with HIV and hepatitis B. Lancet. 1993;342(8880):1175.
24. Zanati SA et al. Hepatic failure due to fibrosing cholestatic hepatitis in a patient with pre-surface mutant hepatitis B virus and mixed connective tissue disease treated with prednisolone and chloroquine. J Clin Virol. 2004;31(1):53–7.
25. Lau JY et al. High-level expression of hepatitis B viral antigens in fibrosing cholestatic hepatitis. Gastroenterology. 1992;102(3):956–62.
26. Angus PW et al. Hepatitis B virus precore mutant infection is associated with severe recurrent disease after liver transplantation. Hepatology. 1995;21(1):14–8.
27. Montalbano M, Neff GW. Management of recurrent viral hepatitis B and C after liver transplantation. Curr Gastroenterol Rep. 2006;8(1):60–6.
28. Jung S et al. Four cases of hepatitis B virus-related fibrosing cholestatic hepatitis treated with lamivudine. J Gastroenterol Hepatol. 2002;17(3):345–50.
29. Chan TM et al. Treatment of fibrosing cholestatic hepatitis with lamivudine. Gastroenterology. 1998;115(1):177–81.
30. Lai CL et al. A one-year trial of lamivudine for chronic hepatitis B. Asia Hepatitis Lamivudine Study Group. N Engl J Med. 1998;339(2):61–8.
31. Allen MI et al. Identification and characterization of mutations in hepatitis B virus resistant to lamivudine. Lamivudine Clinical Investigation Group. Hepatology. 1998;27(6):1670–7.
32. Lo C-M et al. Fibrosing cholestatic hepatitis secondary to precore/core promoter hepatitis B variant with lamivudine resistance: successful retransplantation with combination adefovir dipivoxil and hepatitis B immunoglobulin. Liver Transpl. 2004;10(4):557–63.
33. Tur-Kaspa R et al. Hepatitis B virus DNA contains a glucocorticoid-responsive element. Proc Natl Acad Sci U S A. 1986;83(6):1627–31.
34. Brind AM, Bennett MK, Bassendine MF. Nucleoside analogue therapy in fibrosing cholestatic hepatitis—a case report in an HBsAg positive renal transplant recipient. Liver. 1998;18(2):134–9.
35. Narang TK, Ahrens W, Russo MW. Post-liver transplant cholestatic hepatitis C: a systematic review of clinical and pathological findings and application of consensus criteria. Liver Transpl. 2010;16(11):1228–35.
36. Verna EC et al. Cholestatic hepatitis C following liver transplantation: an outcome-based histological definition, clinical predictors, and prognosis. Liver Transpl. 2013;19(1):78–88.
37. Wiesner RH, Sorrell M, Villamil F. Report of the first International Liver Transplantation Society expert panel consensus conference on liver transplantation and hepatitis C. Liver Transpl. 2003;9(11):S1–9.
38. McCaughan GW, Bowen DG. Pathogenesis of cholestatic hepatitis C. J Hepatol. 2011;54(2): 392–4.
39. Hanouneh IA et al. Interleukin-28B polymorphisms are associated with fibrosing cholestatic hepatitis in recurrent hepatitis C after liver transplantation. Clin Transplant. 2012;26(4): E335–6.
40. Yosephy A et al. Natural history of fibrosing cholestatic hepatitis C (FCH) after liver transplantation: a single center experience. Mount Laurel, NJ: The International Liver Transplantation Society; 2009. p. S93.
41. Gopal DV, Rosen HR. Duration of antiviral therapy for cholestatic HCV recurrence may need to be indefinite. Liver Transpl. 2003;9(4):348–53.
42. Chau TN et al. Epidemiology and clinical features of sporadic hepatitis E as compared with hepatitis A. Am J Gastroenterol. 2006;101(2):292–6.

43. Khuroo MS. Study of an epidemic of non-A, non-B hepatitis. Possibility of another human hepatitis virus distinct from post-transfusion non-A, non-B type. Am J Med. 1980;68(6):818–24.
44. Moucari R et al. Acute hepatitis E with severe jaundice: report of three cases. Eur J Gastroenterol Hepatol. 2007;19(11):1012–5.
45. Mechnik L et al. Acute hepatitis E virus infection presenting as a prolonged cholestatic jaundice. J Clin Gastroenterol. 2001;33(5):421–2.
46. Khuroo MS et al. Spectrum of hepatitis E virus infection in India. J Med Virol. 1994;43(3):281–6.
47. Jacobson MA, Cello JP, Sande MA. Cholestasis and disseminated cytomegalovirus disease in patients with the acquired immunodeficiency syndrome. Am J Med. 1988;84(2):218–24.
48. Cohen JI, Corey GR. Cytomegalovirus infection in the normal host. Medicine (Baltimore). 1985;64(2):100–14.
49. Takeuchi T et al. Cytomegalic inclusion disease presenting acute intrahepatic cholestasis. Intern Med. 1992;31(12):1376–80.
50. Serna-Higuera C et al. Acute cholestatic hepatitis by cytomegalovirus in an immunocompetent patient resolved with ganciclovir. J Clin Gastroenterol. 1999;29(3):276–7.
51. Munoz de Bustillo E et al. Fibrosing cholestatic hepatitis-like syndrome in hepatitis B virus-negative and hepatitis C virus-negative renal transplant recipients. Am J Kidney Dis. 2001;38(3):640–5.
52. Agarwal SK et al. Fibrosing cholestatic hepatitis in renal transplant recipient with CMV infection: a case report. Int Urol Nephrol. 2004;36(3):433–5.
53. Duseja A et al. Fibrosing cholestatic hepatitis-like syndrome in a hepatitis B virus and hepatitis C virus-negative renal transplant recipient: a case report with autopsy findings. Trop Gastroenterol. 2003;24(1):31–4.
54. Cohen JI. Epstein-Barr virus infection. N Engl J Med. 2000;343(7):481–92.
55. Kofteridis DP et al. Epstein Barr virus hepatitis. Eur J Intern Med. 2011;22(1):73–6.
56. Mendez-Sanchez N et al. Hepatic manifestations of Epstein-Barr viral infection. Ann Hepatol. 2005;4(3):205–9.
57. Hinedi TB, Koff RS. Cholestatic hepatitis induced by Epstein-Barr virus infection in an adult. Dig Dis Sci. 2003;48(3):539–41.
58. Mallory FB. Cirrhosis of the liver. Five different types of lesions from which it may arise. Bull Johns Hopkins Hosp. 1911;22:69–75.
59. Tung BY, Carithers Jr RL. Cholestasis and alcoholic liver disease. Clin Liver Dis. 1999;3(3):585–601.
60. Glover SC, McPhie JL, Brunt PW. Cholestasis in acute alcoholic liver disease. Lancet. 1977;2(8052–8053):1305–7.
61. Maddrey WC et al. Corticosteroid therapy of alcoholic hepatitis. Gastroenterology. 1978;75(2):193–9.
62. Phillips GB, Davidson CS. Acute hepatic insufficiency of the chronic alcoholic. AMA Arch Intern Med. 1954;94:585–603.
63. Nissenbaum M, Chedid A, Mendenhall C. Prognostic significance of cholestatic alcoholic hepatitis. Dig Dis Sci. 1990;35:891–6.
64. Spahr L et al. Early liver biopsy, intraparenchymal cholestasis, and prognosis in patients with alcoholic steatohepatitis. BMC Gastroenterol. 2011;11:115.

Chapter 8
Cholestasis Related to Systemic Disorders

Anitha Yadav and Elizabeth J. Carey

Abbreviations

ABC11	ATP-binding cassette, subfamily B member 11
ABC4	ATP-binding cassette
AIDS	Acquired immune deficiency syndrome
BSEP	Bile salt export pump
CF	Cystic fibrosis
CFTR	Cystic fibrosis transmembrane conductance receptor
FXR	Farnesoid X receptor
GVHD	Graft-versus-host disease
HD	Hodgkin's disease
HIV	Human immunodeficiency virus
ICP	Intrahepatic cholestasis of pregnancy
IL6	Interleukin-6
LPS	Lipopolysaccharides
MDR3	Multidrug resistance 3
MRP2	Multidrug resistance-associated protein 2
NHL	Non-Hodgkin's lymphoma
NTCP	Sodium taurocholate cotransporting polypeptide
TNF	Tumor necrosis factor
TPN	Total parenteral nutrition
UDCA	Ursodeoxycholic acid
UNOS/OPTN	United Network for organ sharing/organ procurement and transplantation network

A. Yadav, M.D. (✉)
Transplant Hepatology, Mayo Clinic Arizona, 5777 E. Mayo Blvd, Phoenix, AZ 85054, USA
e-mail: Yadav.anitha@mayo.edu

E.J. Carey, M.D.
Division of Gastroenterology and Hepatology, Mayo Clinic, 5777 E. Mayo Blvd, Phoenix, AZ USA
e-mail: Carey.Elizabeth@mayo.edu

E.J. Carey and K.D. Lindor (eds.), *Cholestatic Liver Disease*, Clinical Gastroenterology,
DOI 10.1007/978-1-4939-1013-7_8,

Table 8.1 Cholestasis due to systemic disorders

Canalicular impairment
Sepsis
Hormone mediated cholestasis (intrahepatic cholestasis of pregnancy)
Congestive hepatopathy
Paraneoplastic cholestasis
Systemic amyloidosis
Sickle cell disease
Small intrahepatic bile ducts obstruction
Sarcoidosis
Rheumatological diseases
Cystic fibrosis
Graft versus host disease
Extrahepatic malignancies
Large intrahepatic bile duct obstruction
HIV cholangiopathy

Introduction

Cholestasis due to primary liver diseases such as primary biliary cirrhosis, primary sclerosing cholangitis and autoimmune hepatitis are highlighted in other chapters. The aim of this chapter is to discuss the epidemiology, pathophysiology, clinical and biochemical presentation, and potential management strategies of major systemic diseases causing cholestasis.

Systemic disorders can secondarily affect the liver and biliary tract by different pathogenic mechanisms resulting in cholestasis. Major systemic conditions with potential anatomic sites of interrupted bile flow such as bile canaliculus, small intralobular bile ducts, and large intrahepatic bile ducts will be discussed (Table 8.1). Conditions causing disruption of bile flow in the biliary canaliculi including sepsis, hormonally influenced cholestasis of pregnancy and congestive cardiac failure will be reviewed. Processes that disrupt bile flow within the small intralobular ducts such as sarcoidosis, connective tissue disorders, and cystic fibrosis and lastly conditions that disrupt bile flow in large intrahepatic bile ducts will also be reviewed.

Cholestasis Due to Impaired Canalicular Function

Sepsis

After malignant biliary obstruction, extrahepatic infections and sepsis-associated cholestasis are the second most common cause of jaundice in hospitalized patients [1]. Cholestasis has been reported in 10–20 % of patients with sepsis; both gram-positive and gram-negative organisms are identified as etiologic agents [1, 2].

Cholestasis may occur early in the course of systemic infection, even before documented bacteriological diagnosis is made, or may not appear until clinical signs of active infection have resolved [3]. Sepsis-associated cholestasis is associated predominantly with jaundice (conjugated bilirubin level usually 5–10 mg/dL), in the setting of normal or moderately elevated alkaline phosphatase and aminotransferases. The mechanisms of cholestasis in sepsis have been studied in experimental models. Circulating bacterial lipopolysaccharides (LPS) induce Kupffer cells to release excessive pro-inflammatory cytokines including tumor necrosis factor (TNF), interleukin-1β, and interleukin-6 (IL-6) into the bloodstream [4]. These pro-inflammatory cytokines are potent inhibitors of hepatocellular transport mechanisms and cause down regulation of key bile acid transporters such as sodium taurocholate cotransporting polypeptide (NTCP), multidrug resistance-associated protein 2 (MRP2) and bile salt export pump (BSEP) resulting in the impairment of bile flow [5–7]. Sepsis is also associated with an increased release of nitric oxide by Kupffer and endothelial cells, which in turn disrupts bile canalicular transportation and ductular bile secretion resulting in cholestasis [8, 9].

Diagnosis of sepsis-induced cholestasis can be clinically challenging due to the frequent presence of confounding comorbidities including acalculous cholecystitis, extrahepatic biliary obstruction and drug induced liver injury. Liver biopsy is not routinely recommended and when obtained reveals bland intrahepatic cholestasis without associated inflammation (Fig. 8.1) [10]. The presence of massive dilatation of bile ductules at the margin of portal tracts with inspissated bile (cholangitis lenta) is seen in patients with indolent sepsis and is associated with poor prognosis [11, 12]. Management of sepsis-related cholestasis focuses on the treatment of underlying

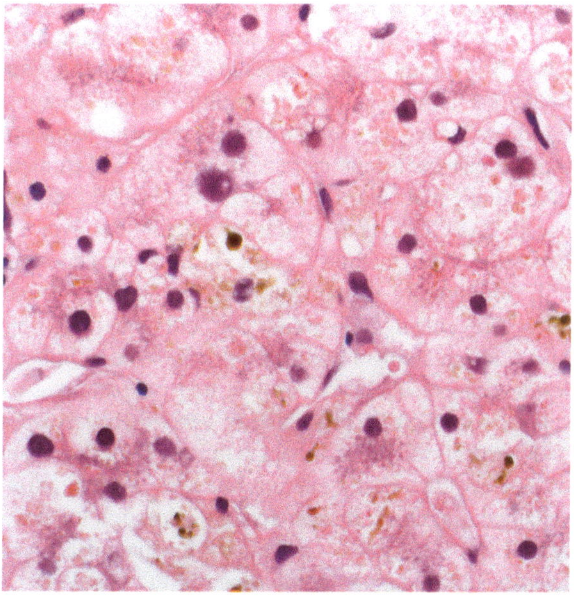

Fig. 8.1 Hepatic lobule showing severe cholestasis within hepatocyte cytoplasm and within bile canaliculi. There is associated ballooning degeneration of hepatocytes secondary to the emulsifier effects of bile. No significant lobular inflammation is in the background. This is the typical appearance of any cholestatic disease, including drug, infection, sepsis, intrahepatic cholestasis of pregnancy, etc. (H&E, 400×)

infection and hemodynamic instability with appropriate antimicrobial therapy and aggressive supportive care. Additionally, corticosteroids may be considered as possible therapeutic options in the treatment of septic shock. Sepsis induced inflammatory cytokines such as TNF-alpha and IL-6 decrease cortisol production from the adrenal gland, inducing corticosteroid resistance and relative adrenal insufficiency [13]. Low-dose steroid therapy is associated with improved blood pressure and duration of vasopressor support but not mortality in patients with septic shock [14, 15].

Hormone Mediated Cholestasis

Estrogen related cholestasis is well known to occur in the setting of oral contraceptive use and in intrahepatic cholestasis of pregnancy (ICP) in susceptible women. In animal models, estrogen glucuronides inhibit canalicular bile secretory processes via interactions with proteins such as BSEP and MRP2 [16, 17]. Estrogens also alter the expression of liver sinusoidal transporters and reduce bile flow [18]. Progesterone and its metabolites can trigger cholestasis by inhibiting bile acid uptake and canalicular transporters as demonstrated in animal studies [19, 20]. Progesterone and its metabolites increase during pregnancy and elevate further in ICP, potentially contributing to the pathogenesis of cholestasis.

ICP, the most common liver disease associated with pregnancy, is characterized by pruritus, elevated bilirubin and alkaline phosphatase and higher serum bile acid concentration. The symptoms usually begin in the second or third trimester of pregnancy and resolve spontaneously within 2–3 weeks after delivery. The incidence of ICP varies from 0.05 to 20 % of pregnancies and genetic, hormonal, and environmental factors may contribute to the pathogenesis [21]. Familial clustering, a higher incidence in certain ethnic groups, and geographic distribution in specific regions of Chile, Bolivia, and Scandinavia support a genetic predisposition for ICP. Heterozygous mutations in the canalicular phospholipid translocator ATP-binding cassette 4/multidrug resistance 3 (ABCB4/MDR3) involved in phosphatidylcholine excretion into the bile have been demonstrated in up to 20 % of women with ICP [22–24]. Mutations in another canalicular transporter, BSEP (ATP-binding cassette, subfamily B member 11 (ABC11) gene) which is critically involved in secretion of bile salts from hepatocytes into the bile, has also been associated with the development of ICP [25, 26]. Additionally, genetic variations in nuclear farnesoid X receptor (FXR), which plays a key role in maintaining bile acid homeostasis by regulating genes involved in bile acid metabolism and transport, have been linked with ICP [27]. Finally, cholestasis can result from estrogen and progesterone metabolites impairing hepatic transporters (BSEP), especially in genetically predisposed women [16, 20].

Pruritus is the predominant symptom in ICP and jaundice is reported in 10–25 % of patients [28]. Fasting serum bile acid concentration greater than 10 mmol/L is a sensitive diagnostic marker for ICP, although this test is not often clinically available. Liver biopsy is not necessary for diagnosis and if performed will show cholestasis and bile plugs predominantly in zone 3 [29]. In 45–70 % of women, ICP recurs in subsequent pregnancies [30]. Maternal prognosis is favorable, but affected women remain at increased lifetime risk of gallstone formation [31]. ICP poses risk for the fetus with an increased risk of premature delivery (60 %) and death [27].

Ursodeoxycholic acid (UDCA, 10–15 mg/kg) is considered the treatment of choice for ICP. UDCA therapy has been shown to reduce pruritus, improve liver test abnormalities [32–35] and also benefit fetal outcomes [36, 37]. Other pharmacologic agents such as cholestyramine, dexamethasone, and S-adenosyl-methionine were found to be ineffective compared to UDCA in patients with ICP [35].

Cholestasis Due to Cardiac Disease

Congestive heart failure, especially right-sided heart failure, is associated with a cholestatic pattern of liver injury [38–41]. Laboratory studies reveal mild to moderate elevation of total bilirubin, moderate increase in alkaline phosphatase and γ-glutamyl transferase with mild alterations in aminotransferases [36]. Prolonged prothrombin time, reduced serum albumin, right upper quadrant pain and ascites can also be seen in some patients with chronic congestive heart failure, making it difficult to distinguish between passive congestion and more advanced liver disease with synthetic dysfunction [37]. Microscopic examination of liver demonstrates sinusoidal dilatation, hemorrhagic necrosis in zone 3, bile thrombi with varying degree of cholestasis, and centrilobular and periportal fibrosis with eventual progression to bridging fibrosis (cardiac sclerosis) [35, 42].

The contributing factors for cholestasis in chronic heart failure are poorly understood. Hemodynamic data suggest that the elevated right atrial pressure and central venous pressure result in backward congestion of hepatic venules and sinusoids leading to hepatocellular dysfunction. Chronic passive congestion triggers sinusoidal collagen formation and fibrosis in the perivenular area leading to disruption of blood flow and hepatocyte atrophy [35, 36]. Animal data suggest that the increase in hepatic intrasinusoidal pressure may potentially disrupt the intrahepatocyte tight junctions (zonula occludens) creating communication between the canaliculus and the sinusoid allowing the bile contents back into systemic circulation [43].

Recent studies demonstrate that the degree of cholestasis is related to the severity of heart failure as assessed by the presence of tricuspid regurgitation and increase in right atrial pressure [39, 41, 44–48]. Cholestasis in heart failure has prognostic significance, as elevated alkaline phosphatase or bilirubin has been found to be an independent predictor of all-cause mortality, cardiovascular death, and hospitalizations in patients with chronic heart failure [40, 41].

Paraneoplastic Cholestasis

Paraneoplastic cholestasis in a patient with renal cell carcinoma (Stauffer's syndrome) was first described in 1961 by M.H Stauffer [49]. The overall incidence of paraneoplastic cholestasis in renal cell carcinoma is estimated at 15 % [50]. Stauffer syndrome is characterized by elevated alkaline phosphatase and γ-glutamyl transferase, with or without jaundice and pruritus in the absence of biliary obstruction or hepatic metastasis [51, 52]. Prolongation of prothrombin time secondary to low grade disseminated intravascular coagulation, thrombocytosis, elevated erythrocyte sedimentation rate, and hepatosplenomegaly are also associated with this syndrome [53]. Histopathology of liver demonstrates prominent sinusoidal dilatation focally in the mid-zone of the hepatic lobules and Kupffer cell hyperplasia with no evidence of hepatocellular necrosis [54, 55]. The pathogenesis of paraneoplastic cholestasis is not fully understood. Inflammatory cytokines such as IL-6 [56, 57], interleukin-1β [58], and other mediators [50, 55] have been implicated. In patients with renal cell carcinoma, serum alkaline phosphatase significantly decreased during anti-IL6 administration, indicating a role of IL-6 in the pathogenesis of Stauffer's syndrome [56].

Appropriate treatment of the primary tumor can lead to complete resolution of cholestasis in Stauffer's syndrome [51, 55, 59–62]. Although paraneoplastic cholestasis is associated primarily with renal cell carcinoma, it has also been described in prostate cancer [62–64], pheochromocytoma [58], medullary thyroid cancer [65], systemic mastocytosis [66, 67] soft tissue sarcoma [68], and lymphoproliferative disorders [69].

Cholestasis Resulting from Obstruction of Small Intrahepatic Ducts

Hepatic Sarcoidosis

Sarcoidosis is a multiorgan granulomatous disease characterized by the presence of noncaseating epithelioid granulomas in the affected organs. Sarcoidosis can affect any age, gender or ethnicity but is more common in young African Americans aged 30–39 years [70, 71].

The etiology of sarcoidosis is uncertain, but environmental agents, microbial triggers, and genetic associations have been implicated in the pathogenesis [72–74]. Hepatic granulomas form as a response to unknown antigenic stimulus in a predisposed host [75]. Activation of CD4 helper T lymphocytes with release of inflammatory cytokines such as IL-2, interferon gamma, interleukin 12, and TNF promote macrophage accumulation and activation resulting in initiation and maintenance of granulomas [76–78]. In response to various proinflammatory cytokines, epithelioid histiocytes, fibroblasts, and lymphocytes accumulate and form clusters resulting in granulomas [79]. De novo sarcoidosis has been reported during and following treatment with pegylated interferon alfa 2b and ribavirin, suggesting the immunomodulatory role of interferon alfa in the initiation of sarcoidosis [80–82].

The diagnosis of hepatic sarcoidosis is based on clinical presentation, biochemical parameters and histology. Most patients with hepatic sarcoid are asymptomatic [83, 84] and only a minority develop cholestasis, portal hypertension, Budd–Chiari syndrome, or cirrhosis [85–90]. Laboratory profile demonstrates elevated alkaline phosphatase [91], moderately elevated total bilirubin, mild increase in aminotransferase levels, and mild hypergammaglobulinemia [92]. Histology reveals noncaseating granulomas found preferentially within the portal triads although they can occasionally be seen in the liver lobules. Accumulation of granulomas in the portal tracts causes destruction of the septal and interlobular bile ducts, eventually leading to chronic cholestasis, ductopenia, and pathology similar to primary biliary cirrhosis [75, 87, 93]. Rarely, sarcoid granulomas affect large bile ducts resulting in severe cholestasis and cholangiographic features similar to primary sclerosing cholangitis [94–97]. In advanced cases, severe ductopenia, dense periportal fibrosis, or cirrhosis can occur [85].

No consensus exists regarding the treatment of hepatic sarcoidosis. Asymptomatic patients with biochemical abnormalities can be observed closely without treatment [98]. Conversely, corticosteroids may be considered in symptomatic patients with hepatic dysfunction [99, 100]. Steroid therapy may result in improvement in liver test abnormalities [101, 102] but does not alter the natural course or progression of disease [103, 104]. Despite steroid therapy, progression of portal hypertension and fibrosis has been noted [88]. Other nonsteroidal therapies reported to have anecdotal efficacy include UDCA [105, 106], methotrexate [107], infliximab [108, 109], and chloroquine [98]. Liver transplantation in advanced sarcoidosis results in good patient and graft outcome [110]. However, the United Network for Organ Sharing/Organ Procurement and Transplantation Network (UNOS/OPTN) analysis showed a slightly worse allograft and patient survival compared to transplantation for other cholestatic liver diseases [111]. Although post-transplant immunosuppression may be helpful to suppress granuloma formation, recurrent disease in the transplanted organ may occur [110–112].

Connective Tissue Diseases

Abnormal liver tests in rheumatologic disorders are highly variable, ranging from asymptomatic elevated liver function tests to cirrhosis [113, 114]. Elevated alkaline phosphatase has been reported in up to 25–50 % of patients with systemic lupus erythematosus [115–117], 18–50 % of rheumatoid arthritis [118, 119], up to 40 % in Felty's syndrome [120], 27–49 % in primary Sjögren's syndrome [121, 122], and 62 % of polymyalgia rheumatica patients [123]. Numerous histological patterns have been reported in systemic rheumatic diseases and findings include nonspecific portal inflammation, granulomas, nodular regenerative hyperplasia, steatosis, fibrosis, and cirrhosis [124]. Clinically significant cholestasis is rare in most of the connective tissue disorders; concomitant primary biliary cirrhosis develops in up to 15 % of patients [118]. Furthermore, nodular regenerative hyperplasia and primary sclerosing cholangitis are also associated with rheumatologic disorders [114, 118].

Cholestasis can also be secondary to drugs used in the treatment of rheumatic diseases. Penicillamine [125, 126], gold salts [127], methotrexate [128], and sulfasalazine [129] are all implicated in drug induced cholestasis in patients with rheumatologic diseases.

Cystic Fibrosis

Cystic fibrosis (CF) is an autosomal recessive disease characterized by mutations in the cystic fibrosis transmembrane conductance receptor (CFTR), a chloride channel transporter localized to the apical membrane of secretory and absorptive epithelial cells within the liver, biliary tree and other organs. Absent or decreased CFTR results in accumulation of inspissated biliary secretions in the intrahepatic bile ducts causing obstruction to the ductular bile flow [130]. Focal obstruction combined with injury to biliary epithelium by endogeneous bile acids results in periportal fibrosis and hepatic dysfunction [131].

Clinically apparent CF-related hepatobiliary disease develops in 15–41 % of CF patients mainly during or before puberty. Disease manifestations include neonatal cholestasis, hepatic steatosis, biliary obstruction eventually leading to biliary cirrhosis in 4.5 % of patients [130, 132]. Development of portal hypertension (7.9 %) leading to ascites and varices as late complications has also been noted in long-term CF survivors [133, 134]. The diagnosis is challenging and a combination of modalities such as clinical symptoms, liver function tests, imaging and histology should be used. There is no definitive therapy for CF-related liver disease. Treatment with high-dose UCDA has been shown to improve liver test abnormalities, histopathology and also to decrease the development of advanced liver disease with long-term use, but no effect on survival has been demonstrated [135–139]. Liver transplantation for CF-related liver disease is uncommon and the adult 5-year survival rate is less than in patients transplanted for other indications [140]. Patients without varices and preserved synthetic function can be managed medically and endoscopically without surgery [141].

Graft Versus Host Disease

Graft-versus-host disease (GVHD) is a major complication of allogenic hematopoietic stem cell transplant. The liver is frequently involved and acute or chronic cholestasis may occur. The pathophysiology of GVHD is complex and involves donor T lymphocytes reacting to host alloantigens, causing a strong cytokine response and eventually end organ damage [142, 143]. Murine GVHD models demonstrate inflammatory cell infiltration in the liver with CD8+ T cells and mononuclear phagocytes causing nonsuppurative destructive cholangitis [144].

Acute GVHD usually occurs within the first 100 days post-transplant and presents with elevation in alkaline phosphatase, gamma glutamyl transpeptidase, and conjugated bilirubin [145]. Chronic GVHD is an indolent cholestatic disease occurring in about 60 % of allograft recipients. However, chronic GVHD with marked elevation of aminotransferases resembling acute hepatitis has also been reported in the literature [146, 147]. Diagnosis of hepatic GVHD can be challenging and biopsy is usually required to confirm the diagnosis. The histologic features noted are endothelialitis, lymphocytic infiltration of the portal areas, immunomodulatory cholangitis, bile duct destruction, and portal fibrosis [148, 149]. Corticosteroids, cyclosporine, and other novel immunomodulatory drugs such as tacrolimus and mycophenolate mofetil are used in the therapy of GVHD. Treatment with UCDA has also been proven to be effective in mild cases with normalization or improvement in liver test abnormalities [150, 151].

Extrahepatic Malignancies

The liver is a common site for metastasis and malignancy. Melanoma and colon, breast, and lung cancers frequently metastasize to the liver [152]. Both Hodgkin's disease (HD) and non-Hodgkin's lymphoma (NHL) can cause cholestatic liver disease secondary to hepatic infiltration, obstruction of small interlobular ducts, or rarely extrahepatic biliary obstruction [153–155]. Liver involvement in HD has been reported in 11–80 % of patients and in 16–43 % in NHL cases [155, 156]. Acute liver failure due to hepatic infiltration has also been described in the literature, more commonly with NHL [157, 158]. Vanishing bile duct syndrome with destruction of small intrahepatic bile ducts is a rare and poorly understood condition seen in HD patients [159–162]. Although the prognosis is poor when vanishing bile duct syndrome occurs, successful treatment with chemotherapy for HD has been reported [160, 163].

Cholestasis from Obstruction of Large Intrahepatic Ducts

Acquired immune deficiency syndrome (AIDS) cholangiopathy is a late complication of human immunodeficiency virus (HIV) infection, commonly seen in advanced stages when CD4 counts are low. Most patients present with epigastric or right upper quadrant pain, fever, and elevated alkaline phosphatase [164]. The pathogenesis is unclear and infectious agents such as cytomegalovirus and cryptosporidium have been attributed as causative agents [165–167]. Intrahepatic or extrahepatic bile duct strictures or papillary stenosis are prominent features noted [164, 166–168]. The diagnosis is based on clinical, biochemical, and imaging evidence of biliary abnormalities. Magnetic resonance cholangiopancreatography will demonstrate biliary dilation [169]; endoscopic retrograde cholangiography is indicated to exclude papillary stenosis and for therapeutic intervention. Liver biopsy demonstrates cholestasis with portal tract edema, neutrophilic infiltration, and bile duct proliferation [170]. In patients with papillary stenosis, endoscopic sphincterotomy relieves pain, but liver enzyme elevation may persist [171]. Antimicrobial therapy for opportunistic infection has been shown to be ineffective. Highly active antiretroviral therapy may recover immune status and potentially improve cholangiographic abnormalities [172]. However, despite aggressive therapy, AIDS cholangiopathy is associated with a dismal prognosis [171, 172].

Cholestasis Due to Other Causes

Hepatic Amyloidosis

Liver involvement is common in both primary (AL) and secondary (AA) amyloidosis. Primary systemic amyloidosis is derived from immunoglobulin light chains and is associated with underlying plasma dyscrasias. Although liver involvement is common in primary amyloidosis (70 %), serious clinical manifestations are rare [173]. Common findings in hepatic amyloidosis include weight loss, abdominal pain, hepatomegaly, hyposplenism, and ascites [174–176]. Common laboratory abnormalities include elevated alkaline phosphatase (>500 U/L), jaundice, and elevated monoclonal protein in serum or urine [174, 176, 177]. Case reports of spontaneous hepatic rupture and massive bleeding have been reported in patients with hepatic amyloidosis [178–180]. Liver histopathology demonstrates amyloid deposition in the sinusoids, parenchyma, and blood vessel walls [181]. Patients with primary amyloidosis have a poor prognosis with median survival of 8–12 months [174, 182]. Treatment may include systemic chemotherapy or hematopoietic stem cell transplantation.

Secondary or AA amyloidosis is commonly seen in the setting of systemic inflammatory diseases or chronic infections. The clinical manifestations in secondary amyloidosis are similar to primary amyloidosis and the management includes treatment of underlying inflammatory disorder.

Sickle Cell Disease

Abnormal liver function tests are common in patients with sickle cell disease. Hepatobiliary complications associated with homozygous sickle cell disease include: acute sickle hepatic crisis, acute hepatic sequestration, sickle cell intrahepatic cholestasis, and extrahepatic cholestasis (cholelithiasis and choledocholithiasis) [183–185]. Acute sickle hepatic crisis occurs in 10 % of patients hospitalized for pain crisis and clinical manifestations include right upper quadrant pain, fever, jaundice, and hepatomegaly [186]. Liver function tests reveal predominantly elevated bilirubin with mild increase in aminotransferases. Sickle cell intrahepatic cholestasis is a rare and severe form of sickle cell crisis with profound conjugated hyperbilirubinemia due to marked intrasinusoidal sickling of erythrocytes and hepatic ischemia [185, 187]. Chronic intrahepatic cholestasis and cirrhosis has also been reported in patients with sickle cell disease [188, 189]. Liver biopsy in sickle cell disease demonstrates sinusoidal dilation, intrasinusoidal sickling, Kupffer cell hyperplasia, and hemosiderosis [190]. Aggressive treatment of sickle cell disease with exchange transfusion [185, 188] and liver transplantation in rare cases [191, 192] has been reported in the literature.

Total Parenteral Nutrition (TPN)

Parenteral nutrition related cholestatic liver disease is discussed in detail elsewhere. TPN induced cholestasis is a multifactorial hepatobiliary complication characterized by progressive increase in conjugated bilirubin (>2 mg/dL) and alkaline phosphatase in both adult and pediatric patients treated with hospital or home parenteral nutrition. Liver biopsy reveals intrahepatic cholestasis, steatohepatitis, varying degrees of fibrosis and cirrhosis [193]. Management includes early resumption of enteral intake, aggressive treatment of sepsis, and bacterial overgrowth. UDCA has been shown to be effective in reducing TPN related intrahepatic cholestasis [194].

Summary

Major systemic disorders can impair biliary function through diverse mechanisms causing varying degrees of cholestasis. In sepsis, Kupffer cell activation by endotoxins and bacteria initiates the cascade of inflammatory cytokines, disrupting the canalicular bile flow and resulting in cholestasis. Sepsis-related cholestasis involves treatment of the underlying infection and aggressive supportive measures. Intrahepatic cholestasis of pregnancy is a complex disorder with heterogeneous etiologies including hormonal, genetic, and environmental factors usually occurring late in pregnancy. ICP is associated with adverse fetal outcomes and UCDA is considered as the mainstay of therapy. Increased central venous pressure due to chronic heart failure results in passive hepatic congestion and cholestasis. The degree of cholestasis is related to the severity of heart failure, and elevated liver function tests have long-term prognostic implications in heart failure patients. Liver involvement in sarcoidosis ranges from asymptomatic cholestatic abnormalities to advanced disease with portal hypertension and cirrhosis. Other disorders such as cystic fibrosis and various rheumatologic conditions also cause cholestasis due to disruption of bile flow in the small intralobular bile ducts. AIDS cholangiopathy occurs in advanced HIV disease with low CD4 counts and is characterized by papillary stenosis, bile duct strictures and sclerosing cholangitis. Treatment includes endoscopic sphincterotomy, biliary stenting, antimicrobial therapy, and HAART regimen. Lastly, systemic amyloidosis and sickle cell disease also involve liver and cause varying degrees of cholestasis.

References

1. Whitehead MW, Hainsworth I, Kingham JG. The causes of obvious jaundice in South West Wales: perceptions versus reality. Gut. 2001;48(3):409–13.
2. Fan HB, Yang DL, Chen AS, Li Z, Xu LT, Ma XJ, et al. Sepsis-associated cholestasis in adult patients: a prospective study. Am J Med Sci. 2013;346:462–6.

3. Franson TR, Hierholzer Jr WJ, LaBrecque DR. Frequency and characteristics of hyperbilirubinemia associated with bacteremia. Rev Infect Dis. 1985;7(1):1–9.
4. Kosters A, Karpen SJ. The role of inflammation in cholestasis: clinical and basic aspects. Semin Liver Dis. 2010;30(2):186–94.
5. Whiting JF, Green RM, Rosenbluth AB, Gollan JL. Tumor necrosis factor-alpha decreases hepatocyte bile salt uptake and mediates endotoxin-induced cholestasis. Hepatology. 1995;22(4 Pt 1):1273–8.
6. Geier A, Fickert P, Trauner M. Mechanisms of disease: mechanisms and clinical implications of cholestasis in sepsis. Nat Clin Pract Gastroenterol Hepatol. 2006;3(10):574–85.
7. Green RM, Beier D, Gollan JL. Regulation of hepatocyte bile salt transporters by endotoxin and inflammatory cytokines in rodents. Gastroenterology. 1996;111(1):193–8.
8. Dufour JF, Turner TJ, Arias IM. Nitric oxide blocks bile canalicular contraction by inhibiting inositol trisphosphate-dependent calcium mobilization. Gastroenterology. 1995;108(3):841–9.
9. Spirli C, Fabris L, Duner E, Fiorotto R, Ballardini G, Roskams T, et al. Cytokine-stimulated nitric oxide production inhibits adenylyl cyclase and cAMP-dependent secretion in cholangiocytes. Gastroenterology. 2003;124(3):737–53.
10. Lefkowitch JH. Histological assessment of cholestasis. Clin Liver Dis. 2004;8(1):27–40. v.
11. Lefkowitch JH. Bile ductular cholestasis: an ominous histopathologic sign related to sepsis and "cholangitis lenta". Hum Pathol. 1982;13(1):19–24.
12. Li MK, Crawford JM. The pathology of cholestasis. Semin Liver Dis. 2004;24(1):21–42.
13. Cooper MS, Stewart PM. Corticosteroid insufficiency in acutely ill patients. N Engl J Med. 2003;348(8):727–34.
14. Patel GP, Balk RA. Systemic steroids in severe sepsis and septic shock. Am J Respir Crit Care Med. 2012;185(2):133–9.
15. Annane D, Bellissant E, Bollaert PE, Briegel J, Confalonieri M, De Gaudio R, et al. Corticosteroids in the treatment of severe sepsis and septic shock in adults: a systematic review. JAMA. 2009;301(22):2362–75.
16. Stieger B, Fattinger K, Madon J, Kullak-Ublick GA, Meier PJ. Drug- and estrogen-induced cholestasis through inhibition of the hepatocellular bile salt export pump (Bsep) of rat liver. Gastroenterology. 2000;118(2):422–30.
17. Huang L, Smit JW, Meijer DK, Vore M. Mrp2 is essential for estradiol-17beta(beta-d-glucuronide)-induced cholestasis in rats. Hepatology. 2000;32(1):66–72.
18. Simon FR, Fortune J, Iwahashi M, Gartung C, Wolkoff A, Sutherland E. Ethinyl estradiol cholestasis involves alterations in expression of liver sinusoidal transporters. Am J Physiol. 1996;271(6 Pt 1):G1043–52.
19. Abu-Hayyeh S, Martinez-Becerra P, Sheikh Abdul Kadir SH, Selden C, Romero MR, Rees M, et al. Inhibition of Na+-taurocholate Co-transporting polypeptide-mediated bile acid transport by cholestatic sulfated progesterone metabolites. J Biol Chem. 2010;285(22): 16504–12.
20. Vallejo M, Briz O, Serrano MA, Monte MJ, Marin JJ. Potential role of trans-inhibition of the bile salt export pump by progesterone metabolites in the etiopathogenesis of intrahepatic cholestasis of pregnancy. J Hepatol. 2006;44(6):1150–7.
21. Geenes V, Williamson C. Intrahepatic cholestasis of pregnancy. World J Gastroenterol. 2009;15(17):2049–66.
22. Schneider G, Paus TC, Kullak-Ublick GA, Meier PJ, Wienker TF, Lang T, et al. Linkage between a new splicing site mutation in the MDR3 alias ABCB4 gene and intrahepatic cholestasis of pregnancy. Hepatology. 2007;45(1):150–8.
23. Wasmuth HE, Glantz A, Keppeler H, Simon E, Bartz C, Rath W, et al. Intrahepatic cholestasis of pregnancy: the severe form is associated with common variants of the hepatobiliary phospholipid transporter ABCB4 gene. Gut. 2007;56(2):265–70.
24. Floreani A, Carderi I, Paternoster D, Soardo G, Azzaroli F, Esposito W, et al. Intrahepatic cholestasis of pregnancy: three novel MDR3 gene mutations. Aliment Pharmacol Ther. 2006;23(11):1649–53.

25. Dixon PH, van Mil SW, Chambers J, Strautnieks S, Thompson RJ, Lammert F, et al. Contribution of variant alleles of ABCB11 to susceptibility to intrahepatic cholestasis of pregnancy. Gut. 2009;58(4):537–44.
26. Meier Y, Zodan T, Lang C, Zimmermann R, Kullak-Ublick GA, Meier PJ, et al. Increased susceptibility for intrahepatic cholestasis of pregnancy and contraceptive-induced cholestasis in carriers of the 1331T>C polymorphism in the bile salt export pump. World J Gastroenterol. 2008;14(1):38–45.
27. Van Mil SW, Milona A, Dixon PH, Mullenbach R, Geenes VL, Chambers J, et al. Functional variants of the central bile acid sensor FXR identified in intrahepatic cholestasis of pregnancy. Gastroenterology. 2007;133(2):507–16.
28. Kondrackiene J, Kupcinskas L. Intrahepatic cholestasis of pregnancy-current achievements and unsolved problems. World J Gastroenterol. 2008;14(38):5781–8.
29. Rolfes DB, Ishak KG. Liver disease in pregnancy. Histopathology. 1986;10(6):555–70.
30. Bacq Y, Sapey T, Brechot MC, Pierre F, Fignon A, Dubois F. Intrahepatic cholestasis of pregnancy: a French prospective study. Hepatology. 1997;26(2):358–64.
31. Ropponen A, Sund R, Riikonen S, Ylikorkala O, Aittomaki K. Intrahepatic cholestasis of pregnancy as an indicator of liver and biliary diseases: a population-based study. Hepatology. 2006;43(4):723–8.
32. Glantz A, Marschall HU, Lammert F, Mattsson LA. Intrahepatic cholestasis of pregnancy: a randomized controlled trial comparing dexamethasone and ursodeoxycholic acid. Hepatology. 2005;42(6):1399–405.
33. Zapata R, Sandoval L, Palma J, Hernandez I, Ribalta J, Reyes H, et al. Ursodeoxycholic acid in the treatment of intrahepatic cholestasis of pregnancy. A 12-year experience. Liver Int. 2005;25(3):548–54.
34. Roncaglia N, Locatelli A, Arreghini A, Assi F, Cameroni I, Pezzullo JC, et al. A randomised controlled trial of ursodeoxycholic acid and S-adenosyl-L-methionine in the treatment of gestational cholestasis. BJOG. 2004;111(1):17–21.
35. Kondrackiene J, Beuers U, Kupcinskas L. Efficacy and safety of ursodeoxycholic acid versus cholestyramine in intrahepatic cholestasis of pregnancy. Gastroenterology. 2005;129(3): 894–901.
36. Bacq Y, Sentilhes L, Reyes HB, Glantz A, Kondrackiene J, Binder T, et al. Efficacy of ursodeoxycholic acid in treating intrahepatic cholestasis of pregnancy: a meta-analysis. Gastroenterology. 2012;143(6):1492–501.
37. Davies MH, da Silva RC, Jones SR, Weaver JB, Elias E. Fetal mortality associated with cholestasis of pregnancy and the potential benefit of therapy with ursodeoxycholic acid. Gut. 1995;37(4):580–4.
38. Giallourakis CC, Rosenberg PM, Friedman LS. The liver in heart failure. Clin Liver Dis. 2002;6(4):947–67. viii–ix.
39. Lau GT, Tan HC, Kritharides L. Type of liver dysfunction in heart failure and its relation to the severity of tricuspid regurgitation. Am J Cardiol. 2002;90(12):1405–9.
40. Allen LA, Felker GM, Pocock S, McMurray JJ, Pfeffer MA, Swedberg K, et al. Liver function abnormalities and outcome in patients with chronic heart failure: data from the Candesartan in heart failure: assessment of reduction in mortality and morbidity (CHARM) program. Eur J Heart Fail. 2009;11(2):170–7.
41. Poelzl G, Ess M, Mussner-Seeber C, Pachinger O, Frick M, Ulmer H. Liver dysfunction in chronic heart failure: prevalence, characteristics and prognostic significance. Eur J Clin Invest. 2012;42(2):153–63.
42. Myers RP, Cerini R, Sayegh R, Moreau R, Degott C, Lebrec D, et al. Cardiac hepatopathy: clinical, hemodynamic, and histologic characteristics and correlations. Hepatology. 2003;37(2):393–400.
43. Cogger VC, Fraser R, Le Couteur DG. Liver dysfunction and heart failure. Am J Cardiol. 2003;91(11):1399.
44. Moller S, Bernardi M. Interactions of the heart and the liver. Eur Heart J. 2013;34:2804–11.

45. Kubo SH, Walter BA, John DH, Clark M, Cody RJ. Liver function abnormalities in chronic heart failure. Influence of systemic hemodynamics. Arch Intern Med. 1987;147(7):1227–30.
46. Batin P, Wickens M, McEntegart D, Fullwood L, Cowley AJ. The importance of abnormalities of liver function tests in predicting mortality in chronic heart failure. Eur Heart J. 1995;16(11):1613–8.
47. Yu SB, Cui HY, Qin M, Liu T, Kong B, Zhao QY, et al. Prevalence and prognostic value of liver function abnormalities in patients with chronic systolic heart failure. Zhonghua Yi Xue Za Zhi. 2011;91(38):2673–7.
48. Ess M, Mussner-Seeber C, Mariacher S, Lorsbach-Koehler A, Pachinger O, Frick M, et al. gamma-Glutamyltransferase rather than total bilirubin predicts outcome in chronic heart failure. J Card Fail. 2011;17(7):577–84.
49. Stauffer MH, Sauer WG, Dearing WH, Baggenstoss AH. The spectrum of cholestatic hepatic disease. JAMA. 1965;191:829–37.
50. Prommer E. Prostate cancer and liver dysfunction: a case of cytokine dysregulation. J Pain Symptom Manage. 2007;34(3):225–6.
51. Dourakis SP, Sinani C, Deutsch M, Dimitriadou E, Hadziyannis SJ. Cholestatic jaundice as a paraneoplastic manifestation of renal cell carcinoma. Eur J Gastroenterol Hepatol. 1997;9(3):311–4.
52. Jacobi GH, Philipp T. Stauffer's syndrome—diagnostic help in hypernephroma. Clin Nephrol. 1975;4(3):113–5.
53. Andrassy K, Gartner H, Siede WH, Ritz E, Riedasch G, Mohring K, et al. Stauffer's syndrome in renal cell carcinoma evidence for intravascular coagulation. Klin Wochenschr. 1980;58(2):91–7.
54. Aoyagi T, Mori I, Ueyama Y, Tamaoki N. Sinusoidal dilatation of the liver as a paraneoplastic manifestation of renal cell carcinoma. Hum Pathol. 1989;20(12):1193–7.
55. Delpre G, Ilie B, Papo J, Streifler C, Gefel A. Hypernephroma with nonmetastatic liver dysfunction (Stauffer's syndrome) and hypercalcemia. Case report and review of the literature. Am J Gastroenterol. 1979;72(3):239–47.
56. Blay JY, Rossi JF, Wijdenes J, Menetrier-Caux C, Schemann S, Negrier S, et al. Role of interleukin-6 in the paraneoplastic inflammatory syndrome associated with renal-cell carcinoma. Int J Cancer. 1997;72(3):424–30.
57. Walther MM, Johnson B, Culley D, Shah R, Weber J, Venzon D, et al. Serum interleukin-6 levels in metastatic renal cell carcinoma before treatment with interleukin-2 correlates with paraneoplastic syndromes but not patient survival. J Urol. 1998;159(3):718–22.
58. Chung CH, Wang CH, Tzen CY, Liu CP. Intrahepatic cholestasis as a paraneoplastic syndrome associated with pheochromocytoma. J Endocrinol Invest. 2005;28(2):175–9.
59. Giannakos G, Papanicolaou X, Trafalis D, Michaelidis I, Margaritis G, Christofilakis C. Stauffer's syndrome variant associated with renal cell carcinoma. Int J Urol. 2005;12(8):757–9.
60. Tomadoni A, Garcia C, Marquez M, Ayala JC, Prado F. Stauffer's syndrome with jaundice, a paraneoplastic manifestation of renal cell carcinoma: a case report. Arch Esp Urol. 2010;63(2):154–6.
61. Morla D, Alazemi S, Lichtstein D. Stauffer's syndrome variant with cholestatic jaundice: a case report. J Gen Intern Med. 2006;21(7):C11–3.
62. Karakolios A, Kasapis C, Kallinikidis T, Kalpidis P, Grigoriadis N. Cholestatic jaundice as a paraneoplastic manifestation of prostate adenocarcinoma. Clin Gastroenterol Hepatol. 2003;1(6):480–3.
63. Nguyen V, Gurney H, van der Poorten D. Paraneoplastic hepatic dysfunction in metastatic prostate cancer: the role of cytokine dysregulation. J Clin Oncol. 2011;29(2):e21–3.
64. Koruk M, Buyukberber M, Savas C, Kadayifci A. Paraneoplastic cholestasis associated with prostate carcinoma. Turk J Gastroenterol. 2004;15(1):53–5.
65. Tiede DJ, Tefferi A, Kochhar R, Thompson GB, Hay ID. Paraneoplastic cholestasis and hypercoagulability associated with medullary thyroid carcinoma. Resolution with tumor debulking. Cancer. 1994;73(3):702–5.

66. Safyan EL, Veerabagu MP, Swerdlow SH, Lee RG, Rakela J. Intrahepatic cholestasis due to systemic mastocytosis: a case report and review of literature. Am J Gastroenterol. 1997;92(7): 1197–200.
67. Kupfer SS, Hart J, Mohanty SR. Aggressive systemic mastocytosis presenting with hepatic cholestasis. Eur J Gastroenterol Hepatol. 2007;19(10):901–5.
68. Sharara AI, Panella TJ, Fitz JG. Paraneoplastic hepatopathy associated with soft tissue sarcoma. Gastroenterology. 1992;103(1):330–2.
69. Barta SK, Yahalom J, Shia J, Hamlin PA. Idiopathic cholestasis as a paraneoplastic phenomenon in Hodgkin's lymphoma. Clin Lymphoma Myeloma. 2006;7(1):77–82.
70. Cox CE, Davis-Allen A, Judson MA. Sarcoidosis. Med Clin North Am. 2005;89(4):817–28.
71. Westney GE, Judson MA. Racial and ethnic disparities in sarcoidosis: from genetics to socioeconomics. Clin Chest Med. 2006;27(3):453–62. vi.
72. Almenoff PL, Johnson A, Lesser M, Mattman LH. Growth of acid fast L forms from the blood of patients with sarcoidosis. Thorax. 1996;51(5):530–3.
73. Brown ST, Brett I, Almenoff PL, Lesser M, Terrin M, Teirstein AS. Recovery of cell wall-deficient organisms from blood does not distinguish between patients with sarcoidosis and control subjects. Chest. 2003;123(2):413–7.
74. Sverrild A, Backer V, Kyvik KO, Kaprio J, Milman N, Svendsen CB, et al. Heredity in sarcoidosis: a registry-based twin study. Thorax. 2008;63(10):894–6.
75. Matheus T, Munoz S. Granulomatous liver disease and cholestasis. Clin Liver Dis. 2004;8(1): 229–46. ix.
76. Lagana SM, Moreira RK, Lefkowitch JH. Hepatic granulomas: pathogenesis and differential diagnosis. Clin Liver Dis. 2010;14(4):605–17.
77. Agostini C, Basso U, Semenzato G. Cells and molecules involved in the development of sarcoid granuloma. J Clin Immunol. 1998;18(3):184–92.
78. Chen ES, Moller DR. Sarcoidosis–scientific progress and clinical challenges. Nat Rev Rheumatol. 2011;7(8):457–67.
79. Denk H, Scheuer PJ, Baptista A, Bianchi L, Callea F, De Groote J, et al. Guidelines for the diagnosis and interpretation of hepatic granulomas. Histopathology. 1994;25(3): 209–18.
80. Adla M, Downey KK, Ahmad J. Hepatic sarcoidosis associated with pegylated interferon alfa therapy for chronic hepatitis C: case report and review of literature. Dig Dis Sci. 2008;53(10):2810–2.
81. Gitlin N. Manifestation of sarcoidosis during interferon and ribavirin therapy for chronic hepatitis C: a report of two cases. Eur J Gastroenterol Hepatol. 2002;14(8):883–5.
82. Gayet AR, Plaisance P, Bergmann JF, Mouly S. Development of sarcoidosis following completion of treatment for hepatitis C with pegylated interferon-{alpha}2a and ribavirin: a case report and literature review. Clin Med Res. 2010;8(3–4):163–7.
83. Kahi CJ, Saxena R, Temkit M, Canlas K, Roberts S, Knox K, et al. Hepatobiliary disease in sarcoidosis. Sarcoidosis Vasc Diffuse Lung Dis. 2006;23(2):117–23.
84. Blich M, Edoute Y. Clinical manifestations of sarcoid liver disease. J Gastroenterol Hepatol. 2004;19(7):732–7.
85. Devaney K, Goodman ZD, Epstein MS, Zimmerman HJ, Ishak KG. Hepatic sarcoidosis. Clinicopathologic features in 100 patients. Am J Surg Pathol. 1993;17(12):1272–80.
86. Ishak KG. Sarcoidosis of the liver and bile ducts. Mayo Clin Proc. 1998;73(5):467–72.
87. Moreno-Merlo F, Wanless IR, Shimamatsu K, Sherman M, Greig P, Chiasson D. The role of granulomatous phlebitis and thrombosis in the pathogenesis of cirrhosis and portal hypertension in sarcoidosis. Hepatology. 1997;26(3):554–60.
88. Valla D, Pessegueiro-Miranda H, Degott C, Lebrec D, Rueff B, Benhamou JP. Hepatic sarcoidosis with portal hypertension. A report of seven cases with a review of the literature. Q J Med. 1987;63(242):531–44.
89. Delfosse V, de Leval L, De Roover A, Delwaide J, Honore P, Boniver J, et al. Budd-Chiari syndrome complicating hepatic sarcoidosis: definitive treatment by liver transplantation: a case report. Transplant Proc. 2009;41(8):3432–4.

90. Russi EW, Bansky G, Pfaltz M, Spinas G, Hammer B, Senning A. Budd-Chiari syndrome in sarcoidosis. Am J Gastroenterol. 1986;81(1):71–5.
91. Cremers J, Drent M, Driessen A, Nieman F, Wijnen P, Baughman R, et al. Liver-test abnormalities in sarcoidosis. Eur J Gastroenterol Hepatol. 2012;24(1):17–24.
92. Ebert EC, Kierson M, Hagspiel KD. Gastrointestinal and hepatic manifestations of sarcoidosis. Am J Gastroenterol. 2008;103(12):3184–92. quiz 93.
93. Rudzki C, Ishak KG, Zimmerman HJ. Chronic intrahepatic cholestasis of sarcoidosis. Am J Med. 1975;59(3):373–87.
94. Alam I, Levenson SD, Ferrell LD, Bass NM. Diffuse intrahepatic biliary strictures in sarcoidosis resembling sclerosing cholangitis. Case report and review of the literature. Dig Dis Sci. 1997;42(6):1295–301.
95. Sotiropoulos GC, Dahmen U, Dirsch O, Antoch G, Freudenberg L, Brokalaki EI, et al. Biliary tract obstruction due to sarcoidosis. Endoscopy. 2005;37(12):1262.
96. Rezeig MA, Fashir BM. Biliary tract obstruction due to sarcoidosis: a case report. Am J Gastroenterol. 1997;92(3):527–8.
97. Buxbaum J, Papademetriou M, Klipfel N, Selby R, Fong TL, Sharma O. Biliary sarcoidosis: early diagnosis minimizes the need for surgery. Am J Respir Crit Care Med. 2013;187(5): 556–9.
98. Ayyala US, Padilla ML. Diagnosis and treatment of hepatic sarcoidosis. Curr Treat Options Gastroenterol. 2006;9(6):475–83.
99. Judson MA. Hepatic, splenic, and gastrointestinal involvement with sarcoidosis. Semin Respir Crit Care Med. 2002;23(6):529–41.
100. Valla DC, Benhamou JP. Hepatic granulomas and hepatic sarcoidosis. Clin Liver Dis. 2000;4(1):269–85. ix–x.
101. Amarapurkar DN, Patel ND, Amarapurkar AD. Hepatic sarcoidosis. Indian J Gastroenterol. 2003;22(3):98–100.
102. Gerard AG, Roth AL, Becker SM, Shih CS. Regression of sarcoid hepatosplenomegaly on corticosteroid therapy. J Med Soc N J. 1968;65(2):64–7.
103. Kennedy PT, Zakaria N, Modawi SB, Papadopoulou AM, Murray-Lyon I, du Bois RM, et al. Natural history of hepatic sarcoidosis and its response to treatment. Eur J Gastroenterol Hepatol. 2006;18(7):721–6.
104. Vatti R, Sharma OP. Course of asymptomatic liver involvement in sarcoidosis: role of therapy in selected cases. Sarcoidosis Vasc Diffuse Lung Dis. 1997;14(1):73–6.
105. Bakker GJ, Haan YC, de Buy M, Wenniger LJ, Beuers U. Sarcoidosis of the liver: to treat or not to treat? Neth J Med. 2012;70(8):349–56.
106. Becheur H, Dall'osto H, Chatellier G, Charton-Bain MC, Aubertin JM, Attar A, et al. Effect of ursodeoxycholic acid on chronic intrahepatic cholestasis due to sarcoidosis. Dig Dis Sci. 1997;42(4):789–91.
107. Baughman RP, Winget DB, Lower EE. Methotrexate is steroid sparing in acute sarcoidosis: results of a double blind, randomized trial. Sarcoidosis Vasc Diffuse Lung Dis. 2000;17(1):60–6.
108. Korsten P, Mirsaeidi M, Sweiss NJ. Nonsteroidal therapy of sarcoidosis. Curr Opin Pulm Med. 2013;19(5):516–23.
109. Baughman RP, Iannuzzi M. Tumour necrosis factor in sarcoidosis and its potential for targeted therapy. BioDrugs. 2003;17(6):425–31.
110. Lipson EJ, Fiel MI, Florman SS, Korenblat KM. Patient and graft outcomes following liver transplantation for sarcoidosis. Clin Transplant. 2005;19(4):487–91.
111. Vanatta JM, Modanlou KA, Dean AG, Nezakatgoo N, Campos L, Nair S, et al. Outcomes of orthotopic liver transplantation for hepatic sarcoidosis: an analysis of the United Network for organ sharing/organ procurement and transplantation network data files for a comparative study with cholestatic liver diseases. Liver Transpl. 2011;17(9):1027–34.
112. Cengiz C, Rodriguez-Davalos M, deBoccardo G, Fiel MI, Rodriguez G, Kovacevic M, et al. Recurrent hepatic sarcoidosis post-liver transplantation manifesting with severe hypercalcemia: a case report and review of the literature. Liver Transpl. 2005;11(12):1611–4.

113. Youssef WI, Tavill AS. Connective tissue diseases and the liver. J Clin Gastroenterol. 2002;35(4):345–9.
114. Selmi C, De Santis M, Gershwin ME. Liver involvement in subjects with rheumatic disease. Arthritis Res Ther. 2011;13(3):226.
115. Schiavon LL, Carvalho-Filho RJ, Narciso-Schiavon JL, Lanzoni VP, Ferraz ML, Silva AE. Late-onset systemic lupus erythematosus-associated liver disease. Rheumatol Int. 2012;32(9):2917–20.
116. Tomasevic R, Golubovic G, Kiurski M, Pavlovic A. [Cholestatic syndrome in patients with systemic erythematous lupus–differential diagnostic aspects]. Med Pregl. 2008;61(5–6):291–4.
117. Runyon BA, LaBrecque DR, Anuras S. The spectrum of liver disease in systemic lupus erythematosus. Report of 33 histologically-proved cases and review of the literature. Am J Med. 1980;69(2):187–94.
118. Abraham S, Begum S, Isenberg D. Hepatic manifestations of autoimmune rheumatic diseases. Ann Rheum Dis. 2004;63(2):123–9.
119. Webb J, Whaley K, MacSween RN, Nuki G, Dick WC, Buchanan WW. Liver disease in rheumatoid arthritis and Sjogren's syndrome. Prospective study using biochemical and serological markers of hepatic dysfunction. Ann Rheum Dis. 1975;34(1):70–81.
120. Thorne C, Urowitz MB, Wanless I, Roberts E, Blendis LM. Liver disease in Felty's syndrome. Am J Med. 1982;73(1):35–40.
121. Kaplan MJ, Ike RW. The liver is a common non-exocrine target in primary Sjogren's syndrome: a retrospective review. BMC Gastroenterol. 2002;2:21.
122. Montano-Loza AJ, Crispin-Acuna JC, Remes-Troche JM, Uribe M. Abnormal hepatic biochemistries and clinical liver disease in patients with primary Sjogren's syndrome. Ann Hepatol. 2007;6(3):150–5.
123. von Knorring J, Wassatjerna C. Liver involvement in polymyalgia rheumatica. Scand J Rheumatol. 1976;5(4):197–204.
124. Malnick S, Melzer E, Sokolowski N, Basevitz A. The involvement of the liver in systemic diseases. J Clin Gastroenterol. 2008;42(1):69–80.
125. Multz CV. Cholestatic hepatitis caused by penicillamine. JAMA. 1981;246(6):674–5.
126. Jacobs JW, Van der Weide FR, Kruijsen MW. Fatal cholestatic hepatitis caused by D-PENICILLAMINE. Br J Rheumatol. 1994;33(8):770–3.
127. Basset C, Vadrot J, Denis J, Poupon J, Zafrani ES. Prolonged cholestasis and ductopenia following gold salt therapy. Liver Int. 2003;23(2):89–93.
128. Kremer JM, Lee RG, Tolman KG. Liver histology in rheumatoid arthritis patients receiving long-term methotrexate therapy. A prospective study with baseline and sequential biopsy samples. Arthritis Rheum. 1989;32(2):121–7.
129. Mitrane MP, Singh A, Seibold JR. Cholestasis and fatal agranulocytosis complicating sulfasalazine therapy: case report and review of the literature. J Rheumatol. 1986;13(5):969–72.
130. Moyer K, Balistreri W. Hepatobiliary disease in patients with cystic fibrosis. Curr Opin Gastroenterol. 2009;25(3):272–8.
131. Colombo C, Russo MC, Zazzeron L, Romano G. Liver disease in cystic fibrosis. J Pediatr Gastroenterol Nutr. 2006;43 Suppl 1:S49–55.
132. Colombo C, Battezzati PM, Crosignani A, Morabito A, Costantini D, Padoan R, et al. Liver disease in cystic fibrosis: a prospective study on incidence, risk factors, and outcome. Hepatology. 2002;36(6):1374–82.
133. Hodson ME, Simmonds NJ, Warwick WJ, Tullis E, Castellani C, Assael B, et al. An international/multicentre report on patients with cystic fibrosis (CF) over the age of 40 years. J Cyst Fibros. 2008;7(6):537–42.
134. Efrati O, Barak A, Modan-Moses D, Augarten A, Vilozni D, Katznelson D, et al. Liver cirrhosis and portal hypertension in cystic fibrosis. Eur J Gastroenterol Hepatol. 2003;15(10):1073–8.
135. Cheng K, Ashby D, Smyth RL. Ursodeoxycholic acid for cystic fibrosis-related liver disease. Cochrane Database Syst Rev. 2012;10:CD000222.

136. Kappler M, Espach C, Schweiger-Kabesch A, Lang T, Hartl D, Hector A, et al. Ursodeoxycholic acid therapy in cystic fibrosis liver disease—a retrospective long-term follow-up case–control study. Aliment Pharmacol Ther. 2012;36(3):266–73.
137. Colombo C, Battezzati PM, Podda M, Bettinardi N, Giunta A. Ursodeoxycholic acid for liver disease associated with cystic fibrosis: a double-blind multicenter trial. The Italian Group for the Study of Ursodeoxycholic Acid in Cystic Fibrosis. Hepatology. 1996;23(6):1484–90.
138. Siano M, De Gregorio F, Boggia B, Sepe A, Ferri P, Buonpensiero P, et al. Ursodeoxycholic acid treatment in patients with cystic fibrosis at risk for liver disease. Dig Liver Dis. 2010;42(6):428–31.
139. Nousia-Arvanitakis S, Fotoulaki M, Economou H, Xefteri M, Galli-Tsinopoulou A. Long-term prospective study of the effect of ursodeoxycholic acid on cystic fibrosis-related liver disease. J Clin Gastroenterol. 2001;32(4):324–8.
140. Mendizabal M, Reddy KR, Cassuto J, Olthoff KM, Faust TW, Makar GA, et al. Liver transplantation in patients with cystic fibrosis: analysis of United Network for Organ Sharing data. Liver Transpl. 2011;17(3):243–50.
141. Gooding I, Dondos V, Gyi KM, Hodson M, Westaby D. Variceal hemorrhage and cystic fibrosis: outcomes and implications for liver transplantation. Liver Transpl. 2005;11(12):1522–6.
142. Ferrara JL, Levine JE, Reddy P, Holler E. Graft-versus-host disease. Lancet. 2009;373(9674):1550–61.
143. Blazar BR, Murphy WJ, Abedi M. Advances in graft-versus-host disease biology and therapy. Nat Rev Immunol. 2012;12(6):443–58.
144. Murai M, Yoneyama H, Harada A, Yi Z, Vestergaard C, Guo B, et al. Active participation of CCR5(+)CD8(+) T lymphocytes in the pathogenesis of liver injury in graft-versus-host disease. J Clin Invest. 1999;104(1):49–57.
145. Dignan FL, Clark A, Amrolia P, Cornish J, Jackson G, Mahendra P, et al. Diagnosis and management of acute graft-versus-host disease. Br J Haematol. 2012;158(1):30–45.
146. Strasser SI, Shulman HM, Flowers ME, Reddy R, Margolis DA, Prumbaum M, et al. Chronic graft-versus-host disease of the liver: presentation as an acute hepatitis. Hepatology. 2000;32(6):1265–71.
147. Maeng H, Lee JH, Cheong JW, Lee ST, Hahn JS, Ko YW, et al. Chronic graft-versus-host disease of the liver presenting as an acute hepatitis following nonmyeloablative hematopoietic stem cell transplantation. Int J Hematol. 2004;79(5):501–4.
148. Snover DC, Weisdorf SA, Ramsay NK, McGlave P, Kersey JH. Hepatic graft versus host disease: a study of the predictive value of liver biopsy in diagnosis. Hepatology. 1984;4(1):123–30.
149. Shulman HM, Sharma P, Amos D, Fenster LF, McDonald GB. A coded histologic study of hepatic graft-versus-host disease after human bone marrow transplantation. Hepatology. 1988;8(3):463–70.
150. Fried RH, Murakami CS, Fisher LD, Willson RA, Sullivan KM, McDonald GB. Ursodeoxycholic acid treatment of refractory chronic graft-versus-host disease of the liver. Ann Intern Med. 1992;116(8):624–9.
151. Arat M, Idilman R, Soydan EA, Soykan I, Erden E, Karayalcin S, et al. Ursodeoxycholic acid treatment in isolated chronic graft-vs-host disease of the liver. Clin Transplant. 2005;19(6):798–803.
152. Bhattacharya R, Rao S, Kowdley KV. Liver involvement in patients with solid tumors of nonhepatic origin. Clin Liver Dis. 2002;6(4):1033–43. x.
153. Odemis B, Parlak E, Basar O, Yuksel O, Sahin B. Biliary tract obstruction secondary to malignant lymphoma: experience at a referral center. Dig Dis Sci. 2007;52(9):2323–32.
154. Fidias P, Carey RW, Grossbard ML. Non-Hodgkin's lymphoma presenting with biliary tract obstruction. A discussion of seven patients and a review of the literature. Cancer. 1995;75(7):1669–77.
155. Singh MM, Pockros PJ. Hematologic and oncologic diseases and the liver. Clin Liver Dis. 2011;15(1):69–87.

156. Sans M, Andreu V, Bordas JM, Llach J, Lopez-Guillermo A, Cervantes F, et al. Usefulness of laparoscopy with liver biopsy in the assessment of liver involvement at diagnosis of Hodgkin's and non-Hodgkin's lymphomas. Gastrointest Endosc. 1998;47(5):391–5.
157. Lefkowitch JH, Falkow S, Whitlock RT. Hepatic Hodgkin's disease simulating cholestatic hepatitis with liver failure. Arch Pathol Lab Med. 1985;109(5):424–6.
158. Rowbotham D, Wendon J, Williams R. Acute liver failure secondary to hepatic infiltration: a single centre experience of 18 cases. Gut. 1998;42(4):576–80.
159. Hubscher SG, Lumley MA, Elias E. Vanishing bile duct syndrome: a possible mechanism for intrahepatic cholestasis in Hodgkin's lymphoma. Hepatology. 1993;17(1):70–7.
160. Ballonoff A, Kavanagh B, Nash R, Drabkin H, Trotter J, Costa L, et al. Hodgkin lymphoma-related vanishing bile duct syndrome and idiopathic cholestasis: statistical analysis of all published cases and literature review. Acta Oncol. 2008;47(5):962–70.
161. de Medeiros BC, Lacerda MA, Telles JE, da Silva JA, de Medeiros CR. Cholestasis secondary to Hodgkin's disease: report of 2 cases of vanishing bile duct syndrome. Haematologica. 1998;83(11):1038–40.
162. Yalcin S, Kars A, Sokmensuer C, Atahan L. Extrahepatic Hodgkin's disease with intrahepatic cholestasis: report of two cases. Oncology. 1999;57(1):83–5.
163. Leeuwenburgh I, Lugtenburg EP, van Buuren HR, Zondervan PE, de Man RA. Severe jaundice, due to vanishing bile duct syndrome, as presenting symptom of Hodgkin's lymphoma, fully reversible after chemotherapy. Eur J Gastroenterol Hepatol. 2008;20(2):145–7.
164. Cello JP. Acquired immunodeficiency syndrome cholangiopathy: spectrum of disease. Am J Med. 1989;86(5):539–46.
165. Teixidor HS, Godwin TA, Ramirez EA. Cryptosporidiosis of the biliary tract in AIDS. Radiology. 1991;180(1):51–6.
166. Benhamou Y, Caumes E, Gerosa Y, Cadranel JF, Dohin E, Katlama C, et al. AIDS-related cholangiopathy. Critical analysis of a prospective series of 26 patients. Dig Dis Sci. 1993;38(6):1113–8.
167. Bouche H, Housset C, Dumont JL, Carnot F, Menu Y, Aveline B, et al. AIDS-related cholangitis: diagnostic features and course in 15 patients. J Hepatol. 1993;17(1):34–9.
168. Margulis SJ, Honig CL, Soave R, Govoni AF, Mouradian JA, Jacobson IM. Biliary tract obstruction in the acquired immunodeficiency syndrome. Ann Intern Med. 1986;105(2):207–10.
169. Tonolini M, Bianco R. HIV-related/AIDS cholangiopathy: pictorial review with emphasis on MRCP findings and differential diagnosis. Clin Imaging. 2013;37(2):219–26.
170. Lefkowitch JH. Pathology of AIDS-related liver disease. Dig Dis. 1994;12(6):321–30.
171. Ducreux M, Buffet C, Lamy P, Beaugerie L, Fritsch J, Choury A, et al. Diagnosis and prognosis of AIDS-related cholangitis. AIDS. 1995;9(8):875–80.
172. Devarbhavi H, Sebastian T, Seetharamu SM, Karanth D. HIV/AIDS cholangiopathy: clinical spectrum, cholangiographic features and outcome in 30 patients. J Gastroenterol Hepatol. 2010;25(10):1656–60.
173. Buck FS, Koss MN. Hepatic amyloidosis: morphologic differences between systemic AL and AA types. Hum Pathol. 1991;22(9):904–7.
174. Park MA, Mueller PS, Kyle RA, Larson DR, Plevak MF, Gertz MA. Primary (AL) hepatic amyloidosis: clinical features and natural history in 98 patients. Medicine (Baltimore). 2003;82(5):291–8.
175. Rockey DC. Striking cholestatic liver disease: a distinct manifestation of advanced primary amyloidosis. South Med J. 1999;92(2):236–41.
176. Gertz MA, Kyle RA. Hepatic amyloidosis: clinical appraisal in 77 patients. Hepatology. 1997;25(1):118–21.
177. Gertz MA, Kyle RA. Hepatic amyloidosis (primary [AL], immunoglobulin light chain): the natural history in 80 patients. Am J Med. 1988;85(1):73–80.
178. Harrison RF, Hawkins PN, Roche WR, MacMahon RF, Hubscher SG, Buckels JA. 'Fragile' liver and massive hepatic haemorrhage due to hereditary amyloidosis. Gut. 1996;38(1):151–2.

179. Bujanda L, Beguiristain A, Alberdi F, Cosme A, Ruiz de la Hermosa J, Gutierrez S, et al. Spontaneous rupture of the liver in amyloidosis. Am J Gastroenterol. 1997;92(8):1385–6.
180. Naito KS, Ichiyama T, Kawakami S, Kadoya M, Tabata T, Matsuda M, et al. AL amyloidosis with spontaneous hepatic rupture: successful treatment by transcatheter hepatic artery embolization. Amyloid. 2008;15(2):137–9.
181. Chopra S, Rubinow A, Koff RS, Cohen AS. Hepatic amyloidosis. A histopathologic analysis of primary (AL) and secondary (AA) forms. Am J Pathol. 1984;115(2):186–93.
182. Kyle RA, Greipp PR, O'Fallon WM. Primary systemic amyloidosis: multivariate analysis for prognostic factors in 168 cases. Blood. 1986;68(1):220–4.
183. Johnson CS, Omata M, Tong MJ, Simmons Jr JF, Weiner J, Tatter D. Liver involvement in sickle cell disease. Medicine (Baltimore). 1985;64(5):349–56.
184. Hatton CS, Bunch C, Weatherall DJ. Hepatic sequestration in sickle cell anaemia. Br Med J (Clin Res Ed). 1985;290(6470):744–5.
185. Shao SH, Orringer EP. Sickle cell intrahepatic cholestasis: approach to a difficult problem. Am J Gastroenterol. 1995;90(11):2048–50.
186. Schubert TT. Hepatobiliary system in sickle cell disease. Gastroenterology. 1986;90(6): 2013–21.
187. Banerjee S, Owen C, Chopra S. Sickle cell hepatopathy. Hepatology. 2001;33(5):1021–8.
188. O'Callaghan A, O'Brien SG, Ninkovic M, Butcher GP, Foster CS, Walters JR, et al. Chronic intrahepatic cholestasis in sickle cell disease requiring exchange transfusion. Gut. 1995;37(1):144–7.
189. Darbari DS, Kple-Faget P, Kwagyan J, Rana S, Gordeuk VR, Castro O. Circumstances of death in adult sickle cell disease patients. Am J Hematol. 2006;81(11):858–63.
190. Omata M, Johnson CS, Tong M, Tatter D. Pathological spectrum of liver diseases in sickle cell disease. Dig Dis Sci. 1986;31(3):247–56.
191. Mekeel KL, Langham Jr MR, Gonzalez-Peralta R, Fujita S, Hemming AW. Liver transplantation in children with sickle-cell disease. Liver Transpl. 2007;13(4):505–8.
192. Blinder MA, Geng B, Lisker-Melman M, Crippin JS, Korenblat K, Chapman W, et al. Successful orthotopic liver transplantation in an adult patient with sickle cell disease and review of the literature. Hematol Rep. 2013;5(1):1–4.
193. Cavicchi M, Beau P, Crenn P, Degott C, Messing B. Prevalence of liver disease and contributing factors in patients receiving home parenteral nutrition for permanent intestinal failure. Ann Intern Med. 2000;132(7):525–32.
194. Beau P, Labat-Labourdette J, Ingrand P, Beauchant M. Is ursodeoxycholic acid an effective therapy for total parenteral nutrition-related liver disease? J Hepatol. 1994;20(2):240–4.

Chapter 9
Complications of Cholestasis

Abrar Ahmed and Marlyn J. Mayo

Abbreviations

AlkPhos	Alkaline phosphatase
ATX	Autotaxin
BMD	Bone mineral density
CLD	Chronic liver disease
CRH	Corticotropin releasing hormone
DEXA	Dual-energy X-ray absorptiometry
IGF	Insulin growth factor
LCAT	Lecithin-cholesterol acyltransferase
LPA	Lysophosphatidic acid
LP-X	Lipoprotein X
LP-Y	Lipoprotein Y
MARS	Molecular adsorbent recirculating system
OLT	Orthotopic liver transplant
OPG	Osteoprotegerin
PBC	Primary biliary cirrhosis
PROMIS-HQ	Patient-reported outcome measure information system health-assessment questionnaire
PSC	Primary sclerosing cholangitis
PTH	Parathyroid hormone
PXR	Pregnane X receptor

A. Ahmed, M.D. • M.J. Mayo, M.D. (✉)
Division of Digestive & Liver Diseases, University of Texas Southwestern Medical Center,
5323 Harry Hines Boulevard, Room K.5.140C, Dallas, TX 75390-9151, USA
e-mail: marlyn.mayo@utsouthwestern.edu

E.J. Carey and K.D. Lindor (eds.), *Cholestatic Liver Disease*, Clinical Gastroenterology,
DOI 10.1007/978-1-4939-1013-7_9,

RANK	Receptor activator of nuclear factor kappa-B
RANKL	Receptor activator of nuclear factor kappa-B Ligand
RMP	Rifampin
SIBO	Small intestinal bowel overgrowth
UGT	Uridine diphosphate glucuronosyltransferase

Overview

It is important to recognize the complications of cholestasis in patients with chronic cholestatic liver disease. Understanding and treating these conditions can result in a significant impact on morbidity and quality of life in this group of patients. Most of what is known is based on small studies of patients with primary biliary cirrhosis (PBC) and primary sclerosing cholangitis (PSC), which is then extrapolated to patients with other cholestatic diseases. This chapter reviews the pathophysiology and management of

- Osteoporosis
- Pruritus
- Dyslipidemia
- Vitamin deficiencies
- Steatorrhea
- Fatigue

Pruritus

Pruritus is one of the most prominent clinical features of cholestatic liver disease. The term used for this form of itching is cholestatic pruritus because the underlying common denominator is impaired bile flow. It is more common in women as compared to men. Fluctuations are characteristic and may occur over long periods of time, as well as in a daily circadian rhythm, typically worse in the evening [1]. Cholestatic pruritus characteristically involves the palms and feet with no primary skin lesions, although secondary eczema, hyperpigmentation, prurigo nodules, and bacterial infections can complicate the scratch marks. Curiously, pruritus may wane as end-stage liver disease develops. Its prevalence varies depending on the underlying etiology of cholestasis, occurring in about 25–80 % of patients with PBC and PSC and in about 5–15 % of those with chronic hepatitis C. Patients with liver disease due to chronic hepatitis B and steatohepatitis do not usually manifest pruritus [1].

Etiology/Pathophysiology

The molecular mechanisms involved in the pathogenesis of cholestatic pruritus remain unclear, which in turn makes the treatment of these patients clinically challenging. Potential etiologic agents that have been studied include lysophosphatidic acid (LPA), bile salts, steroid hormones and their metabolites, endogenous opioids, histamine, and serotonin.

Some recent studies suggest the role of LPA as a mediator of cholestatic pruritus [2]. LPA is produced from lysophosphatidyl choline by the serum enzyme autotoxin (ATX). It is a potent neuronal activator and also mediates the initiation of neuropathic pain, hair growth and embryo implantation. Serum levels of LPA are increased in patients with cholestasic pruritus. ATX activity also correlates with the intensity of cholestatic pruritus [3]. Intradermal injection of LPA causes a dose dependent scratch response in mice, and serum autotoxin (ATX) levels are specific for pruritus of cholestasis, including PBC, PSC, intrahepatic cholestasis of pregnancy, but not pruritus related to uremia, Hodgkin's disease, or atopic dermatitis. Patients with severe, refractory pruritus treated by the Molecular Adsorbent Recirculating System (MARS) or nasobiliary drainage were found to have improvement in the itch intensity which correlated with the reduction of the ATX levels [3]. Rifampicin, which is used as a second-line agent for this condition, may work, at least in part, by the pregnane X receptor (PXR)-dependent transcriptional inhibition of ATX expression [4]. LPA and autotoxin are potential drug targets for patients with chronic pruritus associated with hepatobiliary diseases.

The observed phenomenon of inducing pruritus via instillation of bile salts led to the theory that the retention and subsequent deposition of bile salts induces pruritus, but the level of serum, urine, and skin bile salts does not correlate with the severity of pruritus [1]. In children with cholestatic liver diseases, however, external diversion of the bile stream does improve pruritus [5]. Composition of bile in the liver and/or gut may be important in the pathogenesis of cholestatic itch, but has been difficult to measure.

Unlike allergic pruritus, studies do not support the role of histamine in cholestatic pruritus. There is no difference in mast cell density, neural density, or the interaction between mast cells and neural cells in patients with cholestatic liver disease and normal patients [6]. This may explain the clinical observation that agents such as antihistamines and capsaicin are largely ineffective in cholestatic pruritus. Their sedating effect, however, may help patients to sleep at night through mild itching. Erythema and urticaria which are associated with histamine release are also not seen in patients with cholestatic pruritus.

Opioid peptides in the CNS have been proposed as important mediators in the perception of itch in cholestatic patients [7]. Centrally administered opioid agonists in animal studies induce generalized pruritus [8]. Patients with cholestatic liver disease have increased plasma concentrations of endogenous opioid peptides, methionine enkephalin and leucine enkephalin, and have downregulated mu opioid receptors [9–12]. Indeed, anti-opioid treatment strategies have proven beneficial [13, 14].

A multitude of endogenous pruritogens have now been identified, including acetylcholine, endothelins, kallilkreins, proteases, leukotrienes, prostaglandins, and more. Recently, gastrin releasing peptide and naturietic polypeptide b have also been shown to be important neurotransmitters specific to itch [15]. What role each of these might have in cholestatic pruritus remains unexplored.

Treatment/Therapy

First-line therapy in the treatment of cholestatic pruritus is the anion exchange resins, such as cholestyramine, because of their efficacy and safety (Table 9.1). They bind bile salts in the bowel lumen, interrupting the enterohepatic circulation and leading to increased synthesis of bile salts from cholesterol in hepatocytes. According to a placebo-controlled trial, 80–85 % of patients completely or partially respond to cholestyramine within 4–11 days, with relief being maintained for up to 32 months [16, 17]. The typical dose is 4–16 g/day in divided doses, with the drug theoretically being most effective when one half of the dose is given 30 min before and the other half is given 30 min after breakfast, to allow for maximal bile acid binding as the gallbladder empties. Treatment with this agent is limited by its interference with absorption of other drugs and gastrointestinal side effects, such as bad

Table 9.1 Therapeutic strategies for pruritus in cholestasis

Drug/therapy	Dosage
Efficacy proven in controlled trials	
Cholestyramine	4–16 g/day (PO)
Rifampicin	300–600 mg/day (PO) adult
	10 mg/kg/day (PO) child
Naltrexone	25–50 mg/day (PO)
Naloxone	0.2 μg/kg/min (IV)
Sertraline	75–100 mg/day (PO)
Contradictory efficacy observed in controlled trials	
Ondansetron	4–24 mg/day (PO)
	4–8 mg/day (IV)
Ursodeoxycholic acid	10–15 mg/kg/day (PO)
Efficacy shown in case series or case reports	
Propofol	10–15 mg (IV bolus)
Lidocaine	100 mg/day (IV)
Dronabinol	15 mg/day (PO)
Butorphanol	1–2 mg/day (intranasal)
Phenobarbitol	2–5 mg/kg/day (PO)
Phototherapy	
Plasmapheresis, extracorporeal albumin dialysis (e.g., MARS), plasma separation, anion absorption, nasobiliary drainage, biliary diversion	
Liver transplantation	

taste, bloating, and constipation. Other bile acid binding resins such as colestipol and colesevelam have not been studied to the extent that their use for this indication can be recommended at this time. A double blinded, randomized, placebo-controlled trial published in 2010 found that colesevelam was not effective in cholestatic pruritus, although this study tested colesevelam as a salvage therapy and enrolled patients with previous failure to respond to other bile acid binding resins [18] which may have biased the results towards failure. Clinical investigation of new inhibitors of the apical sodium-dependent bile salt transporter designed to interrupt the enterohepatic circulation of bile acids has begun at the time of writing this chapter.

The second-line therapy for pruritus is the antibiotic rifampin (RMP) [16, 19, 20]. It is a (PXR) agonist in addition to inducing the P450 system. Recent in vitro studies have shown that RMP inhibits ATX expression in human HepG2 hepatoma cells and hepatoma cells overexpressing the PXR, but not in the hepatoma cells in which PXR was knocked down [3]. Hence, the beneficial antipruritic action of RMP may be explained, at least partly, by the PXR dependent transcriptional inhibition of ATX expression. Other mechanisms through which RMP might exert its antipruritic actions include induction of the phase I (P450 system), phase II (1A1) biotransformation enzymes and phase III export pumps, such as canalicular conjugate export pump MRP2 [21]. This enables RMP to accelerate detoxification and excretion of numerous compounds, such as bilirubin, bile acids, steroids and drugs. These mechanisms could lead to enhanced metabolism and/or increased secretion of direct or indirect pruritogens [22, 23]. Phenobarbital, an equally potent inducer of the P450 system, does not decrease pruritus as much as rifampin, suggesting that the observed clinical effect of rifampin may not be entirely due to induction of the P450 system [24]. Rifampin has also been shown to be both safe and effective in children with cholestatic disease, with a greater effect in those with intrahepatic cholestasis compared to those with extrahepatic causes [25]. The typical dose is 300–600 mg/day in divided doses in adults, and 10 mg/kg/day in children. Meta-analysis of prospective, randomized, controlled trials has shown RMP to be an effective and safe short-term treatment of pruritus. About 13 % of patients develop hepatotoxicity which can occur as early 3 months after starting therapy [16]. Hence, serum aminotransferases should be monitored at regular intervals when taking RMP [26]. In addition, patients should be informed that RMP changes the color of urine and tears to an orange-red color, a benign adverse effect.

Based on experimental evidence that opioids are important mediators of itch [27], opioid antagonists have been studied in the treatment of cholestatic pruritus and may be recommended as third-line agents for the treatment of cholestatic pruritus. Several clinical trials have proven the beneficial effects of opioid receptor antagonists on pruritus in patients with cholestasis. They significantly reduced itch and/or scratching behavior. Nalmefene, an oral opioid antagonist, improves pruritus as well as plasma bile acid concentrations in patients with cholestatic liver disease. The starting dose is usually 4–10 mg/day, which is then gradually titrated up every 2 days to achieve symptomatic control; the maximum studied dose is 240 mg/day [28, 29]; however, it is not available in most countries. A double blinded, randomized controlled cross over trial of 29 cholestatic patients given naloxone

(0.4 mg intravenous bolus, followed by 0.2 μg/kg per minute), showed significant improvement in pruritus over 4 days [30]. Another double blinded, randomized control trial of naltrexone, (50 mg/day orally) in 16 cholestatic patients showed a significant improvement in pruritus within 4 weeks [31]. Parenterally administered naloxone should be reserved for emergency treatment. Naltrexone was proven to be more effective than placebo in reducing pruritus as well as in improving fatigue and depression [32]. Varying degrees of severity of a withdrawal-like reaction, characterized by anorexia, nausea, colicky abdominal pain, pallor, cool skin, and increased blood pressure have been reported in cholestatic patients treated with opioid antagonists. The reaction may begin within hours of administration, but the effect is temporary and usually subsides within 2–3 days, despite continued treatment. It may be as a result of an enhanced opioidogeric tone in cholestatic patients [14]. Therefore, opioid receptor antagonists should be started at very low doses. A breakthrough phenomenon, the sustained exacerbation of pruritus in the early weeks of treatment after an initial decrease, has been seen in 1 of 16 patients treated with naltrexone and 5 of 14 patients treated with nalmefene [13, 31]. This effect may be due to the reversal of the downregulated opiate receptors in the brain during therapy. Unmasking of chronic pain can also occur with prolonged treatment [33].

The serotonin antagonists and selective reuptake inhibitors (sertraline and paroxetine) have been studied in patients with chronic pruritus. Sertraline, a selective serotonin reuptake inhibitor, was associated with improvement in cholestatic pruritus in one retrospective study [34], and a pilot study of sertraline (75–100 mg/day) demonstrated a significant improvement in visual analog scores, scratching activity, duration and distribution of itch in those treated with sertraline as compared to placebo. Initial studies of ondansetron, a 5-HT-3 antagonist, showed a small, but significant positive effect on pruritus [35], but a subsequent double blinded, randomized control trial showed that there was no difference in effect [36]. The mechanism by which serotonin modulates the perception of itch is still not known. Further studies are needed to further evaluate the role and efficacy of serotonergic agents in the treatment of pruritus before they can be routinely recommended. The pharmacobiology of the apparently paradoxical effect of sertraline (increased serotonin) and ondansetron (decreased serotonin) on itch is unclear, but could be due to dichotomous effects of serotonin on the central nervous system versus the peripheral nervous system, downregulation of excitatory 5-HT3 receptors, or disparate effects on various norepinephrine, serotonin, or opioid receptor subtypes.

Other proposed therapies include grapefruit juice, dronabinol, plasmapheresis, and molecular adsorbent recirculating system (MARS). Small studies of PBC patients treated with 600 cc of daily grapefruit juice show some improvement in pruritic symptoms [37]. However, subsequent studies have been unable to produce similar results [38]. Patients with refractory pruritus treated with plasmapheresis had prompt relief of their symptoms, but the duration of this effect was variable from 1 day to 5 months [39]. Patients with liver failure and cholestasis treated with MARS show an associated improvement in hepatic function and disappearance of pruritus [40]. The duration of effect is highly variable lasting from a few days to several months, even disappearing completely in several case reports and series [41–43].

A small case series of patients treated with dronabinol showed a brief anti-pruritic effect, lasting approximately 4–6 h [44]. Ursodeoxycholic acid and prednisone are associated with little to no relief in pruritus [45] of chronic cholestatic liver diseases, even though UDCA is quite effective in cholestasis of pregnancy. A 2002 Cochrane database systematic review evaluated the beneficial and adverse effects of per oral UDCA in PBC. Pruritus as an outcome was also studied. It identified a total of 16 randomized trials evaluating UDCA against placebo or no intervention in 1,422 patients. The conclusion was that UDCA given in doses of 8-15 mg/kg/day for 3 months to 5 years had no significant effect on pruritus [45]. The pruritus of PBC is almost always cured by liver transplantation, which is a viable option for patients with severe intractable pruritus.

Bone Disease

Osteopenic bone disease with a predisposition to spontaneous fracturing is a common complication of chronic cholestatic liver disease. In North America, osteodystrophy in cholestasis is mainly a result of osteoporosis and less that of osteomalacia. Osteoporosis is defined as defective bone formation, whereas osteomalacia is defective bone mineralization resulting from vitamin D deficiency. Cirrhosis has been linked to increased risk of fracture by approximately twofold higher than non-cirrhotic liver disease including PBC [46–48].

Prevalence

Osteoporosis occurs in chronic liver disease of all etiologies, not just cholestatic liver disease [49]. The severity of osteoporosis varies according to the type, severity, and progression of the underlying liver disease. It has been shown that osteoporosis seems to be more striking in patients with cholestatic liver diseases than other patients with chronic liver disease with increased risk of fracture. The prevalence of osteoporosis in PBC patients as defined by the WHO is between 14.2 and 51.5 %. The difference between studies is probably due to differences in patient selection, liver disease severity or hypogonadism. In the largest controlled study of PBC to date [50], lumbar *Z*-score was reduced and correlated significantly with a calculated risk score based on age, bilirubin level, prothrombin time, serum albumin level, and edema. Women with PBC lose bone mass at a rate approximately twice that seen in age-matched controls, and this accelerated bone loss is the result of mostly decreased formation rather than increased resorption of bone. An important cofactor for the development of osteoporosis in patients with PBC is the menopausal status. Bone mineral density (BMD) is strongly affected by estrogen status, being normal in premenopausal women but deficient in premature menopause [51]. For many years this notion of menopausal patients with PBC being at higher risk of osteoporosis was considered as a controversial subject [46, 49, 52], but two studies confirmed a fourfold increased risk of osteoporosis and a twofold increased risk of fractures in this group of patients compared with the age-matched controls [51]. The reported cumulative frequency of fragility fractures in patients with PBC ranges from 10 to 26 %, with a cumulative frequency of vertebral fractures of 10 % to 20 %. The prevalence of osteoporosis in end-stage PBC patients is 41 % with fractures occurring in 21 % of these patients [28, 48, 53]. BMD in patients diagnosed with PBC before development of cirrhotic state is similar to healthy controls [54]. Similarly, the prevalence of osteoporosis in PSC is 32 % with fractures occurring in 16 % of these patients [28, 55]. The prevalence of osteoporosis is higher in both PBC and PSC patients with stage III and IV disease than stage I and II disease [28, 29, 56]. Children with chronic cholestasis also develop osteopenia proportional to disease severity and progression [57].

One half of patients with PBC who undergo liver transplantation have severe bone disease. Following liver transplantation, there is a rapid loss of bone during the first 3–6 months, which is believed to be related to the immunosuppressive medications and catabolic state in the peri-transplantation period [58]. As a result, one half of patients with PBC experience a pathologic fracture during the first months after liver transplantation. Sometime during the first 4 months, bone formation rates begin to increase; but they do not overtake the increased rate of bone resorption [56] until approximately 12–24 months post-transplantation, when a gradual increase in total bone mass is noted [58]. The incidence of post-transplant fractures is as high as 30-40 % in cholestatic patients [59]. Most of the fractures occur in the first year and fewer beyond 3 years after liver transplantation [60]. Patients at highest risk for post-transplant fracture are those with a low pre-transplant bone mineral density (BMD) and a history of pre-transplant vertebral fracture [61, 62]. Thus, it is imperative to identify and aggressively manage osteopenia and osteoporosis in pre-transplant patients with chronic cholestatic liver disease.

Pathophysiology

Mechanisms of osteoporosis in cholestatic liver disease remain poorly understood but are believed to be multifactorial (Table 9.2). Older age, higher Mayo risk score, lower body mass index, postmenopausal status, and advanced histological stage are all independent risk factors for osteoporosis in PBC patients [51]. Higher serum bilirubin levels, which may be suggestive of more advanced PBC, correlate significantly with a higher rate of bone loss [28]. In PBC, other factors that appear to either directly or indirectly alter bone mass include insulin growth factor-1 (IGF-1) deficiency/gene polymorphisms [63], hypogonadism, and excess alcohol intake. Other factors implicated are subnormal vitamin D levels, vitamin D receptor gene polymorphisms/genotype [59, 64], osteoprotegerin (OPG) deficiency, collagen type Ia1 gene polymorphisms [65], and immunosuppressive therapy before and after transplantation.

IGF-1 plays an important role in the process of bone remodeling and maintenance of bone mass. Reduced bone formation in patients with cirrhosis and advanced

Table 9.2 Factors that alter bone mass in patients with PBC

Older age
Higher Mayo risk score
Lower body mass index
Postmenopausal status
Advanced histological stage
Insulin growth factor-1 deficiency
Hyperbilirubinemia
Hypogonadism
Alcohol intake
Subnormal vitamin D levels
Vitamin D receptor gene polymorphisms/genotype
Osteoprotegerin (OPG) deficiency
Collagen type Ia1 gene polymorphisms
Immunosuppressive therapy

liver disease is thought to be related to low levels of IGF-1, but no direct relationship has been established between IGF-1 and osteoporosis. OPG secreted by osteoblasts is a member of the TNF receptor super family. It has been found to regulate bone turnover and inhibit osteoclast differentiation in vitro and in vivo, but its role in hepatic osteodystrophy, and particularly in PBC, is still not clear [54, 66].

Studies in PBC have suggested that the receptor activation of NF-kB (RANK) and the receptor activation of NF-kB ligand (RANKL) in addition to OPG are involved in osteoclastic bone resorption [66, 67]; but the exact role of RANK/RANKL in the pathogenesis of low bone turnover in chronic liver disease remains unclear, and there are conflicting findings on the levels of these proteins in the serum. Another study of PBC patients showed that vitamin D receptor genotype correlated with lumbar spine BMD with an allele dose effect. In this study, the risk of vertebral fractures increased from two to threefold with the presence of t-allele [64].

Despite the fact that genetic susceptibility for the development of osteoporosis in PBC has been suggested, including vitamin D receptor gene polymorphisms, collagen type Ia1 gene polymorphisms, and insulin-like growth factor-1 gene polymorphisms, contradictory results have been reported and no definitive genetic susceptibility to bone disease in PBC has been confirmed.

Unconjugated bilirubin inhibits osteoblast activity and function in vitro and in animal models [51], but there is no correlation between unconjugated, conjugated, and total bilirubin levels and bone mineral density (BMD) in patients undergoing liver transplantation. One study confirmed that elevated serum bilirubin alone is not a major contributory factor to hepatic osteodystrophy [68].

Hypogonadism is an established risk factor for osteoporosis in patients with PBC. In postmenopausal women, reduced trabecular bone volume correlates with decreased calcium absorption, which is directly related to longer duration of the disease. Male patients with hypogonadism have decreased levels of estrogen which adversely affects their skeletal health [69, 70].

Metabolism of vitamin D is normal in patients with cholestatic liver disease but calcium and vitamin D malabsorption can occur and lead to bone disease. Diamond et al. [71] compared the largest cohort of 107 patients with chronic liver disease

(CLD) including primary cholestatic disorders with 40 age-matched controls, showing normal levels of vitamin D metabolites in the noncirrhotic patients. Cirrhotic patients showed a significant decrease in 25-OH vitamin D and 1, 25-OH2 without histological features of osetomalacia. Hence, these findings point towards a cause of osteoblast dysfunction in CLD that cannot be explained by abnormalities in vitamin D metabolites.

Corticosteroid use in patients with overlap syndrome and in the post-transplant setting has been shown to cause accelerated trabecular bone loss during the first 12 months with doses >7.5 mg/day [49, 72, 73]. Corticosteroids increase osteoclast differentiation and activity by production of interleukins, especially IL-1 and IL-6, and decrease osteoblast differentiation by suppressing differentiation, recruitment, and indirectly reducing the collagen synthesis. As a result, the lowest effective dose of corticosteroid should be used to minimize the deleterious effect on bone metabolism.

Metabolic bone disease, particularly osteoporosis, is becoming a major cause of morbidity in PBC patients post-transplant [49, 74]. Besides corticosteroids, other factors that also contribute include immunosuppressive therapy such a cyclosporine A and tacrolimus (FK506), immobility, and poor nutrition. All these factors contribute to accelerated bone loss after the OLT. Early accelerated bone turnover seen after OLT is not only because of the corticosteroids but has also been attributed to immunosuppressive agents such as calcineurin inhibitors, although their role in bone turnover after OLT is still controversial.

Diagnosis and Monitoring

The AASLD Guidelines [53] suggest that BMD testing should be considered in all patients with PBC at diagnosis and repeated every 2–3 years. There is a clear consensus that BMD should be assessed in all patients with cirrhosis, those receiving long-term corticosteroids (>3 months) or those who have experienced a fragility fracture and before liver transplantation. The severity and progression of bone disease can be assessed by measurement of BMD in different sites. Dual-energy X-ray absorptiometry (DEXA) and dual-photon absorptiometry are noninvasive techniques that quantify bone mass accurately. Common sites used are the lumbar spine (L2–L3) and the superior segment of the femur. This test is quick, precise, reproducible, and minimally invasive. At the time of referral for/diagnosis of PBC, approximately 20 % of patients have osteoporosis, as defined by a *T*-score below –2.5 in either the lumbar spine or the femoral neck, and approximately 10 % have severe bone disease, as defined by a Z-score below –2 [28, 64]. (The *T-score* is the number of standard deviations below the mean peak value in young gender-matched normal subjects, whereas the *Z-score* is the number of standard deviations below mean normal values corrected for age and gender). The risk of osteoporosis (*T*-score below –2.5) is eight times higher in patients with PBC than in a gender-matched population, whereas the risk of severe bone disease (*Z*-score below –2) is four times higher in patients with PBC. In addition to DEXA assessment, serum levels of calcium, phosphate, 25-OH vitamin D, and parathyroid hormone (PTH) need to be assessed when monitoring osteoporosis. These are obtained at the beginning of the assessment and at subsequent intervals (6 months to 3 years) according to the severity of cholestasis [52, 53, 75, 76].

Therapy

Therapy of osteoporosis in patients with chronic cholestasis is based on trial results in patients with postmenopausal osteoporosis. A few small studies were conducted in PBC patients with the primary outcome of improving BMD rather than the more clinically important endpoint of fracture rates [63].

Nonpharmacological measures should be taken into account in addition to pharmacological therapies for the management of osteoporosis in patients with cholestatic liver disease. Reversible factors that accelerate bone loss should be eliminated such as alcohol intake, tobacco, caffeine ingestion, and corticosteroids. Patients should be encouraged to do regular weight bearing exercise and to incorporate lifestyle changes that maintain both muscle and bone mass.

In patients with PBC, 2 studies [77, 78] showed calcium supplementation improved bone mass in patients who were vitamin D deficient. High-dose supplemental vitamin D, or 25-hydroxy vitamin D, increased bone mass [79, 80] and reversed some of the osteomalacic changes of bone mass in patients with hepatic osteodystrophy. Further studies of calcium and vitamin D supplements are warranted in patients with cholestatic diseases.

The National Institute of Health guidelines suggest prophylaxis with calcium supplementation of 1,000 mg/day for all adults and 1,500 mg/day for those at risk for osteoporosis, and vitamin D supplementation of 800 IU/day for all adults and 50,000 IU given 2 to 3 times per week for those found to be deficient or at risk for osteoporosis [81]. Treatment can be initiated if T score ≤ -2.5, Z score ≤ -1.5, or as clinically indicated.

Therapies can be divided into anti-resorptive and hormone replacement. Bisphosphonates, which are used for treating postmenopausal osteoporosis, are the main therapy for treating cholestatic patients with osteoporosis and are usually given with calcium and vitamin D. This class of drugs was studied in a small number of patients with CLD and especially patients with PBC [80]. Although etidronate was no better than placebo in one randomized controlled study [82], alendronate (70 mg/week) was found to improve bone mass significantly after 2 years of treatment in 13 patients with PBC when compared with etidronate [83] and in 15 patients with PBC when compared with 13 patients treated with placebo [84]. Alendronate was not able to show an effect on fracture rate [84]. After OLT, PBC patients are usually treated with bisphosphonates, which have been studied in seven studies in an attempt to reduce the high fracture rate observed in these patients. Intravenous pamidronate has shown no effect on fracture risk in five studies. With respect to the BMD, 3 studies showed an increase in the bone mass but it was mainly limited to trabecular bone (lumbar spine) [85, 86]. Zoledronic acid given within 7 days of transplantation and then 1, 3, 6, and 9 months reduced bone loss in the first 3 months. Lack of effect on the fracture rate is probably related to small size of the studies [86].

Hormone replacement therapy is considered the second-line therapy after bisphosphonates for the treatment of osteoporosis in women with cholestatic liver disease. This is in part because of the risk of thromboembolic disease and malignancy, as well as heart disease in late postmenopausal women. Treatment with estrogens significantly prevents loss of bone mass in postmenopausal patients with PBC [62] and was not associated with worsening cholestasis in a series of 46 patients with PBC who received estrogen treatment for a mean period of almost 5 years [87]. Estrogens were studied in two small-randomized controlled trials of patients with PBC. They were shown to improve BMD after 2 years but no effect on the fracture rate was seen in the first trial [88]. In another study of 18 patients with PBC, only one patient had to stop the transdermal estrogen because of rising aminotransferases [89]. Because of the carcinogenic properties of estrogens, their lack of protective cardiovascular effects, a possible increased risk of dementia, and resumption of menses, however, many postmenopausal women are not enthusiastic about taking estrogens.

Raloxifene, a selective estrogen receptor modulator, has shown some promise as an alternative to estrogen replacement therapy for postmenopausal osteoporosis. In the MORE trial in non-cholestatic, postmenopausal women with osteoporosis, raloxifene (a selective estrogen receptor modulator) in combination with calcium and cholecalciferol, increased BMD in the spine and femoral neck and reduced the risk of vertebral fracture [90]. Raloxifene was evaluated in a pilot study of nine postmenopausal women with PBC who showed a significant increase in bone mass after 1 year of treatment; this improvement in bone mass was not seen in an age and menopausal status-matched control group [91]. Raloxifene and other selective estrogen receptor modulating agents may eventually have a role in cholestatic patients with osteoporosis, but further studies targeting these patients are needed.

Testosterone is used in hypogonadal male patients to stabilize hormone levels. Transdermal testosterone is preferred to prevent any liver side effects from surges in testosterone levels seen with oral or depot preparations.

Other treatments that have been used are sodium fluoride, strontium ranelate, vitamin K derivatives, and recombinant parathyroid hormone.

Sodium fluoride stimulates bone formation, and it prevented bone loss in a 2-year, prospective, double-blind trial of PBC patients [92]. Though very effective at preventing bone loss and reducing the risk of fractures, side effects of severe dyspepsia limit its use. One randomized trial compared cyclical etidronate to fluoride and showed etidronate to be better tolerated and more effective than fluoride at preventing bone loss in PBC [93]. However, a subsequent randomized controlled trial of etidronate in PBC subjects with established osteopenia (T-score <-2.0) found that etidronate was no more effective than placebo [82].

Strontium ranelate has been approved in Europe since 2004 for the treatment of osteoporosis to reduce the risk for vertebral and hip fractures in postmenopausal women [94]. In 2012 the indication was expanded to include men at increased risk for fracture. Recently the European Medicines Agency has restricted the use of this drug because of concerns about its risk for cardiac adverse events. It is not currently approved in the USA, and there have been no studies on its effect in cholestatic patients with osteoporosis.

Vitamin K derivatives, phytonadione and menaquinone may be effective for the prevention and treatment of osteoporosis due to cholestasis [95]. A randomized, control trial showed a higher BMD in patients receiving vitamin K when compared to placebo [96]. Given the low incidence of side effects and demonstrated efficacy, vitamin K should be considered as part of osteoporosis treatment in cholestatic liver disease.

There are several medications available for the treatment of postmenopausal osteoporosis which have not shown efficacy in trials of cholestatic patients. For example, parenterally administered calcitonin did not stop the progression of bone disease in a cohort of PBC subjects [77]. Another study evaluating subcutaneous calcitonin therapy given during the first 6 months after liver transplantation showed that calcitonin did not prevent or reduce accelerated bone loss or spontaneous fractures [97]. Though there are trials showing benefit from PTH in patients with postmenopausal osteoporosis [98], there are no trials with PTH in patients with cholestatic liver disease. Recombinant parathyroid hormone is reserved for patients intolerant of bisphosphonates to prevent fragility fractures.

Dyslipidemia

Cholestatic disorders manifest a distinct pattern of dyslipoproteinemia due to the retention of cholesterol, phospholipids, and bile salts that are normally secreted in bile [99].

Prevalence

Lipid abnormalities are found in 85 % of patients with PBC. At the time of the first visit, approximately 75 % of PBC patients have a total cholesterol above 200 mg/dl. A cross-sectional study in patients with PBC showed that patients with early and intermediate histologic stages have mild elevations of very low density lipoproteins and low density lipoproteins, and marked increases in high density lipoproteins. Within the LDL fraction of the serum of cholestatic patients, three distinct lipoproteins can be identified: β2-lipoprotein (triglyceride rich), also known as lipoprotein Y (LP-Y); lipoprotein X (LP-X), and normal LDL. LP-Y appears to be a remnant of a triglyceride-rich lipoprotein that is distinct from IDL. LP-X is a complex composed of equimolar amounts of excess phospholipid and unesterified cholesterol. The main protein component is albumin within the core and apolipoprotein C upon the surface. In contrast, patients with advanced disease have marked elevations in LDLs with the presence of lipoprotein-X, and a significant decrease in HDL [100]. Cholestatic patients with elevated triglyceride levels often have clear (not lipemic) serum because most of the triglycerides are contained in LP-Y and LDL.

Pathophysiology

Lp-X is about 50 nm in diameter and its major component bile acid is lithocholic acid. Early studies reported the presence of Lp-X in the serum of patients with cholestasis [101, 102]. Cholestatic patients have elevated levels of lipoprotein X, which may be protective against atherogenesis [103]. However, lipoprotein X may also contribute to hypercholesterolemia in cholestatic patients by not effectively downregulating hepatic hydroxymethylglutaryl coenzyme A reductase [104]. The presence of serum Lp-X does not facilitate the distinction between intrahepatic and extrahepatic cholestasis. Bile lipoprotein is a precursor of Lp-X and in cholestasis this refluxes into the plasma pool and binds to albumin to form Lp-X. Serum Lp-X usually disappears soon after the cholestasis is relieved. Lp-X is not significantly taken up by macrophages but is taken up by hepatocytes. Sometimes severe and prolonged cholestasis can lead to very high serum Lp-X concentrations, resulting in severe hypercholesterolemia and tendon xanthomata [105]. LP-X is also found in patients with lecithin-cholesterol acyltransferase (LCAT) deficiency, an enzyme responsible for cholesterol esterification in plasma. In addition to cholestasis and LCAT deficiency, Lp-X may also be found in the plasma after intravenous infusion of intralipid emulsion such as occurs with total parenteral nutrition. Pseudohyponatremia has also been described in some patients with severe hypercholesterolemia secondary to raised Lp-X. Thus the presence of Lp-X should be considered in pseudohyponatremia associated with cholestasis [106]. Lp-X possesses strong aggregatory properties and can bind to alkaline phosphatase (AlkPhos) producing an Lp-X-AlkPhos complex. This complex may be found in cholestasis; typically that evoked by hepatic malignancy.

Clinical Significance

Usually in patients without cholestasis, the risk of atheroma formation is raised if the level of HDL cholesterol is low and the LDL cholesterol is high. Xanthoma formation can occur in patients with PBC as a result of prolonged increase in total serum cholesterol and lipid levels. The implications of this finding with respect to coronary artery disease, cerebrovascular disease, and overall morbidity and mortality are poorly understood. Despite marked hypercholesterolemia, excess mortality from cardiovascular disease has not been associated with PBC [107]. Studies investigating the risk of dyslipidemia in PBC [108] have shown that hypercholesterolemia in chronic cholestasis is not associated with increased clinical or subclinical

Table 9.3 Treatment options for osteoporosis

Calcium	1,500 mg/day
Alendronate	70 mg/week
Hormone replacement therapy	Various[a]
Fluoride	50 mg/day
Vitamin K [phytonadione]	1 mg/day

[a]Transdermal estradiol 50 μg/day two times per week + medroxyprogesterone 2.5 mg/day; other regimens have been studied and are presumed to be equally efficacious

atherosclerosis. A prospective observational study of 312 PBC patients followed for 7.4 years showed no statistical difference in the incidence of atherosclerotic death when compared to age and sex matched controls [109]. The reason for the observed lack of cardiovascular events in patients with cholestatic dyslipidemia may be related to this difference in composition of the low density lipoproteins. The three factors with protective effects regarding the risk of atheroma formation in hyperlipidemia are: LP-X, HDL cholesterol, and adiponectin, all of which are raised in patients with chronic cholestasis.

Therapy

As is evident from the above discussion, only patients with chronic cholestasis having other risk factors for atheroma formation are likely to benefit from therapy [100, 108, 110]. Treatment includes lifestyle changes and medical therapy (Table 9.3). A small study of 6 PBC patients treated with simvastatin, a 3-hydroxy-3-methylglutaryl coenzyme A reductase inhibitor, showed a significant reduction in total cholesterol, LDL cholesterol, alkaline phosphatase, gamma-glutamyltransferase, and immunoglobulin M [111]. Pravastatin, another HMG-coA reductase inhibitor, at 20 mg/day showed marked decrease in cholesterol and total bile acid levels, with pronounced decreases in cholic acid and chenodeoxycholic acid [112]. The use of reductase inhibitors is increasing in patients with cholestatic liver disease without subsequent reports of hepatotoxicity. However, further studies regarding clinical benefit and risk are needed before HMG-coA reductase inhibitors can be routinely recommended in cholestatic patients. Therapy with UDCA has been shown to lower the LDL levels in patients with PBC and has been useful in some patients with xanthelasmas. Fibrates have not been shown to be efficacious in dyslipidemias seen in chronic cholestasis [107]. Ezetimibe, which inhibits the intestinal absorption of cholesterol (Neiman Pick C1 like protein), was investigated in patients with PBC [104]. Alone or in combination with a statin, ezetemibe reduces LDL cholesterol in cholestasis [103, 104, 109]. Statin therapy is relatively ineffective in lowering Lp-X [113]. Complete regression of xanthomata has been described by treatment with apheresis, which has been suggested by some as the first-choice treatment for patients with massive Lp-X accumulation due to cholestasis [113, 114].

Another promising therapeutic target for cholestatic dyslipidemia is the nuclear receptor inhibitors which regulate cholesterol metabolism, synthesis of bile acids, and hepatic detoxification [111, 112]. As a result of cholestatic injury, a variety of adaptive hepatoprotective mechanisms come into play, including alterations in bile acid transport, synthesis and detoxification. These processes are mediated mainly at a transcriptional level via a complex network involving nuclear receptors including the farnesoid X receptor, pregnane X receptor, vitamin D receptor, and constitutive androstane receptor [111]. Since the intrinsic adaptive response to bile acids cannot fully prevent liver injury in cholestasis, therapeutic targeting of these receptors may further enhance the hepatic defense against the toxic agents found in the serum of patients with cholestatic liver disease.

Vitamin Deficiencies

Prevalence

Patients with cholestatic liver disease rarely present with symptoms of vitamin deficiencies. However, in a trial evaluating the efficacy of ursodeoxycholic acid in 180 patients with PBC at the Mayo Clinic, the proportion of patients with vitamin A, D, E, and K deficiency was 33.5, 13.2, 1.9, and 7.8 %, respectively [115]. Significant underlying disease, represented by advanced histologic stages, elevated Mayo risk score, and low cholesterol levels in a multivariate analysis, is associated with vitamin A deficiency. Similarly, low vitamin D levels are associated with a low serum albumin [115]. Data regarding the prevalence of vitamin E deficiency are conflicting. One study comprised of 42 patients with PBC found 43.5 % to have vitamin E deficiency, all of whom exhibited clinically evident neurologic abnormalities manifested by poor scores on neuropsychological testing measuring psychomotor capacity [116]. Another study evaluating the vitamin E status of patients with chronic liver disease showed 44 % of PBC patients and 32 % of patients with other cholestatic conditions to be deficient in vitamin E. Five of the 12 patients with both PBC and vitamin E deficiency demonstrated a mixed sensorimotor peripheral neuropathy, not characteristic of vitamin E deficiency [117]. In this study, those with very low levels of vitamin E were not readily corrected with oral, or even parenteral, repletion, although those with less severe deficiencies could be repleted.

Pathophysiology

Patients with cholestatic liver disease are at risk for fat-soluble vitamin deficiencies due to the decreased availability of bile salts required for their absorption. Vitamin deficiencies usually occur well before overt symptoms of fat malabsorption. Poor absorption may be exacerbated by bile acid binding resins given for pruritus.

Therapy

Patients with early stage disease should be advised to consume a diet or multivitamin containing at least the RDA for the fat-soluble vitamins (Table 9.4). Patients with advanced cholestatic liver disease at risk for fat-soluble vitamin deficiencies and should be tested annually to identify deficiencies and treated with replacement doses followed by maintenance therapy (Table 9.4).

Vitamin D deficiency should be excluded by measurement of 25-hydroxyvitamin D, a major metabolite of vitamin D. When vitamin D deficiency is encountered, vitamin D in a dose of 25,000–50,000 IU, given once or twice per week, usually is sufficient to achieve a normal serum vitamin D level. Because 25-hydroxylation of vitamin D is normal in patients with PBC, vitamin D (rather than the more expensive 25-hydroxyvitamin D or 1,25-hydroxyvitamin D) can be prescribed.

Symptomatic deficiency of vitamin A is unusual in patients with cholestasis. Assessment of vitamin A deficiency in patients with cholestasis requires measurement of serum retinol levels. Asymptomatic deficit is corrected by giving a dose of 25,000–50,000 IU two to three times per week or 10,000–20,000 IU orally daily for 2 months Symptomatic patients should receive 100,000 U of retinyl palmitate IM every 2 weeks for 6 months, followed by oral vitamin A supplementation of 45–50,000 U twice weekly. Vitamin E aids the intestinal absorption of other fat-soluble vitamins and is recommended as an adjunct in vitamin A deficiency. The adequacy of replacement therapy is assessed by repeating serum vitamin A assays and evaluating the patient for darkness adaptation, if indicated. Of note, serum for vitamin A levels must be drawn into a light-proof vial.

Vitamin K deficiency occurs with severe cholestasis and can be clinically important. It is manifested by a prolonged prothrombin time, so measuring serum vitamin K level or clotting factors II, VII, IX, and X is rarely necessary. A trial of oral vitamin K, 5–10 mg daily, should be given to determine if the prothrombin time improves. If it does, the patient should be maintained on a water-soluble vitamin K, 5 mg per day. Those with active hemorrhage should be treated with IV, IM, or SC vitamin K: 10 mg/day for 2–3 days.

Table 9.4 Fat-soluble vitamins: recommended daily allowance (RDA) and oral treatment options for deficiency

Vitamin	RDA	Replacement	Maintenance	Conversion
Vitamin A	3,000 IU (male) 2,300 IU (female)	15,000 IU/day	10,000 IU/day	10,000 IU = 3,000 mcg retinol or 6,000 mcg beta carotene
Vitamin D	600 IU (age 51–70) 800 IU age 71+)	50,000–100,000 IU/week	800 IU/day	1,000 IU = 25 mcg
Vitamin E	33 IU (synthetic) 22 IU (natural)	10 IU/kg/day	33 IU/day	10 IU = 9 mg DL alpha tocopherol or 6.7 mg D-ALPHA-TOCOPHEROL
Vitamin K	120 mcg (male) 90 mcg (female)	50 mg/day	5 mg/day	N/A

Deficiency of vitamin E has also been reported in patients with cholestatic liver disease. Serum concentration of vitamin E is used to measure the levels. Hyperlipidemia may result in falsely elevated levels as vitamin E is bound to lipoproteins. Hence, the vitamin–total lipid level ratio is a better reflection of the vitamin E level. A ratio of <0.8 mcg/g is considered deficient. Typically, vitamin E deficiency causes a neurologic abnormality that affects the posterior columns and is characterized by areflexia, loss of proprioception, and ataxia. Motor neurological system degenerative changes occur only after 5–10 years of deficiency. In patients with chronic cholestasis and low serum levels of vitamin E, oral replacement therapy with high-dose vitamin E may halt progression of neuropathy. Therapy continues for the duration of the cholestasis, aiming to maintain a vitamin E–total lipid ratio of >0.8. Overall, clinical manifestations of fat-soluble vitamin deficiencies occur only in advanced cholestatic disease. The degree of vitamin deficit is proportional to the severity and evolution of the disease.

Steatorrhea

Steatorrhea can occur in patients with advanced cholestasis, but is uncommon. One potential cause is decreased bile acid delivery with insufficient micellar concentration of bile acids in the small intestine, although pancreatic exocrine insufficiency, celiac disease, and small intestinal bacterial overgrowth (SIBO) due to scleroderma should be excluded. Patients with decreased intestinal bile acid concentrations usually benefit from substitution of medium-chain triglycerides (which do not require bile salts for absorption) for long-chain triglycerides in their diets and decrease in total fat intake (40–50 g/day). Those with concomitant exocrine pancreatic insufficiency should be treated with pancreatic replacement therapy. Patients with celiac disease require gluten withdrawal from the diet and those with SIBO should receive intermittent broad spectrum oral antibiotic therapy.

Fatigue

Fatigue, like pruritus, is a common symptom in chronic cholestasis. It has been mainly studied in PBC [118]. Fatigue in chronic cholestasis is not related to the severity of chronic liver disease and is not usually improved by liver transplantation [119, 120]. A prospective study performed by Carbone et al. [120] to evaluate the role of liver transplantation for the relief of fatigue in patients with PBC showed that a substantial proportion of patients continue to suffer from significant fatigue after 2 years. Before one can attribute fatigue to chronic cholestasis, other medical problems like anemia, hypothyroidism, electrolyte abnormalities, diabetes, and depression, need to be excluded.

Fatigue may be related to changes in the central serotonergic neurotransmitters [75]. Other mechanisms that have been proposed include: aberrant release of corticotrophin releasing factors (CRH) and accumulation of magnesium in the globus pallidus [118]. In PBC, fatigue is associated with changes in the autonomic nervous system (postural hypotension) and sleep disturbances, especially during the day [121]. Functional status was assessed in a representative cohort of 75 patients with PBC using the Patient-Reported Outcome Measure Information System Health-Assessment Questionnaire (PROMIS-HAQ) [121]. The study showed that PBC was associated with substantial functional impairment and PBC symptom distribution evolved over time, with cognitive symptoms making an ever-greater contribution to overall symptom burden. The major potentially modifiable determinant responsible for the functional impairment appeared to be orthostatic symptoms.

Therapy

Currently there is no specific therapy for fatigue associated with chronic cholestasis. In PBC, studies have shown a reduction in daytime somnolence and objective tiredness (quantified through various scales and questionnaires) by using modafenil 100–200 mg/day [122, 123], although long term use carries a risk of dependence. Avoiding coffee consumption in the late afternoon which can lead to sleep disturbances [75, 124] and careful monitoring of antihypertensive medications which can exacerbate dysfunction of the autonomic nervous system are helpful. Exercise has also been show to play a role in fatigue associated with PBC [125]. A randomized, double-blind controlled trial studied fluoxetine for the treatment of fatigue in PBC patients, but showed no benefit [126]. Lastly, psychological support plays an important role as well.

Summary

Though cholestasis is a common clinical problem, it is important to understand that recommendations regarding the management of complications of cholestasis are based on trials consisting of small numbers of patients, predominantly with PBC, and are thus based largely on clinical experience. Osteoporosis is very common in patients with cholestatic liver disease when compared to the general population. Treatment goals are to prevent further bone loss, thereby reducing the risk of fracture. Bisphosphonates, hormone replacement therapy, and vitamin K all increase BMD and prevent further bone loss in cholestatic patients. Management of pruritus resulting from cholestasis remains challenging because of incomplete understanding of the mechanisms involved and the limited array of effective therapies. Recent experimental evidence suggests that the elevated serum levels of lysophosphatidic acid (LPA) and the enzyme autotaxin, which cleaves choline from lysophosphatidylcholine to form LPA, are specific for the pruritus of cholestasis and correlate with the severity of pruritus. LPA and autotaxin are potential drug targets for patients with chronic pruritus associated with hepatobiliary diseases. Previous treatments aimed at reducing bile acid concentration have not been found to be effective. This was shown by the double-blind, randomized, placebo-controlled trial where colesevelam was no better than placebo in alleviating the severity of cholestatic pruritus, even though colesevelam lowers serum bile acid levels. Though patients with cholestatic liver disease exhibit dyslipidemia and these levels can be reduced with the use of HMG-coA reductase inhibitors, the long-term impact of therapy on vascular events remains controversial. Another promising therapeutic target for cholestatic dyslipidemia is the nuclear receptor inhibitors which regulate cholesterol metabolism, synthesis of bile acids and hepatic detoxification. Finally, patients with advanced cholestatic liver disease are at risk for vitamin deficiencies, particularly vitamins A and D, and thus should be screened and treated when found to be deficient. Vitamin E aids the intestinal absorption of other fat-soluble vitamins and is recommended as an adjunct in vitamin A deficiency.

References

1. Franco J. Pruritus. Curr Treat Options Gastroenterol. 1999;2(6):451–6. PubMed PMID: 11097728.
2. Kremer AE, Martens JJ, Kulik W, Rueff F, Kuiper EM, Buuren HR, et al. Lysophosphatidic acid is a potential mediator of cholestatic pruritus. Gastroenterology. 2010;139(3):1008–18. 18 e1. PubMed PMID: 20546739.
3. Kremer AE, van Dijk R, Leckie P, Schaap FG, Kuiper EM, Mettang T, et al. Serum autotaxin is increased in pruritus of cholestasis, but not of other origin, and responds to therapeutic interventions. Hepatology. 2012;56(4):1391–400. PubMed PMID: 22473838.
4. Kremer AE, Beuers U, Oude-Elferink RP, Pusl T. Pathogenesis and treatment of pruritus in cholestasis. Drugs. 2008;68(15):2163–82. PubMed PMID: 18840005.
5. Yang H, Porte RJ, Verkade HJ, De Langen ZJ, Hulscher JB. Partial external biliary diversion in children with progressive familial intrahepatic cholestasis and Alagille disease. J Pediatr Gastroenterol Nutr. 2009;49(2):216–21. PubMed PMID: 19561545. Epub 2009/06/30. eng.
6. O'Keeffe C, Baird AW, Nolan N, McCormick PA. Cholestatic pruritus—the role of cutaneous mast cells and nerves. Aliment Pharmacol Ther. 2004;19(12):1293–300. PubMed PMID: 15191511.
7. Jones EA, Zylicz Z. Treatment of pruritus caused by cholestasis with opioid antagonists. J Palliat Med. 2005;8(6):1290–4. PubMed PMID: 16351546.
8. Koenigstein H. Experimental study of itch stimuli in animals. Arch Derm Syphilol. 1948;57(5):828–49. PubMed PMID: 18888064.
9. Swain MG, Rothman RB, Xu H, Vergalla J, Bergasa NV, Jones EA. Endogenous opioids accumulate in plasma in a rat model of acute cholestasis. Gastroenterology. 1992;103(2):630–5. PubMed PMID: 1634078.
10. Nelson L, Vergnolle N, D'Mello C, Chapman K, Le T, Swain MG. Endogenous opioid-mediated antinociception in cholestatic mice is peripherally, not centrally, mediated. J Hepatol. 2006;44(6):1141–9. PubMed PMID: 16466825.
11. Kuraishi Y, Yamaguchi T, Miyamoto T. Itch-scratch responses induced by opioids through central mu opioid receptors in mice. J Biomed Sci. 2000;7(3):248–52. PubMed PMID: 10810244.

12. Bergasa NV, Rothman RB, Vergalla J, Xu H, Swain MG, Jones EA. Central mu-opioid receptors are down-regulated in a rat model of cholestasis. J Hepatol. 1992;15(1–2):220–4. PubMed PMID: 1324272.
13. Bergasa NV, Alling DW, Talbot TL, Wells MC, Jones EA. Oral nalmefene therapy reduces scratching activity due to the pruritus of cholestasis: a controlled study. J Am Acad Dermatol. 1999;41(3 Pt 1):431–4. PubMed PMID: 10459118.
14. Thornton JR, Losowsky MS. Opioid peptides and primary biliary cirrhosis. BMJ. 1988;297(6662):1501–4. PubMed PMID: 3147046. Pubmed Central PMCID: 1835218.
15. Sun YG, Chen ZF. A gastrin-releasing peptide receptor mediates the itch sensation in the spinal cord. Nature. 2007;448(7154):700–3. PubMed PMID: 17653196.
16. Bachs L, Pares A, Elena M, Piera C, Rodes J. Effects of long-term rifampicin administration in primary biliary cirrhosis. Gastroenterology. 1992;102(6):2077–80. PubMed PMID: 1587427.
17. Datta DV, Sherlock S. Cholestyramine for long term relief of the pruritus complicating intrahepatic cholestasis. Gastroenterology. 1966;50(3):323–32. PubMed PMID: 5905351.
18. Kuiper EM, van Erpecum KJ, Beuers U, Hansen BE, Thio HB, de Man RA, et al. The potent bile acid sequestrant colesevelam is not effective in cholestatic pruritus: results of a double-blind, randomized, placebo-controlled trial. Hepatology. 2010;52(4):1334–40. PubMed PMID: 20683930.
19. Price TJ, Patterson WK, Olver IN. Rifampicin as treatment for pruritus in malignant cholestasis. Support Care Cancer. 1998;6(6):533–5. PubMed PMID: 9833303.
20. Podesta A, Lopez P, Terg R, Villamil F, Flores D, Mastai R, et al. Treatment of pruritus of primary biliary cirrhosis with rifampin. Dig Dis Sci. 1991;36(2):216–20. PubMed PMID: 1988266.
21. LeCluyse EL. Pregnane X, receptor: molecular basis for species differences in CYP3A induction by xenobiotics. Chem Biol Interact. 2001;134(3):283–9. PubMed PMID: 11336976.
22. Miguet JP, Mavier P, Soussy CJ, Dhumeaux D. Induction of hepatic microsomal enzymes after brief administration of rifampicin in man. Gastroenterology. 1977;72(5 Pt 1):924–6. PubMed PMID: 849823.
23. Galeazzi R, Lorenzini I, Orlandi F. Rifampicin-induced elevation of serum bile acids in man. Dig Dis Sci. 1980;25(2):108–12. PubMed PMID: 7353456.
24. Bachs L, Pares A, Elena M, Piera C, Rodes J. Comparison of rifampicin with phenobarbitone for treatment of pruritus in biliary cirrhosis. Lancet. 1989;1(8638):574–6. PubMed PMID: 2564110.
25. Yerushalmi B, Sokol RJ, Narkewicz MR, Smith D, Karrer FM. Use of rifampin for severe pruritus in children with chronic cholestasis. J Pediatr Gastroenterol Nutr. 1999;29(4):442–7. PubMed PMID: 10512405.
26. Prince MI, Burt AD, Jones DE. Hepatitis and liver dysfunction with rifampicin therapy for pruritus in primary biliary cirrhosis. Gut. 2002;50(3):436–9. PubMed PMID: 11839728. Pubmed Central PMCID: 1773130.
27. Summerfield JA. Naloxone modulates the perception of itch in man. Br J Clin Pharmacol. 1980;10(2):180–3. PubMed PMID: 7000110. Pubmed Central PMCID: 1430035.
28. Menon KV, Angulo P, Weston S, Dickson ER, Lindor KD. Bone disease in primary biliary cirrhosis: independent indicators and rate of progression. J Hepatol. 2001;35(3):316–23. PubMed PMID: 11592591.
29. Hay JE, Lindor KD, Wiesner RH, Dickson ER, Krom RA, LaRusso NF. The metabolic bone disease of primary sclerosing cholangitis. Hepatology. 1991;14(2):257–61. PubMed PMID: 1860683.
30. Bergasa NV, Alling DW, Talbot TL, Swain MG, Yurdaydin C, Turner ML, et al. Effects of naloxone infusions in patients with the pruritus of cholestasis. A double-blind, randomized, controlled trial. Ann Intern Med. 1995;123(3):161–7.
31. Wolfhagen FH, Sternieri E, Hop WC, Vitale G, Bertolotti M, Van Buuren HR. Oral naltrexone treatment for cholestatic pruritus: a double-blind, placebo-controlled study. Gastroenterology. 1997;113(4):1264–9. PubMed PMID: 9322521.

32. Terg R, Coronel E, Sorda J, Munoz AE, Findor J. Efficacy and safety of oral naltrexone treatment for pruritus of cholestasis, a crossover, double blind, placebo-controlled study. J Hepatol. 2002;37(6):717–22. PubMed PMID.
33. McRae CA, Prince MI, Hudson M, Day CP, James OF, Jones DE. Pain as a complication of use of opiate antagonists for symptom control in cholestasis. Gastroenterology. 2003;125(2):591–6. PubMed PMID: 12891561.
34. Browning J, Combes B, Mayo MJ. Long-term efficacy of sertraline as a treatment for cholestatic pruritus in patients with primary biliary cirrhosis. Am J Gastroenterol. 2003;98(12): 2736–41. PubMed PMID: 14687826.
35. Muller C, Pongratz S, Pidlich J, Penner E, Kaider A, Schemper M, et al. Treatment of pruritus in chronic liver disease with the 5-hydroxytryptamine receptor type 3 antagonist ondansetron: a randomized, placebo-controlled, double-blind cross-over trial. Eur J Gastroenterol Hepatol. 1998;10(10):865–70. PubMed PMID: 9831410.
36. O'Donohue JW, Pereira SP, Ashdown AC, Haigh CG, Wilkinson JR, Williams R. A controlled trial of ondansetron in the pruritus of cholestasis. Aliment Pharmacol Ther. 2005;21(8):1041–5. PubMed PMID: 15813840.
37. Horsmans Y, Geubel AP. Pruritus associated with cholestatic liver disease. Ann Intern Med. 1996;125(8):701. PubMed PMID: 8849172.
38. Cadranel JF, DiMartino V, Devergie B. Grapefruit juice for the pruritus of cholestatic liver disease. Ann Intern Med. 1997;126(11):920–1. PubMed PMID: WOS:A1997XA91100029. English.
39. Lauterburg BH, Pineda AA, Burgstaler EA, Taswell HF, Dickson ER, Carlson GL. Treatment of pruritus of cholestasis by plasma perfusion through usp-charcoal-coated glass-beads. Lancet. 1980;2(8185):53–5. PubMed PMID: WOS:A1980JZ01000002. English.
40. Stange J, Hassanein TI, Mehta R, Mitzner SR, Bartlett RH. The molecular adsorbents recycling system as a liver support system based on albumin dialysis: a summary of preclinical investigations, prospective, randomized, controlled clinical trial, and clinical experience from 19 centers. Artif Organs. 2002;26(2):103–10. PubMed PMID: 11879237.
41. Acevedo Ribo M, Moreno Planas JM, Sanz Moreno C, Rubio Gonzalez EE, Rubio Gonzalez E, Boullosa Grana E, et al. Therapy of intractable pruritus with MARS. Transplant Proc. 2005;37(3):1480–1. PubMed PMID: 15866646.
42. Bellmann R, Graziadei IW, Feistritzer C, Schwaighofer H, Stellaard F, Sturm E, et al. Treatment of refractory cholestatic pruritus after liver transplantation with albumin dialysis. Liver Tranpl. 2004;10(1):107–14. PubMed PMID: 14755786.
43. Pares A, Cisneros L, Salmeron JM, Caballeria L, Mas A, Torras A, et al. Extracorporeal albumin dialysis: a procedure for prolonged relief of intractable pruritus in patients with primary biliary cirrhosis. Am J Gastroenterol. 2004;99(6):1105–10. PubMed PMID: 15180733.
44. Neff GW, O'Brien CB, Reddy KR, Bergasa NV, Regev A, Molina E, et al. Preliminary observation with dronabinol in patients with intractable pruritus secondary to cholestatic liver disease. Am J Gastroenterol. 2002;97(8):2117–9. PubMed PMID: 12190187.
45. Gluud C, Christensen E. Ursodeoxycholic acid for primary biliary cirrhosis. Cochrane Database Syst Rev. 2002;1, CD000551. PubMed PMID: 11869580.
46. Collier JD, Ninkovic M, Compston JE. Guidelines on the management of osteoporosis associated with chronic liver disease. Gut. 2002;50 Suppl 1:i1–9. PubMed PMID: 11788576. Pubmed Central PMCID: 1867644.
47. Pares A, Guanabens N. Osteoporosis in primary biliary cirrhosis: pathogenesis and treatment. Clin Liver Dis. 2008;12(2):407–24. x. PubMed PMID: 18456188.
48. Solaymani-Dodaran M, Card TR, Aithal GP, West J. Fracture risk in people with primary biliary cirrhosis: a population-based cohort study. Gastroenterology. 2006;131(6):1752–7. PubMed PMID: 17087953.
49. Leslie WD, Bernstein CN, Leboff MS, American Gastroenterological Association Clinical Practice C. AGA technical review on osteoporosis in hepatic disorders. Gastroenterology. 2003;125(3):941–66. PubMed PMID: 12949738.

50. Eastell R, Dickson ER, Hodgson SF, Wiesner RH, Porayko MK, Wahner HW, et al. Rates of vertebral bone loss before and after liver transplantation in women with primary biliary cirrhosis. Hepatology. 1991;14(2):296–300. PubMed PMID: 1860.
51. Guanabens N, Pares A, Ros I, Caballeria L, Pons F, Vidal S, et al. Severity of cholestasis and advanced histological stage but not menopausal status are the major risk factors for osteoporosis in primary biliary cirrhosis. J Hepatol. 2005;42(4):573–7. PubMed PMID: 15763344.
52. Collier J. Bone disorders in chronic liver disease. Hepatology. 2007;46(4):1271–8. PubMed PMID: 17886.
53. Lindor KD, Gershwin ME, Poupon R, Kaplan M, Bergasa NV, Heathcote EJ, et al. Primary biliary cirrhosis. Hepatology. 2009;50(1):291–308. PubMed PMID: 19554543.
54. Szalay F, Hegedus D, Lakatos PL, Tornai I, Bajnok E, Dunkel K, et al. High serum osteoprotegerin and low RANKL in primary biliary cirrhosis. J Hepatol. 2003;38(4):395–400. PubMed PMID: 12663228.
55. Angulo P, Grandison GA, Fong DG, Keach JC, Lindor KD, Bjornsson E, et al. Bone disease in patients with primary sclerosing cholangitis. Gastroenterology. 2011;140(1):180–8. PubMed PMID: 20955707. Pubmed Central PMCID: 3043598.
56. Guichelaar MM, Malinchoc M, Sibonga JD, Clarke BL, Hay JE. Bone histomorphometric changes after liver transplantation for chronic cholestatic liver disease. J Bone Miner Res. 2003;18(12):2190–9. PubMed PMID: 14672354.
57. Argao EA, Specker BL, Heubi JE. Bone mineral content in infants and children with chronic cholestatic liver disease. Pediatrics. 1993;91(6):1151–4. PubMed PMID: 8502519.
58. Xu H, Eichstaedt H. Assessment of serial changes of bone mineral density at lumbar spine and femoral neck before and after liver transplantation. Chin Med J (Engl). 1999;112(4):379–81. PubMed PMID: 11593545.
59. Hay JE, Guichelaar MM. Evaluation and management of osteoporosis in liver disease. Clin Liver Dis. 2005;9(4):747–66. viii. PubMed PMID: 16207574.
60. Guichelaar MM, Schmoll J, Malinchoc M, Hay JE. Fractures and avascular necrosis before and after orthotopic liver transplantation: long-term follow-up and predictive factors. Hepatology. 2007;46(4):1198–207. PubMed PMID: 17654700.
61. Navasa M, Monegal A, Guanabens N, Peris P, Rimola A, Munoz-Gomez J, et al. Bone fractures in liver transplant patients. Br J Rheumatol. 1994;33(1):52–5. PubMed PMID: 8162459.
62. Rust C, Rau H, Gerbes AL, Pape GR, Haller M, Kramling H, et al. Liver transplantation in primary biliary cirrhosis: risk assessment and 11-year follow-up. Digestion. 2000;62(1):38–43. PubMed PMID: 10899724.
63. Lakatos PL, Bajnok E, Tornai I, Folhoffer A, Horvath A, Lakatos P, et al. Insulin-like growth factor I gene microsatellite repeat, collagen type Ialpha1 gene Sp1 polymorphism, and bone disease in primary biliary cirrhosis. Eur J Gastroenterol Hepatol. 2004;16(8):753–9. PubMed PMID: 15256976.
64. Springer JE, Cole DE, Rubin LA, Cauch-Dudek K, Harewood L, Evrovski J, et al. Vitamin D-receptor genotypes as independent genetic predictors of decreased bone mineral density in primary biliary cirrhosis. Gastroenterology. 2000;118(1):145–51.
65. Pares A, Guanabens N, Alvarez L, De Osaba MJ, Oriola J, Pons F, et al. Collagen type Ialpha1 and vitamin D receptor gene polymorphisms and bone mass in primary biliary cirrhosis. Hepatology. 2001;33(3):554–60. PubMed PMID: 11230734.
66. Moschen AR, Kaser A, Stadlmann S, Millonig G, Kaser S, Muhllechner P, et al. The RANKL/OPG system and bone mineral density in patients with chronic liver disease. J Hepatol. 2005;43(6):973–83. PubMed PMID: 16143421.
67. Boyle WJ, Simonet WS, Lacey DL. Osteoclast differentiation and activation. Nature. 2003;423(6937):337–42. PubMed PMID: 12748652.
68. Smith DL, Shire NJ, Watts NB, Schmitter T, Szabo G, Zucker SD. Hyperbilirubinemia is not a major contributing factor to altered bone mineral density in patients with chronic liver disease. J Clin Densitom. 2006;9(1):105–13. PubMed PMID: 16731439.
69. Rouillard S, Lane NE. Hepatic osteodystrophy. Hepatology. 2002;33:301–7.

70. Bell H, Raknerud N, Falch JA, Haug E. Inappropriately low levels of gonadotrophins in amenorrhoeic women with alcoholic and non-alcoholic cirrhosis. Eur J Endocrinol. 1995;132(4):444–9. PubMed PMID: 7711882.
71. Diamond T, Stiel D, Mason R, Lissner D, Bikle D, Wilson S, et al. Serum vitamin D metabolites are not responsible for low turnover osteoporosis in chronic liver disease. J Clin Endocrinol Metab. 1989;69:1234–9.
72. Angulo P, Batts KP, Jorgensen RA, LaRusso NA, Lindor KD. Oral budesonide in the treatment of primary sclerosing cholangitis. Am J Gastroenterol. 2000;95(9):2333–7. PubMed.
73. Angulo P, Jorgensen RA, Keach JC, Dickson ER, Smith C, Lindor KD. Oral budesonide in the treatment of patients with primary biliary cirrhosis with a suboptimal response to ursodeoxycholic acid. Hepatology. 2000;31(2):318–23. PubMed PMID: 10655252.
74. Cheung AM. Post-liver transplantation osteoporosis. J Hepatol. 2001;34(2):337–8. PubMed PMID: 11281566.
75. European Association for the Study of the L. EASL clinical practice guidelines: management of cholestatic liver diseases. J Hepatol. 2009;51(2):237–67. PubMed PMID: 19501929.
76. Pereira SP, Bray GP, Pitt PI, Li F, Moniz C, Williams R. Non-invasive assessment of bone density in primary biliary cirrhosis. Eur J Gastroenterol Hepatol. 1999;11(3):323–8. PubMed PMID: 103332.
77. Camisasca M, Crosignani A, Battezzati PM, Albisetti W, Grandinetti G, Pietrogrande L, et al. Parenteral calcitonin for metabolic bone disease associated with primary biliary cirrhosis. Hepatology. 1994;20(3):633–7. PubMed.
78. Rosen H. Primary biliary cirrhosis and bone disease. Hepatology. 1995;21(1):253–5. PubMed PM.
79. Mobarhan SA, Russell RM, Recker RR, Posner DB, Iber FL, Miller P. Metabolic bone disease in alcoholic cirrhosis: a comparison of the effect of vitamin D2, 25-hydroxyvitamin D, or supportive treatment. Hepatology. 1984;4(2):266–73. PubMed PMID: 6608483.
80. Pares A, Guanabens N. Treatment of bone disorders in liver disease. J Hepatol. 2006;45(3):445–53. PubMed PMID: 16844255.
81. Optimal calcium intake. NIH consensus statement. 1994;12(4):1-31. PubMed PMID: 7599655.
82. Lindor KD, Jorgensen RA, Tiegs RD, Khosla S, Dickson ER. Etidronate for osteoporosis in primary biliary cirrhosis: a randomized trial. J Hepatol. 2000;33(6):878–82. PubMed PMID: 11131448.
83. Guanabens N, Pares A, Ros I, Alvarez L, Pons F, Caballeria L, et al. Alendronate is more effective than etidronate for increasing bone mass in osteopenic patients with primary biliary cirrhosis. Am J Gastroenterol. 2003;98(10):2268–74. PubMed PMID: 14572578.
84. Zein CO, Jorgensen RA, Clarke B, Wenger DE, Keach JC, Angulo P, et al. Alendronate improves bone mineral density in primary biliary cirrhosis: a randomized placebo-controlled trial. Hepatology. 2005;42(4):762–71. PubMed PMID: 16175618.
85. Monegal A, Guanabens N, Suarez MJ, Suarez F, Clemente G, Garcia-Gonzalez M, et al. Pamidronate in the prevention of bone loss after liver transplantation: a randomized controlled trial. Transpl Int. 2009;22(2):198–206. PubMed PMID: 18796000.
86. Bodingbauer M, Pakrah B, Kristo I, Marschalek J, Burghuber C, Gyori G, et al. Nonpersistent effect of short-term bisphosphonate treatment in preventing fractures after liver transplantation. Transpl Int. 2010;23(1):118–20. PubMed PMID: 19624497.
87. Menon KV, Angulo P, Boe GM, Lindor KD. Safety and efficacy of estrogen therapy in preventing bone loss in primary biliary cirrhosis. Am J Gastroenterol. 2003;98(4):889–92. PubMed PMID: 12738473.
88. Pereira SP, O'Donohue J, Moniz C, Phillips MG, Abraha H, Buxton-Thomas M, et al. Transdermal hormone replacement therapy improves vertebral bone density in primary biliary cirrhosis: results of a 1-year controlled trial. Aliment Pharmacol Ther. 2004;19(5):563–70. PubMed PMID: 14987325.
89. Ormarsdottir S, Mallmin H, Naessen T, Petren-Mallmin M, Broome U, Hultcrantz R, et al. An open, randomized, controlled study of transdermal hormone replacement therapy on the rate of bone loss in primary biliary cirrhosis. J Intern Med. 2004;256(1):63–9. PubMed PMID: 15189367.

90. Ettinger B, Black DM, Mitlak BH, Knickerbocker RK, Nickelsen T, Genant HK, et al. Reduction of vertebral fracture risk in postmenopausal women with osteoporosis treated with raloxifene: results from a 3-year randomized clinical trial. Multiple outcomes of raloxifene evaluation (MORE) investigators. JAMA. 1999;282(7):637–45.
91. Levy C, Harnois DM, Angulo P, Jorgensen R, Lindor KD. Raloxifene improves bone mass in osteopenic women with primary biliary cirrhosis: results of a pilot study. Liver Int. 2005;25(1):117–21. PubMed PMID: 15698408.
92. Guanabens N, Pares A, del Rio L, Roca M, Gomez R, Munoz J, et al. Sodium fluoride prevents bone loss in primary biliary cirrhosis. J Hepatol. 1992;15(3):345–9. PubMed PMID: 1447501.
93. Guanabens N, Pares A, Monegal A, Peris P, Pons F, Alvarez L, et al. Etidronate versus fluoride for treatment of osteopenia in primary biliary cirrhosis: preliminary results after 2 years. Gastroenterology. 1997;113(1):219–24. PubMed PMID: 9207281.
94. Yamaguchi M, Weitzmann MN. The intact strontium ranelate complex stimulates osteoblastogenesis and suppresses osteoclastogenesis by antagonizing NF-kappaB activation. Mol Cell Biochem. 2012;359(1–2):399–407. PubMed PMID: 21874315.
95. Adams J, Pepping J. Vitamin K in the treatment and prevention of osteoporosis and arterial calcification. Am J Health Syst Pharm. 2005;62(15):1574–81. PubMed PMID: 16030366.
96. Nishiguchi S, Shimoi S, Kurooka H, Tamori A, Habu D, Takeda T, et al. Randomized pilot trial of vitamin K2 for bone loss in patients with primary biliary cirrhosis. J Hepatol. 2001;35(4):543–5. PubMed PMID: 11682046.
97. Hay JE, Malinchoc M, Dickson ER. A controlled trial of calcitonin therapy for the prevention of post-liver transplantation atraumatic fractures in patients with primary biliary cirrhosis and primary sclerosing cholangitis. J Hepatol. 2001;34(2):292–8. PubMed PMID: 11281559.
98. Potts JT. Parathyroid hormone: past and present. J Endocrinol. 2005;187(3):311–25. PubMed PMID: 16423810.
99. Solaymani-Dodaran M, Aithal GP, Card T, West J. Risk of cardiovascular and cerebrovascular events in primary biliary cirrhosis: a population-based cohort study. Am J Gastroenterol. 2008;103(11):2784–8. PubMed PMID: 18759822.
100. Su TC, Hwang JJ, Kao JH. Hypercholesterolemia in primary biliary cirrhosis. N Engl J Med. 2007;357(15):1561–2. PubMed PMID: 17928612.
101. Seidel D, Alaupovic P, Furman RH. A lipoprotein characterizing obstructive jaundice. I. Method for quantitative separation and identification of lipoproteins in jaundiced subjects. J Clin Invest. 1969;48(7):1211–23. PubMed PMID: 4978447. Pubmed Central PMCID: 322342.
102. Ross A, Murphy GM, Wilkinson PA, Mills GL, Sherlock S. Occurrence of an abnormal lipoprotein in patients with liver disease. Gut. 1970;11(12):1035–7. PubMed PMID: 5511783. Pubmed Central PMCID: 1553163.
103. Ritzel U, Leonhardt U, Nather M, Schafer G, Armstrong VW, Ramadori G. Simvastatin in primary biliary cirrhosis: effects on serum lipids and distinct disease markers. J Hepatol. 2002;36(4):454–8. PubMed PMID: 11943414.
104. Abu Rajab M, Kaplan MM. Statins in primary biliary cirrhosis: are they safe? Dig Dis Sci. 2010;55(7):2086–8. PubMed PMID: 19795210.
105. Chang PY, Lu SC, Su TC, Chou SF, Huang WH, Morrisett JD, et al. Lipoprotein-X reduces LDL atherogenicity in primary biliary cirrhosis by preventing LDL oxidation. J Lipid Res. 2004;45(11):2116–22. PubMed PMID: 15314101.
106. Sivakumar T, Chaidarun S, Lee HK, Cervinski M, Comi R. Multiple lipoprotein and electrolyte laboratory artifacts caused by lipoprotein X in obstructive biliary cholestasis secondary to pancreatic cancer. J Clin Lipidol. 2011;5(4):324–8. PubMed PMID: 21784379.
107. Nakamuta M, Enjoji M, Kotoh K, Shimohashi N, Tanabe Y. Long-term fibrate treatment for PBC. J Gastroenterol. 2005;40(5):546–7. PubMed PMID: 15942724.
108. Sorokin A, Brown JL, Thompson PD. Primary biliary cirrhosis, hyperlipidemia, and atherosclerotic risk: a systematic review. Atherosclerosis. 2007;194(2):293–9. PubMed PMID: 17240380.

109. Tandra S, Vuppalanchi R. Use of statins in patients with liver disease. Curr Treat Options Cardiovasc Med. 2009;11(4):272–8. PubMed PMID: 19627660.
110. Allocca M, Crosignani A, Gritti A, Ghilardi G, Gobatti D, Caruso D, et al. Hypercholesterolaemia is not associated with early atherosclerotic lesions in primary biliary cirrhosis. Gut. 2006;55(12):1795–800. PubMed PMID: 16632556. Pubmed Central PMCID: 1856484.
111. Zollner G, Trauner M. Nuclear receptors as therapeutic targets in cholestatic liver diseases. Br J Pharmacol. 2009;156(1):7–27. PubMed PMID: 19133988. Pubmed Central PMCID: 2697779.
112. Zollner G, Marschall HU, Wagner M, Trauner M. Role of nuclear receptors in the adaptive response to bile acids and cholestasis: pathogenetic and therapeutic considerations. Mol Pharm. 2006;3(3):231–51. PubMed PMID: 16749856.
113. Franceschini G, Busnach G, Chiesa G, Sirtori CR. Management of lipoprotein-X accumulation in severe cholestasis by semi-selective LDL-apheresis. Am J Med. 1991;90(5):633–8. PubMed PMID: 2029022.
114. Kojima S, Toyota Y, Shiba M, Tsushima M, Matsuoka H, Yamamoto A. Different apheresis methods in the treatment of hypercholesterolemia in primary biliary cirrhosis: a case report. Artif Organs. 1995;19(9):938–41. PubMed PMID: 8687302.
115. Phillips JR, Angulo P, Petterson T, Lindor KD. Fat-soluble vitamin levels in patients with primary biliary cirrhosis. Am J Gastroenterol. 2001;96(9):2745–50. PubMed PMID: 11569705.
116. Arria AM, Tarter RE, Warty V, Van Thiel DH. Vitamin E deficiency and psychomotor dysfunction in adults with primary biliary cirrhosis. Am J Clin Nutr. 1990;52(2):383–90. PubMed PMID: 1973868.
117. Jeffrey GP, Muller DP, Burroughs AK, Matthews S, Kemp C, Epstein O, et al. Vitamin E deficiency and its clinical significance in adults with primary biliary cirrhosis and other forms of chronic liver disease. J Hepatol. 1987;4(3):307–17. PubMed PMID: 3036938.
118. Newton JL, Gibson GJ, Tomlinson M, Wilton K, Jones D. Fatigue in primary biliary cirrhosis is associated with excessive daytime somnolence. Hepatology. 2006;44(1):91–8. PubMed PMID: 16800007.
119. Zenouzi R, Weiler-Normann C, Lohse AW. Is fatigue in primary biliary cirrhosis cured by transplantation? J Hepatol. 2013;59(3):418–9. PubMed PMID: 23742911.
120. Carbone M, Bufton S, Monaco A, Griffiths L, Jones DE, Neuberger JM. The effect of liver transplantation on fatigue in patients with primary biliary cirrhosis: a prospective study. J Hepatol. 2013;59(3):490–4. PubMed PMID: 23628322.
121. Newton JL, Elliott C, Frith J, Ghazala C, Pairman J, Jones DE. Functional capacity is significantly impaired in primary biliary cirrhosis and is related to orthostatic symptoms. Eur J Gastroenterol Hepatol. 2011;23(7):566–72. PubMed PMID: 21593676.
122. Czeisler CA, Walsh JK, Roth T, Hughes RJ, Wright KP, Kingsbury L, et al. Modafinil for excessive sleepiness associated with shift-work sleep disorder. N Engl J Med. 2005;353(5):476–86. PubMed PMID: 16079371.
123. Ian Gan S, de Jongh M, Kaplan MM. Modafinil in the treatment of debilitating fatigue in primary biliary cirrhosis: a clinical experience. Dig Dis Sci. 2009;54(10):2242–6. PubMed PMID: 19082890.
124. Watson JP, Jones DE, James OF, Cann PA, Bramble MG. Case report: oral antioxidant therapy for the treatment of primary biliary cirrhosis: a pilot study. J Gastroenterol Hepatol. 1999;14(10):1034–40. PubMed PMID: 10530501.
125. Cerri G, Cocchi CA, Montagna M, Zuin M, Podda M, Cavallari P, et al. Patients with primary biliary cirrhosis do not show post-exercise depression of cortical excitability. Clin Neurophysiol. 2010;121(8):1321–8. PubMed PMID: 20363183.
126. Talwalkar JA, Donlinger JJ, Gossard AA, Keach JC, Jorgensen RA, Petz JC, et al. Fluoxetine for the treatment of fatigue in primary biliary cirrhosis: a randomized, double-blind controlled trial. Dig Dis Sci. 2006;51(11):1985–91. PubMed PMID: 17053955.

Chapter 10
Cholestasis Post-Liver Transplantation

Denise M. Harnois and Kymberly D.S. Watt

Cholestasis is common after a liver transplant and occurs when the process of bile production or bile flow is impeded. This can happen within the extrahepatic biliary system or at the intrahepatic or the cellular level. Depending on the underlying reason for the cholestasis, the short- and long-term consequences can range from minimal to severe.

The differential diagnosis of post-transplant cholestasis is broad. It is commonly interpreted in terms of "early cholestatic syndrome" (<6 months) and "late cholestatic syndrome" (>6 months) relative to the operative procedure, but considerable overlap can occur. Within these timeframes, both intrahepatic and extrahepatic causes exist. Table 10.1 outlines these concepts.

Biliary Complications

Biliary complications following liver transplant occur in 10–50 % of transplants with associated mortality rates of 0–20 %, anastomosis revision rates of 12–25 %, and re-transplantation rates of 6–12 % [1–4]. The spectrum of biliary tract complications in the post-transplant setting may include biliary leaks, strictures, choledocholithiasis, cast formation, and other less commonly seen complications such as papillary stenosis [1]. Higher rates of biliary complications after a Roux-en-Y anastomosis are thought to be representative of its more complicated procedures (i.e., re-transplantation and diffuse extrahepatic diseases such as primary sclerosing cholangitis [PSC]) [3].

D.M. Harnois, D.O. (✉)
Department of Transplant, Mayo Clinic, 4500 San Pablo Road, Jacksonville, FL 32224, USA
e-mail: Harnois.denise@mayo.edu

K.D.S. Watt, M.D.
Gastroenterology and Hepatology, Mayo Clinic,
200 First Street SW, Rochester, MN 55905, USA
e-mail: watt.kymberly@mayo.edu

E.J. Carey and K.D. Lindor (eds.), *Cholestatic Liver Disease*, Clinical Gastroenterology,
DOI 10.1007/978-1-4939-1013-7_10,

Table 10.1 Causes of cholestasis after liver transplantation

Early (<6 months)	Late (>6 months)
Extrahepatic:	*Extrahepatic:*
Stricture—single (anastomotic, external compression)	Benign stricture—single (anastomotic)
Stricture—multiple (HAT/ischemic)	Multiple (HAT/ischemic, rPSC)
Biliary leak	Stones
Cholangitis	
Intrahepatic:	*Intrahepatic:*
Preservation/reperfusion injury	Acute cellular rejection
ABO incompatibility	Chronic rejection
HAT	Drug induced
Small-for-size graft	Recurrent disease (PBC, PSC, viral)
Drug induced	De novo viral hepatitis, autoimmune disease
Acute cellular rejection	
Sepsis	
Infection—CMV, bacterial, fungal, Hepatitis BCRC or HCV/HBV	

The most common biliary complications in the early postoperative setting include biliary leak and biliary obstruction related to both anastomotic and nonanastomotic strictures, with secondary cholangitis as a possible consequence. Biliary leaks can occur at the anastomosis, as a result of ischemic bile duct injury, or from the cut surface of the liver, particularly after a living donor or split liver transplant. The presence of bile in the output of operative drains is an early indicator of a bile leak, which can be confirmed with further testing radiographically or endoscopically. The benefit and use of T-tubes in reducing these complications are still debated [1–4].

Early intervention in biliary complications is important to graft survival. Biliary leaks or biliary strictures can often be treated nonsurgically. Endoscopic and percutaneous biliary stenting for strictures has the highest success rate (60–75 %) when biliary stents are placed following dilatation, as opposed to dilatation alone [5]. These procedures are most successful in early strictures (<6 months) rather than late strictures (>6 months) [3]. Traditionally, endoscopic biliary access was not possible in patients with Roux-en-Y hepaticojejunostomy, but advances in endoscopy technology—such as single- and double-balloon enteroscopy and overtube-assisted enteroscopy—have increasingly allowed for successful endoscopic diagnosis and treatment of biliary complications in these patients [1].

Nonanastomotic strictures occur at a frequency of 2–20 % [6]. They tend to be multifocal, can be both intrahepatic and extrahepatic, and are more likely to require re-transplantation. They can occur early (<6 months) or late (>6 months) and are associated with several underlying causes, including hepatic artery thrombosis (HAT), warm and cold/ischemic injury, ABO incompatibility, recurrent PSC, and possible viral infections such as cytomegalovirus (CMV) or even hepatitis C (HCV). These are discussed in more detail in later sections [6, 7]. Graft survival appears to be significantly lower in patients with nonanastomotic strictures when compared to matched patients without strictures [6]. Other important donor factors in patients receiving cadaveric organs may influence the development of biliary strictures [8–12].

Traditionally, cadaveric organs for liver transplants were donated after brain death (DBD). However, there are not sufficient numbers of these donors for patients currently waiting on liver transplant lists. Donation after cardiac death (DCD) is recognized as an important source of organs to increase the availability of donors for liver transplant. In DCD donors, declaration of death is based on cardiopulmonary criteria rather than cessation of brain and brainstem function and these organs are harvested after cardiopulmonary arrest in contrast to organs procured after established brain death. The reported outcomes of vascular (hepatic artery thrombosis) and biliary complications in DCD donors are more frequent than in DBD donors, resulting in an increased risk of graft loss [13]. In particular, these grafts appear to have a higher incidence of diffuse ischemic biliary strictures and cholangiopathy (IC).

The etiology of these higher rates of stricture seems to be related to increased donor warm ischemic times [14]. Other relevant operative features, such as the time from asystole to cross clamp, may also predict the development of biliary strictures [15]. As donor procurement techniques improve, the rate of biliary stricturing in these grafts will undoubtedly improve. While the rate of graft loss is higher in DCD than in DBD donors, the presence of biliary ischemic cholangiopathy does not necessarily result in graft loss. Many of these patients can be managed endoscopically in the early postoperative period with resolution of their biliary complications. It is, however, still too early to know the long-term complications and survival of these grafts.

Impacted biliary stones generally occur later post-transplant and are often associated with biliary strictures and impaired bile flow. Medications including cyclosporine may increase the risk of stone formation in the transplant setting [16]. These biliary stones can respond to endoscopic treatment [1].

Preservation/Reperfusion Injury and ABO Incompatibility

Preservation injury has been reported from approximately 17 % of transplants to as high as 50 % of transplants [17, 18]. Extrahepatic biliary complications, such as nonanastomotic strictures, occur with increasing frequency as the cold ischemia time reaches over 10–12 h [17, 18]. Preservation injury also occurs at the cellular level, involving nonparenchymal cells (sinusoidal endothelial cell injury and Kupffer cell activation with accumulating inflammatory cells and platelets) as well as parenchymal cells, including biliary epithelial cells [19, 20]. Histological findings of preservation/reperfusion injury include neutrophilic infiltration, microvesicular steatosis, hepatocyte cytoaggregation occurring early and progressing to centrilobular necrosis, hepatocyte swelling, and cholestasis later in the process [18]. Mild cases resolve spontaneously, but more severe cases may cause residual damage or result in primary graft nonfunction [18].

Blood group-related antigens (ABO) are expressed on the epithelial cells of large bile ducts and periductular hepatocytes [21]. Thus, the hepatic allograft may be more susceptible to immunologic bile duct injury after transplantation across the ABO barrier. Complication rates for biliary strictures, HAT, and cellular rejection were significantly higher in these patients [7]. Graft survival and patient survival have been inferior to ABO-matched transplants in retrospective studies [7].

Small-for-Size Syndrome

Small-for-size syndrome (SFSS) is a recognized complication occurring when the recipient receives inadequate functional tissue. It is thought to occur at a graft-to-recipient body weight ratio less than 0.8. The presentation can vary from mild isolated hyperbilirubinemia to graft failure. Within the first week of transplant the patient may develop cholestasis, prolonged coagulation, ascites, and variceal bleeding [22]. Histologic examination shows bilirubin plugs and cholestasis with patchy areas of necrosis and regenerative tissue [22]. The physiologic mechanisms of SFSS are not clear but seem to be related to portal hyperperfusion and arterial hypoperfusion resulting in endothelial disruption and subsequent molecular derangements on the hepatic regeneration process [22].

Hepatic Artery Thrombosis (HAT)

HAT is described in 3–9 % of transplants, with another 3 % of patients experiencing nonthrombotic complications such as hepatic artery stenosis, redundancy, and pseudoaneurysm [23]. In the transplanted liver, HAT results in more significant biliary damage than in a non-transplanted liver because the surgical excision interrupts smaller peripheral arteries that normally supply collateral flow [23]. One-third of HAT cases occurs within the first month and may present with cholestasis [24]. Because the main blood supply to the biliary system stems from the hepatic artery, later complications tend to include bile duct stricturing with subsequent cholangitis, liver abscess, biloma, and/or biliary necrosis with bile leak. Both early and late presentation of HAT can progress to severe liver failure [24, 25]. Re-transplantation rates of 50–80 % and mortality rates of up to 50–70 % have been described in patients with HAT [24–26].

Risk factors of HAT include vascular surgical technique, biliary anastomosis (Roux-en-Y), biliary leaks, cold and warm ischemic injury, antibody cross-match status, coagulation abnormalities, infections (particularly CMV), and possible immunologic factors [25, 26]. An increased risk has been associated with cigarette smoking in both the pre-transplant setting and the post-transplant setting [27]. Interventional radiology procedures (such as angioplasty and fibrinolysis) or immediate surgical revascularization are often needed to avoid re-transplantation [25, 28].

Infectious Complications

Bacterial and Fungal

Cholestasis with or without hyperbilirubinemia is frequently associated with extrahepatic bacterial or fungal infections and sepsis [29]. Evidence suggests that proinflammatory cytokines and endotoxin release are potent inhibitors of hepatobiliary transporter gene expression, resulting in hyperbilirubinemia and cholestasis [30]. Although seldom necessary, histological assessment may reveal nonspecific cholestasis and hepatitis or a neutrophilic infiltration of the bile ducts, biliary proliferation, and bile plugs termed "cholangitis lenta" [31].

Viral

Cytomegalovirus (CMV) is a common viral pathogen in liver transplant recipients and is reported in 30–80 % of transplant patients, with up to 30 % of patients developing CMV disease and 12–17 % CMV hepatitis. The highest risk is within the first 3–4 months post-transplant [29, 32]. CMV can infect and injure not only hepatocytes but also biliary epithelium and vascular endothelium [33, 34]. Thus, it can present as cholestasis. Histologic findings can range from lymphocytic infiltration, ballooned hepatocytes, cholangitis, cholestasis, endothelitis, and Kupffer cell reaction to more specific findings of microabscesses or, rarely, viral inclusions [35]. CMV has been implicated in vanishing bile duct syndrome and both acute and chronic rejection [33, 35].

Human herpesvirus-6 and -7 (HHV-6 and -7) activations are common and are usually associated with CMV infection and rejection in liver transplant patients [36]. They may present with cholestasis in a manner similar to CMV. Herpes simplex virus (HSV), as well as toxoplasmosis, should be considered with the immunosuppressed patient in appropriate settings [29]. Hepatitis C and hepatitis B viral (HBV) infections are discussed below.

Drug Induced

Drugs and toxins are common causes of cholestasis and can be the result of either a direct injury to the cells or an idiosyncratic reaction to a drug. Many of the commonly used drugs following transplant should be considered in the work-up of cholestasis. These drugs include immunosuppressive drugs, antibiotics, and antifungal agent. Table 10.2 outlines some of the more common post-transplant drugs that can contribute to cholestasis. In this chapter, we focus on a review of immunosuppressive medications.

Table 10.2 Common causes of drug-induced cholestasis after liver transplantation

Immunosuppression	*Other*
Cyclosporine	Verapamil
Tacrolimus	Seizure medications
Sirolimus	Tricyclic antidepressants
Everolimus	Oral glycemic agents
Azathioprine	Hydrochlorothiazides
Antibiotics:	
Sulfa (trimethoprim/sulfamethoxazole)	
Cephalosporins	
Amoxicillin-clavulanate	
Macrolide antibiotics	
Isoniazid	
Antifungal agents:	
Fluconazole	
Itraconazole	

Cyclosporine induces cholestasis by decreasing both bile flow and bile salt secretion. This suppression of bile salt synthesis reduces the bile salt pool size [37]. The drug inhibits bile salt and phospholipid secretion without a corresponding change in cholesterol secretion, thus elevating cholesterol saturation in bile and raising the potential risk for stone formation [16, 37]. In contrast to cyclosporine, tacrolimus shows higher bile flow rates and more rapid recovery of bile flow post-transplantation [38]. Cholestasis has also been attributed to tacrolimus, which may be the result of deranged bile acid transport or of impaired glutathione and bicarbonate excretion [38, 39]. Sirolimus and everolimus also have cholestatic effects through the retention of toxic metabolites within the hepatocytes [39, 40]. Azathioprine can cause hepatotoxicity of a variety of mechanisms, including cholestasis [41].

Acute Cellular Rejection and Chronic Rejection (CR)

The mechanism by which patients with acute cellular rejection (ACR) develop cholestasis is multifactorial. It is related to lymphocytic destruction of the small intrahepatic bile ducts or apoptosis of the biliary epithelial cell, and to impaired bile secretions related to Kupffer cell-induced cytokine release [42–44]. If early ACR is not treated or responds inadequately to treatment, progression to irreversible injury or chronic rejection occurs.

Chronic "ductopenic" rejection occurs in 2–5 % of patients and generally presents as cholestasis within 6 weeks to 12 months of transplantation. However, it has been noted as early as 2–3 weeks post-operation [45, 46]. It is characterized by progressive loss of intrahepatic, interlobular, and septal bile ducts (ductopenia) with lipid-laden vasculopathy in 50 % of portal tracts (Fig. 10.1) [46]. Risk factors for the development of chronic rejection include CMV infection and pre-transplant disease etiology. Immune-related diseases such as PSC, primary biliary cirrhosis [PBC], and

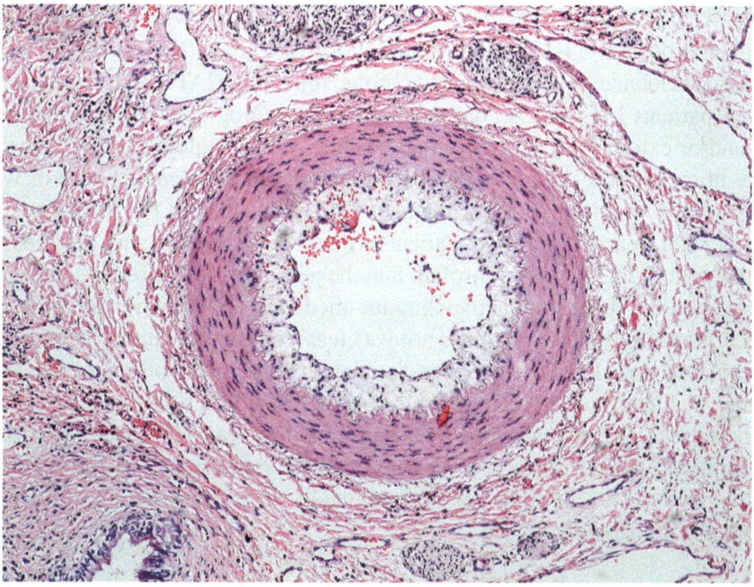

Fig 10.1 This liver biopsy demonstrates foam cell arteriopathy characteristic of chronic allograft rejection

autoimmune hepatitis [AIH] have the highest incidence. Human leukocyte antigen (HLA) mismatching, donor male to recipient female matching, and the number and/or severity of acute rejection episodes have also been linked to chronic rejection [34, 45]. Whether the pathogenesis is related to an immune-mediated injury or to an ischemic injury resulting from the obliterative arteritis is unclear [23, 47]. Undoubtedly the processes are linked, and it is the combination and severity of each component that results in the clinical manifestation of chronic ductopenic rejection.

Recurrent Disease

Primary Biliary Cirrhosis (PBC) and Primary Sclerosing Cholangitis (PSC)

PBC recurs in up to 17 % of patients by 36 months and 30–50 % of patients within 10 years following liver transplant [48–50]. The diagnosis is confirmed by histologic findings of florid duct lesions or destructive lymphocytic cholangitis within a dense portal mononuclear inflammatory infiltrate or by the formation of lymphoid aggregates and epithelioid granulomas [48]. Clear risk factors for recurrence have not been defined. The choice of immunosuppression was initially thought to be a risk factor, but recent studies are inconclusive. Interestingly, recurrent PBC does not demonstrate any significant influence on patient survival, and PBC-related graft loss is rare (1–5%) [50].

Recurrent PSC is thought to occur in 9–20 % of patients within 5 years after liver transplantation [51–54]. It is not a straightforward diagnosis, as there is also an increased incidence of both acute and chronic rejection, HAT, and biliary stricturing in these patients [51–54]. A combination of cholangiographic findings of intrahepatic and/or extrahepatic strictures and beading, plus histologic findings, including biliary fibrosis/cirrhosis, fibro-obliterative lesions, and cholangitis with or without ductopenia, is required for the diagnosis [51]. Risk factors for recurrent disease have not been clearly delineated. Patients who received maintenance corticosteroids or orthoclone (OKT3) post-transplant may be at higher risk of recurrent PSC. This may suggest that those with active immune-mediated inflammation are more at risk for recurrent disease, though this is not yet clear from the literature [54]. Coexistent inflammatory bowel disease was associated with higher rates of recurrence, but this also may be due to steroid requirements [54]. In addition, a single-center experience has shown that patients who had a colectomy before transplant were less likely to develop recurrence of disease [55]. The need for retransplantion for graft failure resulting from recurrent disease is approximately 12 %. These patients will often do well with re-transplant.

Viral Hepatitis

Recurrent viral hepatitis of any severity can present with cholestasis. Fibrosing cholestatic hepatitis (FCH) is a severe form of HBV and HCV recurrence or reactivation in the allograft. It manifests clinically within weeks to months of transplantation as cholestasis and progresses rapidly to liver failure, if left untreated. The frequency of this entity in HBV-infected patients has decreased significantly since the introduction of prophylactic therapies to prevent HBV recurrence, but it continues to occur in approximately 5–8 % of patients transplanted for HCV and 20 % of HIV/HCV co-infected individuals [56, 57]. It is thought to be a result of virus-specific cytopathic injury rather than immunologic injury. FCH is characterized histologically by periportal fibrosis, prominent cholestasis, and hepatocyte swelling that progresses to centrilobular balloon degeneration and bridging fibrosis/cirrhosis [56, 58]. Early treatment with antiviral medications may delay the progression of disease and improve prognosis. Emerging evidence indicates success in treating FCH secondary to HCV with newer antiviral therapy [59].

Summary

Cholestasis is a frequent finding in liver post-transplantation with a very broad differential diagnosis. Timing of the cholestatic presentation may help to narrow the possibilities, but significant overlap exists. Careful diagnostic imaging of the biliary tree is an important first step in the work-up, followed by liver biopsy, if clinically indicated.

References

1. Arain MA, Attam R, Freeman ML. Advances in endoscopic management of biliary tract complications after liver transplantation. Liver Transpl. 2013;19:482–98.
2. Seehofer D, Eurich D, Veltzke-Schlieker W, Neuhaus P. Am J Transplant. 2013;13:253–65.
3. Thethy S, Thomson BNJ, Pleass H, et al. Management of biliary tract complications after orthotopic liver transplantation. Clin Transplant. 2004;18(6):647–53.
4. Scatton O, Meunier B, Cherqui D, et al. Randomized trial of choledocho-choledochostomy with or without a T-tube in orthotopic liver transplantation. Ann Surg. 2001;233(3):432–7.
5. Zoepf T, Maldonado-Lopez EJ, Hilgard P, et al. Balloon dilatation vs balloon dilatation plus bile duct endoprostheses for treatment of anastomotic biliary strictures after liver transplantation. Liver Transpl. 2006;12(1):88–94.
6. Guichelaar MM, Benson JT, Malinchoc M, et al. Risk factors for and clinical course of non-anastomotic biliary strictures after liver transplantation. Am J Transplant. 2003;3(7):885–90.
7. Sanchez-Urdazpal L, Batts KP, Gores GJ, et al. Increased bile duct complications in liver transplantation across the ABO barrier. Ann Surg. 1993;218(2):152–8.
8. Muiesan P, Girlanda R, Jassem W, Melendez HV, O'Grady J, Bowles M, Rela M, Heaton N. Single-center experience with liver transplantation from controlled non-heartbeating donors. Ann Surg. 2005;242(5):732–8.
9. Nguyen JH, Bonatti H, Dickson RC, Hewitt WR, Grewall HP, Willingham DL, Harnois DM, Schmitt TM, Machicao VI, Ghabril MS, Keaveny AP, Aranda-Michel J, Satyanarayana R, Rosser BG, Hinder RA, Steers JL, Hughes CB. Long-term outcomes of donation after cardiac death liver allografts from a single center. Clin Transplant. 2009;23:168–73.
10. DeOliveira ML, Jassem W, Valente R, Khorsandi SE, Santori G, Prachalias A, Sirinivasan P, Rela M, Heaton N. Biliary complications after liver transplantation using grafts from donors after cardiac death: Results from a matched control study in a single large volume center. Ann Surg. 2011;254(5):716–23.
11. Foley DP, Fernandez LA, Leverson G, Anderson M, Mezrich J, Sollinger HW, D'Alessandro A. Biliary complications after liver transplantation from donation after cardiac death donors: An analysis of risk factors and long term outcomes from a single center. Ann Surg. 2011;253(4):817–25.
12. Van der Hilst CS, Ijtsma AJC, Bottema JT, van Hoek B, Dubbeld J, Metelaar HJ, Kazemier G, van den Berg AP, Porte RJ, Slooff MJH. The price of donation after cardiac death in liver transplantation: a prospective cost-effectiveness study. Transpl Int 2013.
13. Taner CB, Bulatao LG, Willingham DL, Perry DK, Siblesky L, Pungapong S, Aranda-Michel J, Keaveny AP, Kramer DJ, Nguyen JH. Events in procurement as risk factors to ischemic cholangiopathy in liver transplantation using donation after cardiac death donors. Liver Transpl. 2012;18:101–12.
14. Abt P, Crawford M, Desai N, et al. Liver transplantation from controlled non-heart-beating donors: an increased incidence of biliary complications. Transplantation. 2003;75(10):1659–63.
15. Taner CB, Bulatao IG, Perry DK, Sibulesky L, Willingham DL, Kramer DJ, Nguyen JH. Asystole to cross-clamp period predicts development of biliary complications in liver transplantation using donation after cardiac death donors. Transplant Int. 2012;25:838–46.
16. Cadranel JF, Erlinger S, Desruenne M, et al. Chronic administration of cyclosporine A induces a decrease in hepatitis excretory function in man. Dig Dis Sci. 1992;37(10):1473–6.
17. Buquets J, Figueras J, Serrano T, et al. Post reperfusion biopsies are useful in predicting complications after liver transplantation. Liver Transpl. 2001;7(5):432–5.
18. Lee YM, Obrien CB, Yamashiki N, et al. Preservation injury patterns in liver transplantation associated with poor prognosis. Transplant Proc. 2003;35:2964–6.
19. Cutrin JC, Cantino D, Biasi F, et al. Reperfusion damage to the bile canaliculi in transplanted human liver. Hepatology. 1996;24(5):1053–7.
20. Kukan M, Haddad PS. Role of hepatocytes and bile duct cells in preservation-reperfusion injury of liver grafts. Liver Transpl. 2001;7(5):381–400.

21. Nakanuma Y, Sasaki M. Expression of blood group-related antigens in the intrahepatic biliary tree and hepatocytes in normal livers and various hepatobiliary diseases. Hepatology. 1989;10(2):174–8.
22. Dahm F, Georgiev P, Clavien PA. Small-for-size syndrome after partial liver transplantation: definition, mechanisms of disease and clinical implications. Am J Transplant. 2005;5(11):2605–10.
23. Deltenre P, Valla DC. Ischemic cholangiopathy. J Hepatol. 2006;44:806–17.
24. Jain A, Costa G, Marsh W, et al. Thrombotic and nonthrombotic hepatic artery complications in adults and children following primary liver transplantation with long-term follow-up in 1000 consecutive patients. Transpl Int. 2006;19(1):27–37.
25. Silva MA, Jambulingam PS, Gunson BK, et al. Hepatic artery thrombosis following orthotopic liver transplantation: a 10-year experience from a single Centre in the United Kingdom. Liver Transpl. 2006;12(1):146–51.
26. Pastacaldi S, Teixeira R, Montalto P, Rolles K, Burroughs AK. Hepatic artery thrombosis after orthotopic liver transplantation: a review of nonsurgical causes. Liver Transpl. 2001;7:75–81.
27. Levy GA, Marsden PA. Cigarette smoking—association with hepatic artry thrombosis. Liver Transpl. 2002;8(7):588–90.
28. Pinna AD, Smith CV, Furukawa H, Starzl TE, Fung JJ. Urgent revascularization of liver allografts after early hepatic artery thrombosis. Transplantation. 1996;62:1584–7.
29. Kusne S, Blair JE. Viral and fungal infections after liver transplantation—part II. Liver Transpl. 2006;12(1):2–11.
30. Trauner M, Fickert P, Stauber RE. Inflammation-induced cholestasis. J Gastroenterol Hepatol. 1999;14(10):946–59.
31. Lefkowich JH. Bile ductular cholestasis: an ominous histopathologic sign related to sepsis and "cholangitis lenta". Hum Pathol. 1982;13(1):19–24.
32. Paya CV, Hermans PE, Wiesner RH, et al. Cytomegalovirus hepatitis in liver transplantation: prospective analysis of 93 consecutive orthotopic liver transplantations. J Infect Dis. 1989;160(5):752–8.
33. Martelius T, Krogerus L, Hockerstedt K, Bruggeman C, Lautenschlager I. Cytomegalovirus infection is associated with increased inflammation and severe bile duct damage in rat liver allografts. Hepatology. 1998;27(4):996–1002.
34. Evans PC, Coleman N, Wreghitt TG, Wright DG, Alexander GJ. Cytomegalovirus infection of bile duct epithelial cells, hepatic artery and portal venous endothelium in relation to chronic refection of liver grafts. J Hepatol. 1999;31(5):913–20.
35. Lautenschlager I, Hockerstedt K, Taskinen E. Histologic findings associated with CMV infection in liver transplantation. Transplant Proc. 2003;35(2):819.
36. Lautenschlager I, Lappalainen M, Linnavuori K, Suni J, Hockerstedt K. CMV infection is usually associated with concurrent HHV-6 and HHV-7 antigenemia in liver transplant patients. J Clin Virol. 2002;25 Suppl 2:S57–61.
37. Chan FK, Shaffer EA. Cholestatic effects of cyclosporine in the rat. Transplantation. 1997;63(11):1574–8.
38. Deters M, Klabunde T, Kirchner G, Resch K, Kaever V. Sirolimus/cyclosporine/tacrolimus interactions on bile flow and biliary excretion of immunosuppressants in a subchronic bile fistula rat model. Br J Pharmacol. 2002;136(4):604–12.
39. Sanchez-Campos S, Lopez-Acebo R, Gonzalez P, et al. Cholestasis and alteration of glutathione metabolism induced by tacrolimus (FK506) in the rat. Transplantation. 1998;66(1):84–8.
40. Deters M, Kirchner G, Koal T, Rech K, Kaever V. Everolimus/cyclosporine interactions on bile flow and biliary excretion of bile salts and cholesterol in rats. Dig Dis Sci. 2004;49(1):30–7.
41. Romagnuolo J, Sadowski DC, Lalor E, Jewell L, Thomson AB. Cholestatic hepatocellular injury with azathioprine: a case report and review of the mechanisms of hepatotoxicity. Can J Gastroenterol. 1998;12(7):479–83.
42. Vierling JM, Fennell Jr RH. Histopathology of early and late human hepatic allograft rejection: evidence of progressive destruction of interlobular bile ducts. Hepatology. 1985;5(6):1076–82.
43. Nawaz S, Fennell RH. Apoptosis of bile duct epithelial cells in hepatic allograft rejection. Histopathology. 1994;25(2):137–42.

44. Savier E, Lemasters JJ, Thurman RG. Kupffer cells participate in rejection following liver transplantation in the rat. Transpl Int. 1994;7 Suppl 1:S183–6.
45. Neuberger J. Incidence, timing, and risk factors for acute and chronic rejection. Liver Transpl Surg. 1999;5(4 Suppl 1):S30–6.
46. Batts KP. Acute and chronic hepatic allograft rejection; pathology and classification. Liver Transpl Surg. 1999;5(4 Suppl 1):S21–9.
47. Demetris AJ, Murase N, Ye Q, et al. Analysis of chronic rejection and obliterative arteriopathy. Possible contributions of donor antigen-presenting cells and lymphatic disruption. Am J Pathol. 1997;150(2):563–78.
48. Neuberger J. Recurrent primary biliary cirrhosis. Liver Transpl. 2003;9(6):539–46.
49. Sylvestre PB, Batts KP, Burgart LJ, Poterucha JJ, Wiesner RH. Recurrence of primary biliary cirrhosis after liver transplantation: histologic estimate of incidence and natural history. Liver Transpl. 2003;9(10):1086–93.
50. Jacob DA, Neumann UP, Bahra M, Langrehr JM, Nauhaus P. Liver transplantation for primary biliary cirrhosis: influence of primary immunosuppression on survival. Transplant Proc. 2005;37(4):1691–2.
51. Fosby B, Karlsen TH, Melum E. Recurrence and rejection in liver transplantation for primary sclerosing cholangitis. World J Gastroenterol. 2012;18(1):1–15.
52. Goss JA, Shackleton CR, Farmer DG, et al. Orthotopic liver transplantation for primary biliary sclerosing cholangitis. A 12-year single center experience. Ann Surg. 1997;225(5):472–81.
53. Brandsaeter B, Schrumpf E, Bentdal O, et al. Recurrent primary sclerosing cholangitis after liver transplantation: a magnetic resonance cholangiography study with analysis of predictive factors. Liver Transpl. 2005;11(11):1361–9.
54. Kugelmas M, Spiegelman P, Osgood MJ. Different immunosuppressive regimens and recurrence of primary sclerosing cholangitis after liver transplantation. Liver Transpl. 2003;9(7): 727–32.
55. Alabraba E, Nightingale P, Gunson B, Hubscher S, Olliff S, Mirza D, Neuberger J. A re-evaluation of the risk factors for the recurrence of primary sclerosing cholangitis in liver allografts. Liver Transpl. 2009;15:330–40.
56. Taga SA, Washington MK, Terrault N, et al. Cholestatic hepatitis C in liver allografts. Liver Transpl Surg. 1998;4(4):304–10.
57. Antonini TM, Sebagh M, Roque-Alfonso AM, Sobesky R, Coilly A, Vaghefi P, Adam R, Vittecoq D, Castaing D, Samuel D, Duclos-Vallee JC. Fibrosing Cholestatic hepatitis in HIV/HCV co-infected transplant patients—usefulness of early markers after liver transplantation. Am J Transplant. 2011;11:1686–95.
58. Colter SJ, Taylor SL, Gretch DR, et al. Hyperbilirubinemia and cholestatic liver injury in hepatitis C-infected liver transplant recipients. Am J Gastroenterol. 2000;95(3):753–9.
59. Coilly A, Roche B, Dumortier J, Leroy V, Botta-Fridlund D, Radenne S, Pageaux GP, Si-Ahmed SN, Guillaud O, Antonini TM, Haim-Boukobza S, Roque-Afonso AM, Samuel D, Duclos-Vallee JC. Safety and efficacy of protease inhibitors to treat hepatitis C after liver transplantation, a multicenter experience. J Hepatol. 2013;60:78–86.

Chapter 11
Cholestasis in the Hospitalized Patient

Anne M. Larson

Introduction

Cholestasis with resultant accumulation of bile acids within the liver and serum ultimately leads to hepatic toxicity. There are many potential systemic causes of cholestasis and jaundice [1]. Cholestatic patients may have underlying liver disease which has been previously unrecognized (Table 11.1) or may develop extrahepatic biliary obstruction. Intrahepatic cholestasis may result from parenteral nutrition, sepsis, or drug-induced liver injury. Those causes unique to the hematopoietic stem cell transplantation (HSCT) patient include infections seen in the immunocompromised, graft-versus-host disease (GVHD), and sinusoidal obstruction syndrome [2, 3]. Patients undergoing HSCT commonly develop cholestasis and jaundice during the peri- and posttransplant period. Fortunately, with the institution of preventive measures, the incidence of liver-related complications has declined over the last 10–15 years [2].

Extrahepatic Biliary Obstruction

Biliary obstruction is one of the more common causes of jaundice. It should be ruled out in the cholestatic hospitalized patient. Abdominal imaging and/or endoscopic diagnostic studies are generally sufficient to determine the cause. If obstruction is absent, then true hepatic cholestasis is likely.

A.M. Larson, M.D. (✉)
Swedish Liver Center, Swedish Health Systems, 1101 Madison Street #200,
Seattle, WA 98104, USA
e-mail: anne.larson@swedish.org

E.J. Carey and K.D. Lindor (eds.), *Cholestatic Liver Disease*, Clinical Gastroenterology,
DOI 10.1007/978-1-4939-1013-7_11, © Springer Science+Business Media New York 2014

Table 11.1 Liver diseases associated with jaundice

Primary biliary cirrhosis (PBC)
Primary sclerosing cholangitis (PSC)
Autoimmune sclerosing cholangitis
Granulomatous hepatitis
Hepatic amyloidosis
Congestive hepatopathy
Hepatic sarcoidosis
Systemic viral infections
• Hepatitis Viruses (A, B, C, D, E)
• Cytomegalovirus (CMV)
• Epstein–Barr virus (EBV)
Hemophagocytic syndrome

Cholestasis of Sepsis (Cholangitis Lenta)

Pathogenesis

To understand the pathology of cholestasis of sepsis, one must understand the basics of bile processing. A primary hepatic function is the removal of organic anions (such as bilirubin), cations, and bile acids from the circulation. Hepatic bile salt and anionic steroidal compound uptake is mediated by the sinusoidal Na^+/Taurocholate Co-transporting Polypeptide (NTCP), which is driven by the hepatocyte cellular sodium gradient. Organic anions such as bilirubin and cations are taken across the hepatocyte basolateral membrane in a sodium-independent manner by groups of transport proteins with overlapping specificity—Organic Cation Transporters (OCTs), Organic Anion Transporting Polypeptides (OATPs), and Organic Anion Transporters (OATs) [4, 5]. Thus, the liver plays a crucial role in bile acid metabolism and secretion [6].

Following uptake and processing, the hepatocytes then secrete the bile acids into the bile canaliculus. Bile formation is both bile acid-dependent, related to the bile salt excretion, and bile acid-independent, related to active secretion of the inorganic electrolytes and solutes [7, 8]. The bile canalicular transporters are members of the adenosine triphosphate (ATP)-binding cassette (ABC) superfamily (see Phase III Reactions, below) [9]. Canalicular secretion of bile acids is medicated by the bile salt export pump (BSEP/ABCB11), which transports bile acids across a concentration gradient and is the rate limited step in their secretion [10–15]. Secretion of the non-bile acid organic anions is medicated by the multidrug resistance-associated protein 2 (MRP2/ABCC2), formerly known as the canalicular multispecific organic anion transporter (cMOAT) [15–17]. Organic cations are secreted into the bile by the multidrug resistant P-glycoprotein 1 (MDR1/ABCB1) and MDR3 (ABCB4). These membrane transporters are regulated at the level of gene transcription, RNA translation, and posttranslationally [7, 18].

Cholestasis of sepsis (CoS) has been linked predominantly to gram-negative bacterial infections, although any significant extrahepatic systemic infection can cause it [1, 7, 19–24]. Following malignant biliary obstruction, CoS is the second most common cause of jaundice in the hospitalized patient [1, 25]. Bacterial cell walls contain lipopolysaccharides (LPS), called endotoxins, which are powerful inducers of proinflammatory cytokines, such as interleukin-1 (IL1), interleukin 6 (IL6), and tumor necrosis factor alpha (TNFα). Endotoxins and the proinflammatory cytokines they induce play a key role in the development of CoS.

Endotoxins increase intestinal permeability, leading to escape of bacterial cell wall components and endotoxin into the portal venous system [26]. This results in the accumulation of endotoxin within the liver which ultimately causes significant injury [1, 27–29]. Proinflammatory cytokines subsequently secreted by the Kupffer cells play a central role in further mediating CoS [1, 27, 30]. The cytokines may lead to expression of ligands on the sinusoidal endothelial cells, Kupffer cells, and hepatocytes, stimulating margination of neutrophils with subsequent release of superoxide radicals and enzymes. This promotes further hepatocellular injury [31–36]. Endotoxins act as powerful cholestatic agents by inhibiting both hepatocellular bile acid uptake (via NTCP and OATP) and canalicular bile secretion (via BSEP and MRP2) [31, 37–41]. Endotoxemia reduces the excretion of conjugated bile acids and bilirubin-glucuronides, and decreases bile flow [7, 41]. It severely impairs both bile acid-dependent and bile acid-independent organic anion transport at the sinusoidal and canalicular membranes [37, 42–44]. The reductions in anion transport are correlated with decreased protein and mRNA levels [38, 42, 45, 46]. Bile acid-independent biliary flow and biliary HCO_3 secretion are reduced [37, 47]. Pretreatment with medications which block the LPS-mediated release of cytokines significantly attenuates the reduction in bile acid secretion and bile flow, confirming the critical role of these molecules in the development of CoS [39, 43, 44, 48, 49].

Clinical

The association of jaundice and bacterial infection was described as early as 1837 [50]. Cholestasis of sepsis, historically called cholangitis lenta, should always be considered in the differential diagnosis of any hospitalized patient who develops jaundice [25]. Cholestasis of sepsis is associated with disproportionate elevations in serum alkaline phosphatase and bilirubin compared with serum aminotransferase levels [51]. An isolated elevation in the bilirubin level may be the only abnormality seen [7]. The bilirubin elevation and cholestasis may be even more pronounced in patients with underlying hepatobiliary disease, such as sinusoidal obstruction syndrome, GVHD, or other biliary tract disorders. Bilirubin levels can approach 30 mg/dL in the septic patient in this setting [51]. In the HSCT recipient, fever and infection generally occur during the first month, when the granulocyte counts are at their nadir. Elevations in bilirubin level may even precede positive blood cultures, and a continued rise in a patient with underlying liver disease is correlated with a worse outcome [7, 51]. Treatment is directed at the underlying infection.

Liver biopsy is rarely necessary for the diagnosis of CoS. When performed in the setting of uncomplicated CoS; however, the most prominent histological finding is that of pericentral canalicular or periportal ductular cholestasis [52]. This can be associated with Kupffer cell hyperplasia, portal mononuclear inflammation, focal hepatocyte dropout, and steatosis [7, 22–24, 51]. Those who are immunosuppressed often do not show evidence of the portal inflammation seen in the immunocompetent patient [31]. Patients who are at greatest risk of dying may have a more uncommon form of CoS in which the portal and periportal bile ductules are dilated with inspissated bile [53].

Parenteral Nutrition

The use of parenteral nutrition (PN) is often critical to providing nutritional support to those who are unable to be fed enterally. Its prolonged use, however, can result in multiple complications, including metabolic bone disease, line infections, and PN-associated liver disease (PNLD), particularly cholestasis [28, 54].

Extrahepatic Complications

The most common extrahepatic complications of PN in adults include the development of biliary sludge, gallstones, and acalculous cholecystitis [28, 55–58]. Complete bowel rest decreases the production of cholecystokinin (CCK) resulting in decreased gallbladder contraction, inhibition of sphincter of Oddi relaxation, and decreased biliary flow [28, 59]. This leads to stasis and biliary sludge formation [60]. Biliary sludge has been shown to be present in all patients within 6 weeks of starting PN [56, 58]. Gallstones, which become evident after about 4 months of PN, are generally pigment stones [61]. Both calculous and acalculous cholecystitis have been reported.

Intrahepatic Complications

Many patients will develop mild to moderate liver enzyme elevations upon starting PN; however, these generally stabilize by 1–2 weeks and are not usually associated with histologic findings [62]. The liver disease associated with PN can be extremely severe. It has been assumed that the longer the duration of use of PN, the greater the risk of developing chronic liver disease; however, more recently this dogma has been questioned [63]. Chronic cholestasis has been reported in over 50 % of patients and between 15 and 40 % of patients receiving PN will develop end-stage liver disease [28, 64–66]. PNLD can lead to irreversible liver failure, with mortality rates as high as 51 % [67–69].

Multiple histologic findings are seen in the setting of PNLD. Hepatic steatosis is generally the earliest finding noted in adults and may be associated with excess glucose in the PN [28]. Most patients will have some degree of hepatic steatosis following 3 or more months of PN [55]. Over time, patients develop a pattern of injury which includes cholestasis, steatosis, portal edema and inflammation, ductular reaction and ductopenia, and portal and perivenular fibrosis [63].

The etiology of PNLD is most likely multifactorial; however, the precise cause remains unknown [54, 68, 70, 71]. Multiple factors have been proposed. PN-induced changes in bile composition may lead to biliary injury, bile sludging, bile duct obstruction, and subsequent hepatocyte injury [55, 58, 72, 73]. The use of PN with excess calories, particularly in the form of carbohydrates, leads to fatty acid synthesis and development of hepatic steatosis [28]. In fact, a direct correlation has been reported between total PN calories and fatty infiltration [74]. Hyperinsulinemia subsequently develops which stimulates glycolysis, fatty acid esterification, glycogenolysis, and gluconeogenesis and inhibits fatty acid oxidation [75–77]. Lipids may also play a role in PNLD [64]. Lipid emulsions contain phytosterols and omega-6 fatty acids which have been associated with inhibition of bile acid secretion and bile acid-stimulated bile flow [78–81]. Both serum and tissue levels of antioxidants, including glutathione, β-carotene, and vitamin E, are markedly reduced in patients on PN [28, 82, 83]. Conversely, the products of oxidative injury are increased [84]. Oxidative injury and subsequent hepatocyte apoptosis also play a role in PNLD [85]. Nutrient deficiencies, such as choline, glutamine, and taurine, may also contribute to the development of PNLD [28, 86, 87].

Management

The ideal management is to maximize enteral feeding, although this is not always possible. Multiple attempts have been made to optimize the composition of PN in an effort to prevent or decrease the associated PNLD. The most common of these changes include avoiding excess calories, decreasing amino acid content, or adding lipids, glutamine, choline, and lecithin [55]. The response has been mixed; however, and PNLD remains a significant clinical problem [63, 88]. Allowing a daily PN-free period of time of 8 h or more has also been reported to improve liver enzymes [89]. The use of ursodeoxycholic acid has been shown in small studies to improve liver enzymes [90–92]. Liver transplantation may ultimately be required if the PNLD progresses to liver failure.

Drug-Induced Cholestasis

Drugs must be considered in the differential diagnosis of cholestasis in the hospitalized patient. The liver is responsible for the selective uptake, concentration, metabolism, and excretion of the majority of drugs, toxins, and xenobiotics ("substances") introduced into the body. Each substance has a specific disposal pathway involving one or more of the soluble or membrane-bound enzymes which process these substances. The majority of substances absorbed from the gastrointestinal tract are lipophilic and water-insoluble and they must be rendered water-soluble to be excreted.

Drug Metabolism

Exogenous substances are metabolized mainly via phase I or phase II reactions, or a combination of both (Fig. 11.1) [93–95]. The final products are then moved across the canalicular or sinusoidal membranes via excretory transporters (phase III reactions) [96]. Genetic polymorphisms exist in all of these enzymes, which can lead to either decreased or increased activity, and may predispose to xenobiotic-induced cholestasis or injury [97–105].

Phase I Reactions

Phase I reactions transform lipophilic molecules into more polar, hydrophilic molecules via oxidation, reduction, or hydrolysis. These reactions are catalyzed by the membrane-bound cytochrome P450 (CYP) family of mixed function oxidases

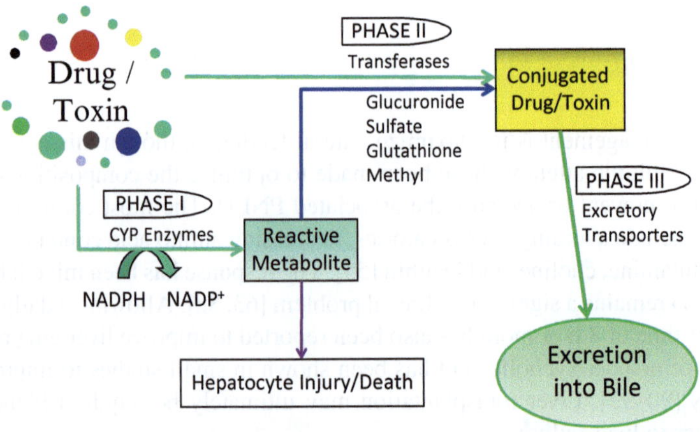

Fig. 11.1 Xenobiotic Metabolism. Exogenous substances are metabolized via phase I or phase II reactions, or a combination of both. The final products are then moved across the canalicular or sinusoidal membranes via excretory transporters (phase III reactions) for disposal

[106–110]. The P450 molecules are hemoproteins composed of an apoprotein and a heme prosthetic group (the oxidizing center). There are over 50 proteins in the CYP group which are organized into 18 families (e.g., CYP2) and 43 subfamilies (e.g., CYP2E1) [111]. Most are located on the cytoplasmic side of the smooth ER membrane (microsomal-type) or the mitochondria (mitochondrial type) [111]. Phase I drug metabolism is performed predominantly via the microsomal-type. There is zonal heterogeneity of these enzymes within the liver—some are more prominent in the perivenular (zone 3) hepatocytes (i.e., P450 2E1), while others are clustered within other acinar zones. Hepatic metabolism of exogenous drugs and toxins is performed mainly by the CYP1, CYP2, and CYP3 families, with a smaller contribution from CYP4 [111–117]. The most important drug metabolizing member within the liver is CYP3A4, which comprises about 60 % of all hepatic cytochromes and catalyzes the biotransformation of over 50 % of commonly used drugs [111, 118]. Free radicals and toxic electrophilic compounds can be produced during this process.

Phase II Reactions

Phase II reactions occur either directly with a parent compound (rare) or with a metabolite formed by a phase I reaction which is still not adequately hydrophilic for excretion. These reactions conjugate the metabolic byproducts to highly polar ligands, such as glucuronate, sulfate, acetate, glycine, glutathione, or a methyl group (Fig. 11.1). The resultant water-soluble substances are nontoxic and readily excreted [95, 119, 120]. Phase II reactions occur primarily within the hepatocyte cytoplasm via the UDP-glucuronyl transferases (UGT1 and UGT2), sulfotransferases, and glutathione S-transferases [93]. Conjugation ordinarily leads to a decrease in pharmacologic activity (detoxification) and phase II enzymes are rarely responsible for toxic metabolite formation; however, exceptions do occur.

Phase III Reactions

Phase III reactions lead to the transport of compounds across the canalicular membranes and into the bile [119]. As noted above, the bile canalicular transporters include multidrug resistant P-glycoprotein 1 (MDR1/ABCB1), MDR3 (ABCB4), multidrug resistant protein 2 (MRP2/ABCC2), and the bile sale export protein (BSEP/ABCB11) [11]. Their predominant role is that of regulation of bile formation and the excretion of xenobiotics [11]. Emerging data suggests that cholestatic drug induced liver injury (DILI) is secondary to drug- or metabolite-mediated inhibition of these transporters [11, 121].

Hepatotoxicity

Because of the liver's central role in detoxification, it is uniquely susceptible to DILI. More than a thousand drugs and herbal products have been reported to cause hepatotoxicity (Table 11.2) [122]. Those most commonly associated with cholestasis in the setting of HSCT include calcineurin inhibitors (particularly cyclosporine), azole antifungal agents, trimethoprim-sulfamethoxazole, ribavirin, busulfan, and bis-chloroethylnitrosourea [2].

Up to 5 % of the jaundice seen in hospitalized patients is caused by drugs [25, 123–125]. Cholestatic and mixed cholestatic/hepatocellular injury account for up to half of all drug-induced liver disease, and are its most severe presentation [121, 126–128]. Drugs dosed at over 50 mg daily are more likely to cause DILI than those with daily doses less than this amount [129, 130]. Additionally, drugs which are significantly hepatically metabolized and excreted into the bile are the most likely to produce cholestatic liver injury [131]. This injury may be manifest at any of the enzyme sites along the metabolism pathway.

Table 11.2 Examples of drugs associated with cholestasis [2, 121]

Anti-infectives	• Amoxicillin–clavulanate • Erythromycin, clarithromycin, and azithromycin • Trimethoprim/sulfamethoxazole • Azole antifungal agents • Flucloxacillin, dicloxacillin • Nitrofurantoin • Isoniazid, rifampin • Ciprofloxacin • Cephalosporins • Terbinafine • HIV antivirals—stavudine, didanosine, nevirapine
Anti-inflammatories	• Azathioprine • Diclofenac • Ibuprofen • Sulindac • Nimesulide
Psychotropics	• Chlorpromazine • Imipramine, amitryptyline • Duloxetine • Risperidone
Chemotherapeutics	• Busulfan • Cytarabine • Bis-chloroethylnitrosourea
Others	• Estrogens/oral contraceptives • Anabolic steroids • Calcineurin inhibitors (i.e., cyclosporine) • ACE Inhibitors • Clopidogrel • Irbesartan • Phenothiazines

Table 11.3 Liver test abnormality classification [143]

Hepatitis (hepatocellular)	Cholestasis	Mixed
ALT $\geq 3 \times$ ULN	AlkPhos $\geq 2 \times$ ULN	ALT $\geq 3 \times$ ULN AlkPhos $\geq 2 \times$ ULN
$R \geq 5$	$R \leq 2$	$R > 2$ to < 5

ALT alanine aminotransferase, *AlkPhos* alkaline phosphatase, *ULN* upper limit of normal, *R*—ALT/ULN divided by AlkPhos/ULN

Cholestasis secondary to DILI is defined as an elevated alkaline phosphatase (AlkPhos) greater than two times the upper limit of normal and/or an alanine aminotransferase (ALT) to AlkPhos ratio of less than 2 (Table 11.3) [121]. Injury is considered to be mixed if the ALT/AlkPhos ratio is greater than 2 but less than 5 and hepatocellular if this ratio is >5. The presence of jaundice (serum bilirubin >2 times the upper limit of normal) in association with an elevation in serum aminotransferases (>3 times the upper limit of normal) is associated with a worse prognosis than that seen in the setting of isolated aminotransferase abnormalities (an observation noted by Hyman Zimmerman and known as "Hy's law") [132, 133]. In this setting, the mortality is as high as 14 % [121, 126, 134–136].

Clinical Features

DILI must remain in the differential diagnosis of all patients presenting with cholestasis. Drug-induced cholestatic liver injury can present either acutely or chronically, mimicking many extrahepatic and intrahepatic liver diseases. Presentation may be weeks to months after beginning the offending agent. Patients may be asymptomatic with only isolated elevations in alkaline phosphatase or they may be frankly jaundiced and symptomatic [122]. Fever, nausea, anorexia, malaise, fatigue, pruritus, and/or abdominal pain or discomfort may also be present. Cholestatic DILI is more common in those over 60 years of age and in those with certain genetic polymorphisms, such as HLA DRB1*15 and HLADQB1*06 [129, 137, 138]. It remains unclear whether underlying liver disease is a predisposing risk factor for cholestatic DILI [121]. Cholestasis and jaundice tend to be prolonged after discontinuation of the offending agent, and can take weeks to months to resolve. If prolonged, patients may develop xanthomas, pruritus, and melanoderma [122].

Diagnosis

The diagnosis of DILI can be difficult. Prior to attributing cholestasis to a certain drug or toxin, a complete evaluation must be undertaken to rule out other causes. Abdominal imaging may be necessary to rule out obstructive disease. Cholestasis secondary to sepsis, TPN or heart failure must be eliminated [121].

Certain infections, such as cholestatic hepatitis A virus, Epstein–Barr virus, typhoid fever, or Q fever can also present with a cholestatic picture [121, 139–141]. Obtaining a careful drug history is important but not always reliable—the relationship between exposure to the drug and cholestasis is not always clear. Hospitalized patients are often taking multiple medications, making identification of a single offending agent difficult. Extrahepatic manifestations caused by the offending agent, such as rash, interstitial nephritis, or other organ toxicity may be helpful in eliciting the diagnosis [122].

There is no gold standard, specific serum biomarker or characteristic histologic feature that reliably identifies a drug as the cause of toxicity [121]. The Council for International Organizations of Medical Sciences (CIOMS) developed a series of standard designations of drug-induced liver disorders and classification of injury [142]. The US FDA Drug Hepatotoxicity Steering Committee proposed modifications to the CIOMS scheme for classifying hepatotoxicity in clinical trials (Table 11.3) [143]. The most commonly used scale to codify causality of drug toxicity is CIOMS Roussel-Uclaf Causality Assessment Method (RUCAM) scale [142, 144, 145]. These assessments do not address all risk factors in all patients, and none are used routinely in clinical practice.

Features which suggest drug toxicity include a lack of illness prior to ingesting the drug, clinical illness or biochemical abnormalities developing after beginning the drug, and improvement after the drug is withdrawn. The illness will generally recur upon reintroduction of the offending substance if the DILI is immunologic; therefore, rechallenge is not advised. Nonspecific symptoms developing after introduction of a drug (such as nausea, anorexia, malaise, fatigue, right upper quadrant pain, or pruritus) may indicate drug toxicity and should prompt evaluation. Key elements for attributing liver injury to a drug include [146]:

- Exposure must precede the onset of liver injury (although the latent period is highly variable)
- Underlying liver disease should be excluded
- Injury may improve when the drug is stopped (although in some cases injury may initially worsen for days or weeks, while in fulminant cases, declining liver biochemical tests may indicate deterioration rather than improvement)
- Liver injury may have recurred more rapidly and severely after repeated exposure

Histologically, drug-induced cholestatic liver injury can be classified as either bland, without associated inflammation, or as cholestatic hepatitis, with inflammatory changes [147]. These changes may include portal inflammation, portal neutrophils and plasma cells, fibrosis, and intracellular cholestasis and can resemble autoimmune hepatitis [148]. DILI most often leads to cholestatic hepatitis [121, 147].

Treatment

No specific therapies have been shown to alter the clinical course of DILI. Most cases of mild cholestatic DILI will resolve with discontinuation of the drug which caused it. Chronic progressive disease can develop; however, potentially leading to vanishing bile duct syndrome, biliary cirrhosis, and ultimately progression to liver failure and death [121, 135, 149]. Patients with cholestatic DILI are more likely to develop chronic liver disease than those with hepatocellular DILI [121, 150]. Liver transplantation can be considered in appropriate patients who develop liver failure.

Lymphoma

Liver involvement with either Hodgkin or, more commonly, non-Hodgkin lymphoma can lead to cholestasis [1]. Primary hepatic lymphoma, in the absence of systemic disease, is rare and accounts for <1 % of cases [151]. Forty to 70 % of patients with hepatic disease will have elevations in serum alkaline phosphatase and bilirubin. Diffuse large cell type B-cell lymphoma is responsible for most cases of primary hepatic lymphoma [151]. A more rare form of hepatosplenic T-cell lymphoma may also cause cholestasis in the afflicted patient [1, 152]. Solid organ and HSCT recipients are at risk for post-transplant lymphoproliferative disorder (PTLD) [153, 154]. This Epstein–Barr virus associated type of non-Hodgkin lymphoma can involve the liver and can lead to either intrahepatic or extrahepatic (obstructive) cholestasis [1].

Graft-Versus-Host Disease

GVHD is a major complication following HSCT which can involve the liver, among many other organ systems [2]. Its incidence has been reported in up to 80 % of transplant recipients, depending on the type of transplant [155]. GVHD presents as either acute—within the first 100 days after HSCT—or chronic disease.

Pathogenesis

GVHD develops when donor-derived T-cells expand within the recipient and recognize host antigens as foreign. Several risk factors predispose to the development of GVHD, including HLA mismatch, gender mismatch, reduced-intensity conditioning, and high number of T-cells transported from the donor [156, 157]. Acute GVHD (aGVHD) results directly from the degree of human leukocyte antigen (HLA) mismatch. The donor cytotoxic T-cells target host hepatocytes, epithelial cells of the small bile ducts and periductal glands [158]. Host cell death is mediated by apoptosis via the Fas/Fas ligand pathway. Histologically, there is lymphocytic infiltration and destruction of bile ducts as well as endothelialitis [159, 160]. Apoptotic bodies are seen [159]. Bile duct injury is also typical of chronic GVHD (cGVHD); however, development of fibrosis is rare unless there is concomitant underlying liver disease.

Clinical

Liver involvement in aGVHD generally follows skin involvement, which consists of a maculopapular rash involving the palms and soles. Acute disease is often a diagnosis of exclusion, the differential including sinusoidal obstruction syndrome, viral infection, drug toxicity, and sepsis [155]. The patient develops cholestatic liver injury and subsequent jaundice. Tender hepatomegaly and fluid retention are common and patients may develop fever, nausea, and anorexia [155]. Serum biochemistries will generally show an elevation in conjugated bilirubin, alkaline phosphatase, and gamma-glutamyltranspeptidase, although a more hepatitic presentation with elevations in alanine aminotransferase has been described [155, 161–163]. Coagulopathy and elevated ammonia levels can be seen. Acute GVHD is considered to be severe if the serum bilirubin level is >6.1 mg/dL, and the prognosis is poor in this setting [164]. The grade of aGVHD severity, generally based upon the modified Seattle Glucksberg criteria, carries prognostic significance (Table 11.4) [165–167].

Chronic GVHD (cGVHD) develops 100 days or more after transplant. Those who develop aGVHD are more likely to develop cGVHD, but this is not a prerequisite. Additionally, older age is a risk factor for its development [157]. Chronic GHVD can have similar clinical findings to aGVHD or presents with overlap features of both acute and chronic disease [155, 168]. Features which are diagnostic of cGVHD include skin poikiloderma, lichen planus, lichen-type changes on mucus membranes, fasciitis, and joint contractures [155]. Distinctive features include alopecia, nail dystrophy, xerostomia, mucoceles, mouth ulceration, keratoconjunctivitis sicca, and myositis. Liver involvement is evidenced by continued or worsening cholestasis. There may be sudden or progressive elevation in the alkaline phosphatase and gamma glutamyl transpeptidase. The development of hyperbilirubinemia is generally late in the course and coincides with the development of cirrhosis and small bile duct destruction [159]. cGVHD is classified as mild, moderate, or severe (Table 11.5) [168, 169]. The differential diagnosis includes viral infection, and liver biopsy

Table 11.4 Grading of acute graft-versus-host disease [165–167]

	Skin rash	Bilirubin (mg/dL)	Gut fluid loss
Grade I	<25 % of body	1.52–3.5	500–1,000 mL/day
Grade II	25–50 %	3.57–8.0	1,000–1,500 mL/day
Grade III	>50 % or erythroderma	8.0–15.0	>1,500 mL/day
Grade IV	Bullae; desquamation of skin	>15	>2,500 mL/day or ileus

Table 11.5 Staging of chronic graft-versus-host disease [168, 169]

Mild	• Involvement of 1 or 2 organs (not lung involvement) with a score of 1
Moderate	• Involvement of 3 organs with a score of 1, or • Involvement of 1 organ with a score of 2, or • Pulmonary involvement with a score of 1
Severe	• Major disability in any site, or • Pulmonary involvement with a score of 2 or 3

Scoring: 0—no involvement; 1—mild involvement but not impairment of daily living; 2—moderate involvement with significant impairment of daily living; 3—severe impairment with major disability should be performed in this setting to establish the diagnosis. Up to 80 % of patients will show improvement with initiation of immunosuppressive therapy—corticosteroids with or without a calcineurin inhibitor. Additionally, ursodeoxycholic acid may be used. Patients who fail to respond have a poor long-term prognosis [2].

Treatment

The use of prophylactic immunosuppression has been associated with a 20–25 % decreased incidence of aGVHD and subsequently cGHVD [155, 170]. Ursodeoxycholic has also been shown to reduce the incidence of hepatic aGVHD and is generally used prophylactically during the first 80 days following HSCT [171, 172].

Grade I aGVHD rarely requires systemic therapy. Corticosteroids and calcineurin inhibitors (i.e., cyclosporin, tacrolimus) form the backbone of therapy for those with grade II–IV aGVHD [157, 165]. Immunosuppression leads to resolution in about 30–50 % of cases, with long-term survival rates of 60 % in this group [165, 173–177]. Patients who fail first-line therapy may require extracorporeal photopheresis, anti-tumor necrosis factor alpha (anti-TNFα) antibodies, mTOR (mammalian target of rapamycin) inhibitors, mycophenolate mofetil, or interleukin-2 receptor antibodies [165, 178–180]. Third-line agents include mesenchymal stem cells, alemtuzumab (Campath 1H), or pentostatin [165]. Long-term survival in this group drops to only 20–35 % [174]. Patients who fail therapy may go on to develop cGVHD [2]. Therapy is similar to that of aGVHD using systemic corticosteroids. Failing that, second-line therapies include extracorporeal photopheresis, mTOR inhibitors, rituximab, pentostatin, methotrexate, or mycophenolate mofetil.

Sinusoidal Obstruction Syndrome (SOS)

Veno-occlusive disease (VOD) was first described in 1920 following ingestion of Senecio tea containing pyrrolizidine alkaloids [181]. It was first described following HSCT in 1979 [182, 183]. The term veno-occlusive disease has fallen out of favor and has been replaced by sinusoidal obstruction syndrome as a better reflection of its pathophysiology [184, 185]. Development of SOS is related to the conditioning regimen used prior to stem cell infusion (myeloablative HSCT) with a variably reported incidence of 5–70 %, with a mean incidence of about 14 % [2, 186–191]. It has a reported mortality of up to 50 %, averaging 15–20 % [184, 192, 193].

Pathogenesis

The primary inciting event is the randomly distributed development of hepatic sinusoidal endothelial injury usually within zone 3 of the hepatic acinus [184, 186, 194–196]. Loss of endothelial cell fenestrations occurs and gaps in the endothelial cell lining form, ultimately leading to frank endothelial denudation and loss of sinusoidal integrity [197]. Involvement of the hepatic venules is not essential to the diagnosis and is present in 50–75 % of cases [184, 194, 198–200]. There is edematous thickening in the subintimal zone of the central and sublobular venules. This leads to concentric luminal narrowing with subsequent increased resistance to blood flow, resulting in hepatic congestion, sinusoidal dilation, and portal hypertension [184]. The congestion is associated with extravasation of red blood cells into the perisinusoidal space (space of Disse) [198]. Fragmented red blood cells, fibrin, and factor VIII have been shown to be present, and contribute further to partial to complete fibrotic obliteration of the venules [2, 195]. Focal ischemia leads to progressive derangements within the liver, with cytokine release [201, 202]. Hepatocyte atrophy, injury and death occur, prominently localized to the centrilobular region. Injury can be potentiated by medications used in the prophylaxis of GVHD such as sirolimus and tacrolimus [203]. SOS may also be associated with other liver lesions, including peliosis hepatis, nodular regenerative hyperplasia, and centrilobular and venular fibrosis [198, 204–206].

Controversy remains as to whether the coagulation pathways play a role in the pathogenesis of SOS [184, 204]. There is evidence that the damaged endothelium elicits activation of the coagulation cascade [2, 193, 207–210]. Levels of anticoagulant proteins are decreased in patients with SOS, while levels of procoagulant proteins are elevated [209–213]. It remains unclear whether this is cause or effect, as the presence of thrombi in the sinusoids and venules is uncommon [184, 194].

The drugs which lead to SOS show preferential toxicity to sinusoidal endothelial cells rather than other cell types within the liver [214, 215]. The incidence of SOS appears to be higher in patients undergoing allogeneic compared with autologous HSCT, although this may be related more to the type of conditioning regimen [184, 188]. Additional risk factors for the development of SOS include preexisting liver disease, hepatic metastases, advanced age, female gender, unrelated or HLA-mismatched related donors, prior use of vancomycin, acyclovir, norethisterone or gemtuzumab ozogamicin, use of the conditioning agents cyclophosphamide, busulfan, melphalan, and/or high dose total body irradiation over 14 Gy, and concomitant sirolimus use [158, 184, 188, 189, 191, 216–224]. Risk may be cumulative if patients require a second HSCT and were previously exposed to these agents. Cyclophosphamide carries the greatest risk for causing SOS. It is metabolized by cytochrome P450 into its therapeutic metabolite, phosphoramide, and the toxic metabolite, acrolein. Acrolein causes injury to the adjacent endothelial cells which can be ameliorated by glutathione [184, 225–228]. Glutathione is then depleted by over 95 % prior to onset of hepatic toxicity [229]. The use of *N*-acetylcysteine has shown mixed results. Toxicity is more likely if cyclophosphamide is combined with total body irradiation over 14 Gy [223, 230]. The incidence of SOS can be decreased by fractionating the total body irradiation dosing or increasing the interval between irradiation and cytotoxic therapy [217, 231, 232]. Busulfan given concurrently with cyclophosphamide potentiates its hepatotoxicity [217, 233]. The risk increases when the area under the curve for busulfan is >1,500 μmol/min/L and thus close monitoring of its serum levels is critical [234, 235]. Gemtuzumab ozogamicin is a monoclonal antibody against CD33. It carries a 15–40 % risk of causing sinusoidal injury, particularly if given prior to cyclophosphamide [236]. This antibody was withdrawn from the US market in 2010.

Clinical

Clinical criteria for the diagnosis of SOS have been developed (Table 11.6) [190, 223]. Patients present within the first 3–4 weeks after HSCT with a wide spectrum of severity, ranging from mild, reversible disease to severe often fatal illness (Table 11.7) [2, 184, 192, 193, 199, 200, 223]. Classically, SOS is characterized by rapid weight gain with or without ascites, tender hepatomegaly, and elevated bilirubin/jaundice. Asymptomatic weight gain precedes the other symptoms, occurring within 6–8 days of the transplant in the majority of patients and results from avid renal sodium and water retention. Within days, an isolated elevation in conjugated bilirubin becomes obvious [184]. Elevations in alkaline phosphatase and serum aminotransferases accompany the progressive increase in bilirubin. Patients complain of right upper quadrant pain, which can be severe enough to require narcotic pain relief. Half of those with severe SOS develop hepatorenal syndrome and 25–50 % require hemodialysis [2]. The fluid overload and thrombocytopenia are refractory to therapy [193, 237]. As disease advances, SOS can lead to prolonged prothrombin time, encephalopathy, and/or multiorgan failure.

Table 11.6 Criteria for diagnosis of sinusoidal obstruction syndrome

Baltimore criteria [190]	Modified Seattle criteria [223]

Within 21 days of transplantation:
• Serum bilirubin > 2 mg/dL (34 μmol/L)
• At least two of the following:
  • Hepatomegaly
  • >5 % weight gain from baseline
  • Ascites
	Within 20 days of transplantation, at least two of the following:
	• Serum bilirubin >2 mg/dL (34 μmol/L)
	• Hepatomegaly with right upper quadrant pain
	• >2 % weight gain from baseline due to fluid retention

Table 11.7 Staging of sinusoidal obstruction syndrome [223]

Mild	• No adverse effects of liver disease, and • No medications required for diuresis or hepatic pain, and • All symptoms, signs and laboratory features reversible
Moderate	• Adverse effects of liver disease present, and • Sodium restriction or diuretics required, or • Medication for hepatic pain required, and • All symptoms, signs and laboratory features reversible
Severe	• Adverse effects of liver disease present, and • Symptoms, signs or laboratory features not resolved by day +100, or • Death

Diagnosis

One must rule out other causes of cholestatic liver injury, including aGVHD, cyclosporine-induced hepatotoxicity, fungal infection, viral hepatitis, cholestasis of sepsis, drug-induced cholestasis, PNLD, and persistent tumor infiltration. Hepatic Doppler imaging often shows ascites, hepatomegaly, hepatic vein dilation and, late in the course of disease, evidence of portal hypertension with reversal of venous flow in the portal veins [238]. Magnetic resonance imaging reveals hepatomegaly, hepatic vein narrowing, periportal cuffing, ascites, and signs of reduced portal venous flow velocity [184]. Liver biopsy remains the gold standard for diagnosis, but may not be needed. When performed, it should be via the transjugular route and hepatic venous pressure gradients should be obtained. A gradient of over 10 mmHg has a specificity of >90 % and a positive predictive value of over 85 % for SOS [239, 240]. Elevated serum markers of endothelial injury, such as plasminogen activator inhibitor type-1 (PAI-1), can be measured and may be useful as a diagnostic and prognostic biomarker of SOS [241].

Treatment

Successful management of SOS involves prevention if possible. Alteration of the conditioning regimen and/or the GVHD prophylaxis may decrease the incidence of SOS [241]. The use of prophylactic ursodeoxycholic acid has been shown to reduce the incidence of SOS [171]. Defibrotide has shown some promise in decreasing the incidence of SOS, but large randomized controlled trials are lacking [242]. No clear evidence of preventive benefit has been shown with prostaglandin E1, tissue plasminogen activator, *N*-acetylcysteine, human antithrombin III concentrate, activated protein C, low-dose heparin, albumin, or prednisone [216, 241, 243, 244]. Low-dose dopamine may be of some benefit in patients with hepatorenal syndrome.

Mild SOS is self-limited, and no treatment is required. Unfortunately, there are no known effective treatments for moderate to severe disease and care remains largely supportive. Severe SOS is heralded by a rapidly rising serum bilirubin and increasing aminotransferase levels, progressing to portal vein thrombosis and multiorgan failure. It carries a mortality rate of over 80 % [186, 193]. The use of systemic anticoagulants and thrombolytics has been mixed, showing no survival advantage, and is associated with significant bleeding complications [216]. Defibrotide has been shown to improve the signs and symptoms of SOS in about 42 % of those afflicted [241, 245].

Summary

Cholestasis in the hospitalized patient has a broad differential given the numerous potential systemic causes [1]. In the HSCT, cholestasis is often an ominous sign of poor outcome, although preventive measures have improved survival. Diagnosis requires a thorough history and evaluation. Patients require aggressive supportive care and removal of the cause of cholestasis if possible.

References

1. Delemos AS, Friedman LS. Systemic causes of cholestasis. Clin Liver Dis. 2013;17(2): 301–17.
2. Tuncer HH, Rana N, Milani C, Darko A, Al-Homsi SA. Gastrointestinal and hepatic complications of hematopoietic stem cell transplantation. World J Gastroenterol. 2012;18(16): 1851–60.
3. Gratwohl A, Baldomero H, Aljurf M, Pasquini MC, Bouzas LF, Yoshimi A, et al. Hematopoietic stem cell transplantation: a global perspective. JAMA. 2010;303(16):1617–24.
4. Kimoto E, Yoshida K, Balogh LM, Bi YA, Maeda K, El-Kattan AF, et al. Characterization of organic anion transporting polypeptide (OATP) expression and its functional contribution to the uptake of substrates in human hepatocytes. Mol Pharm. 2012;9(12):3535–42.
5. Iusuf D, van de Steeg E, Schinkel AH. Functions of OATP1A and 1B transporters in vivo: insights from mouse models. Trends Pharmacol Sci. 2012;33(2):100–8.
6. Vlahcevic ZR, Heuman DM, Hylemon PB. Regulation of bile acid synthesis. Hepatology. 1991;13(3):590–600.
7. Moseley RH. Sepsis and cholestasis. Clin Liver Dis. 2004;8(1):83–94.
8. Trauner M, Boyer JL. Bile salt transporters: molecular characterization, function, and regulation. Physiol Rev. 2003;83(2):633–71.
9. Pauli-Magnus C, Meier PJ. Hepatocellular transporters and cholestasis. J Clin Gastroenterol. 2005;39(4 Suppl 2):S103–10.
10. Kubitz R, Droge C, Stindt J, Weissenberger K, Haussinger D. The bile salt export pump (BSEP) in health and disease. Clin Res Hepatol Gastroenterol. 2012;36(6):536–53.
11. Pauli-Magnus C, Meier PJ. Hepatobiliary transporters and drug-induced cholestasis. Hepatology. 2006;44(4):778–87.
12. Jansen PL, Sturm E. Genetic cholestasis, causes and consequences for hepatobiliary transport. Liver Int. 2003;23(5):315–22.
13. Byrne JA, Strautnieks SS, Mieli-Vergani G, Higgins CF, Linton KJ, Thompson RJ. The human bile salt export pump: characterization of substrate specificity and identification of inhibitors. Gastroenterology. 2002;123(5):1649–58.
14. Noe J, Stieger B, Meier PJ. Functional expression of the canalicular bile salt export pump of human liver. Gastroenterology. 2002;123(5):1659–66.
15. Jansen PL, Muller M. The molecular genetics of familial intrahepatic cholestasis. Gut. 2000;47(1):1–5.
16. Keppler D. Cholestasis and the role of basolateral efflux pumps. Z Gastroenterol. 2011; 49(12):1553–7.
17. Slot AJ, Molinski SV, Cole SP. Mammalian multidrug-resistance proteins (MRPs). Essays Biochem. 2011;50(1):179–207.
18. Karpen SJ. Nuclear receptor regulation of hepatic function. J Hepatol. 2002;36(6):832–50.
19. Tung CB, Tung CF, Yang DY, Hu WH, Hung DZ, Peng YC, et al. Extremely high levels of alkaline phosphatase in adult patients as a manifestation of bacteremia. Hepatogastroenterology. 2005;52(65):1347–50.
20. Franson TR, LaBrecque DR, Buggy BP, Harris GJ, Hoffmann RG. Serial bilirubin determinations as a prognostic marker in clinical infections. Am J Med Sci. 1989;297(3):149–52.
21. Sikuler E, Guetta V, Keynan A, Neumann L, Schlaeffer F. Abnormalities in bilirubin and liver enzyme levels in adult patients with bacteremia. A prospective study. Arch Intern Med. 1989;149(10):2246–8.
22. Zimmerman HJ. Intrahepatic cholestasis. Arch Intern Med. 1979;139(9):1038–45.
23. Miller DJ, Keeton DG, Webber BL, Pathol FF, Saunders SJ. Jaundice in severe bacterial infection. Gastroenterology. 1976;71(1):94–7.

24. Vermillion SE, Gregg JA, Baggenstoss AH, Bartholomew LG. Jaundice associated with bacteremia. Arch Intern Med. 1969;124(5):611–8.
25. Whitehead MW, Hainsworth I, Kingham JG. The causes of obvious jaundice in South West Wales: perceptions versus reality. Gut. 2001;48(3):409–13.
26. Ding LA, Li JS, Li YS, Zhu NT, Liu FN, Tan L. Intestinal barrier damage caused by trauma and lipopolysaccharide. World J Gastroenterol. 2004;10(16):2373–8.
27. Fuchs M, Sanyal AJ. Sepsis and cholestasis. Clin Liver Dis. 2008;12(1):151–72. ix.
28. Raman M, Allard JP. Parenteral nutrition related hepato-biliary disease in adults. Appl Physiol Nutr Metab. 2007;32(4):646–54.
29. Gonnella PA, Helton WS, Robinson M, Wilmore DW. O-side chain of Escherichia coli endotoxin 0111:B4 is transported across the intestinal epithelium in the rat: evidence for increased transport during total parenteral nutrition. Eur J Cell Biol. 1992;59(1):224–7.
30. Sturm E, Zimmerman TL, Crawford AR, Svetlov SI, Sundaram P, Ferrara JL, et al. Endotoxin-stimulated macrophages decrease bile acid uptake in WIF-B cells, a rat hepatoma hybrid cell line. Hepatology. 2000;31(1):124–30.
31. Crawford JM, Boyer JL. Clinicopathology conferences: inflammation-induced cholestasis. Hepatology. 1998;28(1):253–60.
32. Sakamoto S, Okanoue T, Itoh Y, Sakamoto K, Nishioji K, Nakagawa Y, et al. Intercellular adhesion molecule-1 and CD18 are involved in neutrophil adhesion and its cytotoxicity to cultured sinusoidal endothelial cells in rats. Hepatology. 1997;26(3):658–63.
33. Jaeschke H. Chemokines, neutrophils, and inflammatory liver injury. Shock. 1996;6(6):403–4.
34. van Oosten M, van de Bilt E, de Vries HE, van Berkel TJ, Kuiper J. Vascular adhesion molecule-1 and intercellular adhesion molecule-1 expression on rat liver cells after lipopolysaccharide administration in vivo. Hepatology. 1995;22((5):1538–46.
35. Oka Y, Murata A, Nishijima J, Ogawa M, Mori T. The mechanism of hepatic cellular injury in sepsis: an in vitro study of the implications of cytokines and neutrophils in its pathogenesis. J Surg Res. 1993;55(1):1–8.
36. Ayres RC, Neuberger JM, Shaw J, Joplin R, Adams DH. Intercellular adhesion molecule-1 and MHC antigens on human intrahepatic bile duct cells: effect of pro-inflammatory cytokines. Gut. 1993;34(9):1245–9.
37. Trauner M, Arrese M, Soroka CJ, Ananthanarayanan M, Koeppel TA, Schlosser SF, et al. The rat canalicular conjugate export pump (Mrp2) is down-regulated in intrahepatic and obstructive cholestasis. Gastroenterology. 1997;113(1):255–64.
38. Green RM, Beier D, Gollan JL. Regulation of hepatocyte bile salt transporters by endotoxin and inflammatory cytokines in rodents. Gastroenterology. 1996;111(1):193–8.
39. Whiting JF, Green RM, Rosenbluth AB, Gollan JL. Tumor necrosis factor-alpha decreases hepatocyte bile salt uptake and mediates endotoxin-induced cholestasis. Hepatology. 1995;22(4 Pt 1):1273–8.
40. Green RM, Whiting JF, Rosenbluth AB, Beier D, Gollan JL. Interleukin-6 inhibits hepatocyte taurocholate uptake and sodium-potassium-adenosinetriphosphatase activity. Am J Physiol. 1994;267(6 Pt 1):G1094–100.
41. Roelofsen H, van der Veere CN, Ottenhoff R, Schoemaker B, Jansen PL, Oude Elferink RP. Decreased bilirubin transport in the perfused liver of endotoxemic rats. Gastroenterology. 1994;107(4):1075–84.
42. Wagner M, Zollner G, Trauner M. New molecular insights into the mechanisms of cholestasis. J Hepatol. 2009;51(3):565–80.
43. Bolder U, Ton-Nu HT, Schteingart CD, Frick E, Hofmann AF. Hepatocyte transport of bile acids and organic anions in endotoxemic rats: impaired uptake and secretion. Gastroenterology. 1997;112(1):214–25.
44. Roelofsen H, Schoemaker B, Bakker C, Ottenhoff R, Jansen PL, Elferink RP. Impaired hepatocanalicular organic anion transport in endotoxemic rats. Am J Physiol. 1995;269(3 Pt 1):G427–34.
45. Zollner G, Fickert P, Zenz R, Fuchsbichler A, Stumptner C, Kenner L, et al. Hepatobiliary transporter expression in percutaneous liver biopsies of patients with cholestatic liver diseases. Hepatology. 2001;33(3):633–46.

46. Moseley RH. Sepsis-associated jaundice. Hepatology. 1996;24(4):969–70.
47. Spirli C, Nathanson MH, Fiorotto R, Duner E, Denson LA, Sanz JM, et al. Proinflammatory cytokines inhibit secretion in rat bile duct epithelium. Gastroenterology. 2001;121(1):156–69.
48. Warskulat U, Kubitz R, Wettstein M, Stieger B, Meier PJ, Haussinger D. Regulation of bile salt export pump mRNA levels by dexamethasone and osmolarity in cultured rat hepatocytes. Biol Chem. 1999;380(11):1273–9.
49. Kubitz R, Wettstein M, Warskulat U, Haussinger D. Regulation of the multidrug resistance protein 2 in the rat liver by lipopolysaccharide and dexamethasone. Gastroenterology. 1999;116(2):401–10.
50. Garvin IP. Remarks on pneumonia biliosa. S Med Surg J. 1837;1:536.
51. Franson TR, Hierholzer Jr WJ, LaBrecque DR. Frequency and characteristics of hyperbilirubinemia associated with bacteremia. Rev Infect Dis. 1985;7(1):1–9.
52. Phillips MJ, Poucell S, Oda M. Mechanisms of cholestasis. Lab Invest. 1986;54(6):593–608.
53. Lefkowitch JH. Bile ductular cholestasis: an ominous histopathologic sign related to sepsis and "cholangitis lenta". Hum Pathol. 1982;13(1):19–24.
54. Carter BA, Karpen SJ. Intestinal failure-associated liver disease: management and treatment strategies past, present, and future. Semin Liver Dis. 2007;27(3):251–8.
55. Sandhu IS, Jarvis C, Everson GT. Total parenteral nutrition and cholestasis. Clin Liver Dis. 1999;3(3):489–508. viii.
56. Moss RL, Amii LA. New approaches to understanding the etiology and treatment of total parenteral nutrition-associated cholestasis. Semin Pediatr Surg. 1999;8(3):140–7.
57. Balistreri WF, Bove KE. Hepatobiliary consequences of parenteral alimentation. Prog Liver Dis. 1990;9:567–601.
58. Messing B, Bories C, Kunstlinger F, Bernier JJ. Does total parenteral nutrition induce gallbladder sludge formation and lithiasis? Gastroenterology. 1983;84(5 Pt 1):1012–9.
59. Barbier J, Gineste D, Kraimps JL, Benand P, Carretier M, Beau P, et al. [Hepatobiliary complications of total parenteral nutrition]. Chirurgie. 1992;118(1–2):47–53.
60. Nightingale JM. Hepatobiliary, renal and bone complications of intestinal failure. Best Pract Res Clin Gastroenterol. 2003;17(6):907–29.
61. Kwan V, George J. Liver disease due to parenteral and enteral nutrition. Clin Liver Dis. 2004;8(4):893. x.
62. Clarke PJ, Ball MJ, Kettlewell MG. Liver function tests in patients receiving parenteral nutrition. JPEN J Parenter Enteral Nutr. 1991;15(1):54–9.
63. Naini BV, Lassman CR. Total parenteral nutrition therapy and liver injury: a histopathologic study with clinical correlation. Hum Pathol. 2012;43(6):826–33.
64. Cavicchi M, Beau P, Crenn P, Degott C, Messing B. Prevalence of liver disease and contributing factors in patients receiving home parenteral nutrition for permanent intestinal failure. Ann Intern Med. 2000;132(7):525–32.
65. Chan S, McCowen KC, Bistrian BR, Thibault A, Keane-Ellison M, Forse RA, et al. Incidence, prognosis, and etiology of end-stage liver disease in patients receiving home total parenteral nutrition. Surgery. 1999;126(1):28–34.
66. Kelly DA. Liver complications of pediatric parenteral nutrition–epidemiology. Nutrition. 1998;14(1):153–7.
67. Squires RH, Duggan C, Teitelbaum DH, Wales PW, Balint J, Venick R, et al. Natural history of pediatric intestinal failure: initial report from the pediatric intestinal failure consortium. J Pediatr. 2012;161(4):723–8.
68. Willis TC, Carter BA, Rogers SP, Hawthorne KM, Hicks PD, Abrams SA. High rates of mortality and morbidity occur in infants with parenteral nutrition-associated cholestasis. JPEN J Parenter Enteral Nutr. 2010;34(1):32–7.
69. Spencer AU, Yu S, Tracy TF, Aouthmany MM, Llanos A, Brown MB, et al. Parenteral nutrition-associated cholestasis in neonates: multivariate analysis of the potential protective effect of taurine. JPEN J Parenter Enteral Nutr. 2005;29(5):337–43.
70. Andorsky DJ, Lund DP, Lillehei CW, Jaksic T, Dicanzio J, Richardson DS, et al. Nutritional and other postoperative management of neonates with short bowel syndrome correlates with clinical outcomes. J Pediatr. 2001;139(1):27–33.

71. Beath SV, Davies P, Papadopoulou A, Khan AR, Buick RG, Corkery JJ, et al. Parenteral nutrition-related cholestasis in postsurgical neonates: multivariate analysis of risk factors. J Pediatr Surg. 1996;31(4):604–6.
72. Moss RL, Amii LA. New approaches to understanding the etiology and treatment of total parenteral nutrition-associated cholestasis. Semin Pediatr Surg. 1999;8(3):140–7.
73. Fein BI, Holt PR. Hepatobiliary complications of total parenteral nutrition. J Clin Gastroenterol. 1994;18(1):62–6.
74. Campos AC, Oler A, Meguid MM, Chen TY. Liver biochemical and histological changes with graded amounts of total parenteral nutrition. Arch Surg. 1990;125(4):447–50.
75. Meguid MM, Chen TY, Yang ZJ, Campos AC, Hitch DC, Gleason JR. Effects of continuous graded total parenteral nutrition on feeding indexes and metabolic concomitants in rats. Am J Physiol. 1991;260(1 Pt 1):E126–40.
76. Li S, Nussbaum MS, Teague D, Gapen CL, Dayal R, Fischer JE. Increasing dextrose concentrations in total parenteral nutrition (TPN) causes alterations in hepatic morphology and plasma levels of insulin and glucagon in rats. J Surg Res. 1988;44(6):639–48.
77. Kaminski DL, Adams A, Jellinek M. The effect of hyperalimentation on hepatic lipid content and lipogenic enzyme activity in rats and man. Surgery. 1980;88(1):93–100.
78. Premkumar MH, Carter BA, Hawthorne KM, King K, Abrams SA. High rates of resolution of cholestasis in parenteral nutrition-associated liver disease with fish oil-based lipid emulsion monotherapy. J Pediatr. 2013;162(4):793–8.
79. Ellegard L, Sunesson A, Bosaeus I. High serum phytosterol levels in short bowel patients on parenteral nutrition support. Clin Nutr. 2005;24(3):415–20.
80. Iyer KR, Spitz L, Clayton P. BAPS prize lecture: new insight into mechanisms of parenteral nutrition-associated cholestasis: role of plant sterols. British association of paediatric surgeons. J Pediatr Surg. 1998;33(1):1–6.
81. Clayton PT, Bowron A, Mills KA, Massoud A, Casteels M, Milla PJ. Phytosterolemia in children with parenteral nutrition-associated cholestatic liver disease. Gastroenterology. 1993;105(6):1806–13.
82. Matilla B, Ortiz J, Gonzalez P, Garcia-Diez F, Jorquera F, Culebras JM, et al. Effects of parenteral nutrition supplemented with glutamine or glutamine dipeptides on liver antioxidant and detoxication systems in rats. Nutrition. 2000;16(2):125–8.
83. Sokol RJ, Taylor SF, Devereaux MW, Khandwala R, Sondheimer NJ, Shikes RH, et al. Hepatic oxidant injury and glutathione depletion during total parenteral nutrition in weanling rats. Am J Physiol. 1996;270(4 Pt 1):G691–700.
84. Chessex P, Lavoie JC, Laborie S, Rouleau T. Parenteral multivitamin supplementation induces both oxidant and antioxidant responses in the liver of newborn guinea pigs. J Pediatr Gastroenterol Nutr. 2001;32(3):316–21.
85. Cai W, Wu J, Hong L, Xu Y, Tang Q, Shi C. Oxidative injury and hepatocyte apoptosis in total parenteral nutrition-associated liver dysfunction. J Pediatr Surg. 2006;41(10):1663–8.
86. Wu J, Tang Q, Feng Y, Huang J, Tao Y, Wang Y, et al. Nutrition assessment in children with short bowel syndrome weaned off parenteral nutrition: a long-term follow-up study. J Pediatr Surg. 2007;42(8):1372–6.
87. Buchman AL, Ament ME, Sohel M, Dubin M, Jenden DJ, Roch M, et al. Choline deficiency causes reversible hepatic abnormalities in patients receiving parenteral nutrition: proof of a human choline requirement: a placebo-controlled trial. JPEN J Parenter Enteral Nutr. 2001;25(5):260–8.
88. Misra S, Ament ME, Vargas JH, Skoff C, Reyen L, Herzog F. Chronic liver disease in children on long-term parenteral nutrition. J Gastroenterol Hepatol. 1996;11(5):S4–6.
89. Hwang TL, Lue MC, Chen LL. Early use of cyclic TPN prevents further deterioration of liver functions for the TPN patients with impaired liver function. Hepatogastroenterology. 2000;47(35):1347–50.
90. Trauner M, Wagner M, Fickert P, Zollner G. Molecular regulation of hepatobiliary transport systems: clinical implications for understanding and treating cholestasis. J Clin Gastroenterol. 2005;39(4 Suppl 2):S111–24.

91. Chen CY, Tsao PN, Chen HL, Chou HC, Hsieh WS, Chang MH. Ursodeoxycholic acid (UDCA) therapy in very-low-birth-weight infants with parenteral nutrition-associated cholestasis. J Pediatr. 2004;145(3):317–21.
92. Kumar D, Tandon RK. Use of ursodeoxycholic acid in liver diseases. J Gastroenterol Hepatol. 2001;16(1):3–14.
93. Sugatani J. Function, genetic polymorphism, and transcriptional regulation of human UDP-glucuronosyltransferase (UGT) 1A1. Drug Metab Pharmacokinet. 2012;28:83–92.
94. Park K, Williams DP, Naisbitt DJ, Kitteringham NR, Pirmohamed M. Investigation of toxic metabolites during drug development. Toxicol Appl Pharmacol. 2005;207(2 Suppl):425–34.
95. Park BK, Pirmohamed M, Kitteringham NR. The role of cytochrome P450 enzymes in hepatic and extrahepatic human drug toxicity. Pharmacol Ther. 1995;68(3):385–424.
96. Gunawan BK, Kaplowitz N. Mechanisms of drug-induced liver disease. Clin Liver Dis. 2007;11(3):459–75. v.
97. Possuelo LG, Castelan JA, de Brito TC, Ribeiro AW, Cafrune PI, Picon PD, et al. Association of slow N-acetyltransferase 2 profile and anti-TB drug-induced hepatotoxicity in patients from Southern Brazil. Eur J Clin Pharmacol. 2008;64(7):673–81.
98. Leiro V, Fernandez-Villar A, Valverde D, Constenla L, Vazquez R, Pineiro L, et al. Influence of glutathione S-transferase M1 and T1 homozygous null mutations on the risk of antituberculosis drug-induced hepatotoxicity in a Caucasian population. Liver Int. 2008;28(6):835–9.
99. Lucena MI, Andrade RJ, Martinez C, Ulzurrun E, Garcia-Martin E, Borraz Y, et al. Glutathione S-transferase m1 and t1 null genotypes increase susceptibility to idiosyncratic drug-induced liver injury. Hepatology. 2008;48(2):588–96.
100. Daly AK, Aithal GP, Leathart JB, Swainsbury RA, Dang TS, Day CP. Genetic susceptibility to diclofenac-induced hepatotoxicity: contribution of UGT2B7, CYP2C8, and ABCC2 genotypes. Gastroenterology. 2007;132(1):272–81.
101. Choi JH, Ahn BM, Yi J, Lee JH, Lee JH, Nam SW, et al. MRP2 haplotypes confer differential susceptibility to toxic liver injury. Pharmacogenet Genomics. 2007;17(6):403–15.
102. Lang C, Meier Y, Stieger B, Beuers U, Lang T, Kerb R, et al. Mutations and polymorphisms in the bile salt export pump and the multidrug resistance protein 3 associated with drug-induced liver injury. Pharmacogenet Genomics. 2007;17(1):47–60.
103. Cho HJ, Koh WJ, Ryu YJ, Ki CS, Nam MH, Kim JW, et al. Genetic polymorphisms of NAT2 and CYP2E1 associated with antituberculosis drug-induced hepatotoxicity in Korean patients with pulmonary tuberculosis. Tuberculosis (Edinb). 2007;87(6):551–6.
104. Roy B, Chowdhury A, Kundu S, Santra A, Dey B, Chakraborty M, et al. Increased risk of antituberculosis drug-induced hepatotoxicity in individuals with glutathione S-transferase M1 'null' mutation. J Gastroenterol Hepatol. 2001;16(9):1033–7.
105. Ohno M, Yamaguchi I, Yamamoto I, Fukuda T, Yokota S, Maekura R, et al. Slow N-acetyltransferase 2 genotype affects the incidence of isoniazid and rifampicin-induced hepatotoxicity. Int J Tuberc Lung Dis. 2000;4(3):256–61.
106. Werck-Reichhart D, Feyereisen R. Cytochromes P450: a success story. Genome Biol. 2000;1(6):REVIEWS3003.
107. Peterson JA, Graham SE. A close family resemblance: the importance of structure in understanding cytochromes P450. Structure. 1998;6(9):1079–85.
108. Smith G, Stubbins MJ, Harries LW, Wolf CR. Molecular genetics of the human cytochrome P450 monooxygenase superfamily. Xenobiotica. 1998;28(12):1129–65.
109. Nelson DR, Koymans L, Kamataki T, Stegeman JJ, Feyereisen R, Waxman DJ, et al. P450 superfamily: update on new sequences, gene mapping, accession numbers and nomenclature. Pharmacogenetics. 1996;6(1):1–42.
110. Gonzalez FJ. Molecular genetics of the P-450 superfamily. Pharmacol Ther. 1990;45(1): 1–38.
111. Danielson PB. The cytochrome P450 superfamily: biochemistry, evolution and drug metabolism in humans. Curr Drug Metab. 2002;3(6):561–97.
112. Lehmann DE. Enzymatic shunting: resolving the acetaminophen-warfarin controversy. Pharmacotherapy. 2000;20(12):1464–8.

113. Ehrenpreis ED, Ehrenpreis S. Cytochrome P450: role in drug-induced hepatotoxicity. Clin Liver Dis. 1998;2:457.
114. Wrighton SA, Vandenbranden M, Ring BJ. The human drug metabolizing cytochromes P450. J Pharmacokinet Biopharm. 1996;24(5):461–73.
115. Wilkinson GR. Cytochrome P4503A (CYP3A) metabolism: prediction of in vivo activity in humans. J Pharmacokinet Biopharm. 1996;24(5):475–90.
116. Ketter TA, Flockhart DA, Post RM, Denicoff K, Pazzaglia PJ, Marangell LB, et al. The emerging role of cytochrome P450 3A in psychopharmacology. J Clin Psychopharmacol. 1995;15(6):387–98.
117. Watkins PB. Drug metabolism by cytochromes P450 in the liver and small bowel. Gastroenterol Clin North Am. 1992;21(3):511–26.
118. Waxman DJ. P450 gene induction by structurally diverse xenochemicals: central role of nuclear receptors CAR, PXR, and PPAR. Arch Biochem Biophys. 1999;369(1):11–23.
119. Ho RH, Kim RB. Transporters and drug therapy: implications for drug disposition and disease. Clin Pharmacol Ther. 2005;78(3):260–77.
120. Murray M. Mechanisms and significance of inhibitory drug interactions involving cytochrome P450 enzymes (review). Int J Mol Med. 1999;3(3):227–38.
121. Bjornsson ES, Jonasson JG. Drug-induced cholestasis. Clin Liver Dis. 2013;17(2):191–209.
122. Padda MS, Sanchez M, Akhtar AJ, Boyer JL. Drug-induced cholestasis. Hepatology. 2011;53(4):1377–87.
123. Bjornsson E, Ismael S, Nejdet S, Kilander A. Severe jaundice in Sweden in the new millennium: causes, investigations, treatment and prognosis. Scand J Gastroenterol. 2003;38(1): 86–94.
124. Malchow-Moller A, Matzen P, Bjerregaard B, Hilden J, Holst-Christensen J, Staehr JT, et al. Causes and characteristics of 500 consecutive cases of jaundice. Scand J Gastroenterol. 1981;16(1):1–6.
125. Bjorneboe M, Iversen O, Olsen S. Infective hepatitis and toxic jaundice in a municipal hospital during a five-year period. Incidence and prognosis. Acta Med Scand. 1967;182(4):491–501.
126. Chalasani N, Fontana RJ, Bonkovsky HL, Watkins PB, Davern T, Serrano J, et al. Causes, clinical features, and outcomes from a prospective study of drug-induced liver injury in the United States. Gastroenterology. 2008;135(6):1924–34. 1934.
127. Bohan A, Boyer JL. Mechanisms of hepatic transport of drugs: implications for cholestatic drug reactions. Semin Liver Dis. 2002;22(2):123–36.
128. Sgro C, Clinard F, Ouazir K, Chanay H, Allard C, Guilleminet C, et al. Incidence of drug-induced hepatic injuries: a French population-based study. Hepatology. 2002;36(2):451–5.
129. Lucena MI, Andrade RJ, Kaplowitz N, Garcia-Cortes M, Fernandez MC, Romero-Gomez M, et al. Phenotypic characterization of idiosyncratic drug-induced liver injury: the influence of age and sex. Hepatology. 2009;49(6):2001–9.
130. Lammert C, Einarsson S, Saha C, Niklasson A, Bjornsson E, Chalasani N. Relationship between daily dose of oral medications and idiosyncratic drug-induced liver injury: search for signals. Hepatology. 2008;47(6):2003–9.
131. Lammert C, Bjornsson E, Niklasson A, Chalasani N. Oral medications with significant hepatic metabolism at higher risk for hepatic adverse events. Hepatology. 2010;51(2):615–20.
132. Bjornsson E. Drug-induced liver injury: Hy's rule revisited. Clin Pharmacol Ther. 2006;79(6):521–8.
133. Reuben A. Hy's law. Hepatology. 2004;39(2):574–8.
134. Chalasani N, Bjornsson E. Risk factors for idiosyncratic drug-induced liver injury. Gastroenterology. 2010;138(7):2246–59.
135. Bjornsson E, Olsson R. Outcome and prognostic markers in severe drug-induced liver disease. Hepatology. 2005;42(2):481–9.
136. Andrade RJ, Lucena MI, Fernandez MC, Pelaez G, Pachkoria K, Garcia-Ruiz E, et al. Drug-induced liver injury: an analysis of 461 incidences submitted to the Spanish registry over a 10-year period. Gastroenterology. 2005;129(2):512–21.

137. Andrade RJ, Lucena MI, Alonso A, Garcia-Cortes M, Garcia-Ruiz E, Benitez R, et al. HLA class II genotype influences the type of liver injury in drug-induced idiosyncratic liver disease. Hepatology. 2004;39(6):1603–12.
138. Hautekeete ML, Horsmans Y, Van WC, Demanet C, Henrion J, Verbist L, et al. HLA association of amoxicillin-clavulanate–induced hepatitis. Gastroenterology. 1999;117(5):1181–6.
139. Maggio MC, Liotta A, Cardella F, Corsello G. Stevens-Johnson syndrome and cholestatic hepatitis induced by acute Epstein-Barr virus infection. Eur J Gastroenterol Hepatol. 2011;23(3):289.
140. Ratnayake EC, Shivanthan C, Wijesiriwardena BC. Cholestatic hepatitis in a patient with typhoid fever—a case report. Ann Clin Microbiol Antimicrob. 2011;10:35.
141. Choi HC, Lee SH, Kim J, Kim SH, Hwang JH, Kim JW, et al. A case of acute q Fever with severe acute cholestatic hepatitis. Gut Liver. 2009;3(2):141–4.
142. Benichou C, Danan G, Flahault A. Causality assessment of adverse reactions to drugs–II. An original model for validation of drug causality assessment methods: case reports with positive rechallenge. J Clin Epidemiol. 1993;46(11):1331–6.
143. USFDA. Guidance for industry drug-induced liver injury: premarketing clinical evaluation. 2007. Ref type: online source.
144. Kaplowitz N. Causality assessment versus guilt-by-association in drug hepatotoxicity. Hepatology. 2001;33(1):308–10.
145. Danan G, Benichou C. Causality assessment of adverse reactions to drugs–I. A novel method based on the conclusions of international consensus meetings: application to drug-induced liver injuries. J Clin Epidemiol. 1993;46(11):1323–30.
146. Navarro VJ, Senior JR. Drug-related hepatotoxicity. N Engl J Med. 2006;354(7):731–9.
147. Kleiner DE. The pathology of drug-induced liver injury. Semin Liver Dis. 2009;29(4):364–72.
148. Suzuki A, Brunt EM, Kleiner DE, Miquel R, Smyrk TC, Andrade RJ, et al. The use of liver biopsy evaluation in discrimination of idiopathic autoimmune hepatitis versus drug-induced liver injury. Hepatology. 2011;54(3):931–9.
149. Moradpour D, Altorfer J, Flury R, Greminger P, Meyenberger C, Jost R, et al. Chlorpromazine-induced vanishing bile duct syndrome leading to biliary cirrhosis. Hepatology. 1994;20(6):1437–41.
150. Andrade RJ, Lucena MI, Kaplowitz N, Garcia-Munoz B, Borraz Y, Pachkoria K, et al. Outcome of acute idiosyncratic drug-induced liver injury: long-term follow-up in a hepatotoxicity registry. Hepatology. 2006;44(6):1581–8.
151. Noronha V, Shafi NQ, Obando JA, Kummar S. Primary non-Hodgkin's lymphoma of the liver. Crit Rev Oncol Hematol. 2005;53(3):199–207.
152. Kotlyar DS, Osterman MT, Diamond RH, Porter D, Blonski WC, Wasik M, et al. A systematic review of factors that contribute to hepatosplenic T-cell lymphoma in patients with inflammatory bowel disease. Clin Gastroenterol Hepatol. 2011;9(1):36–41.
153. Green M, Michaels MG. Epstein-Barr virus infection and posttransplant lymphoproliferative disorder. Am J Transplant. 2013;13 Suppl 3:41–54.
154. Rasche L, Kapp M, Einsele H, Mielke S. EBV-induced post transplant lymphoproliferative disorders: a persisting challenge in allogeneic hematopoetic SCT. Bone Marrow Transplant. 2013;49:163–7.
155. Dignan FL, Scarisbrick JJ, Cornish J, Clark A, Amrolia P, Jackson G, et al. Organ-specific management and supportive care in chronic graft-versus-host disease. Br J Haematol. 2012;158(1):62–78.
156. Chen GL, Zhang Y, Hahn T, Abrams S, Ross M, Liu H, et al. Acute GVHD prophylaxis with standard-dose, micro-dose or no MTX after fludarabine/melphalan conditioning. Bone Marrow Transplant. 2013;49:248–53.
157. Ferrara JL, Levine JE, Reddy P, Holler E. Graft-versus-host disease. Lancet. 2009;373(9674):1550–61.
158. Strasser SI, Shulman HM, McDonald GB. Cholestasis after hematopoietic cell transplantation. Clin Liver Dis. 1999;3(3):651–68. x.

159. Shulman HM, Sharma P, Amos D, Fenster LF, McDonald GB. A coded histologic study of hepatic graft-versus-host disease after human bone marrow transplantation. Hepatology. 1988;8(3):463–70.
160. Snover DC. Acute and chronic graft versus host disease: histopathological evidence for two distinct pathogenetic mechanisms. Hum Pathol. 1984;15(3):202–5.
161. Akpek G, Boitnott JK, Lee LA, Hallick JP, Torbenson M, Jacobsohn DA, et al. Hepatitic variant of graft-versus-host disease after donor lymphocyte infusion. Blood. 2002;100(12):3903–7.
162. Fujii N, Takenaka K, Shinagawa K, Ikeda K, Maeda Y, Sunami K, et al. Hepatic graft-versus-host disease presenting as an acute hepatitis after allogeneic peripheral blood stem cell transplantation. Bone Marrow Transplant. 2001;27(9):1007–10.
163. Strasser SI, Shulman HM, Flowers ME, Reddy R, Margolis DA, Prumbaum M, et al. Chronic graft-versus-host disease of the liver: presentation as an acute hepatitis. Hepatology. 2000;32(6):1265–71.
164. Gooley TA, Rajvanshi P, Schoch HG, McDonald GB. Serum bilirubin levels and mortality after myeloablative allogeneic hematopoietic cell transplantation. Hepatology. 2005;41(2):345–52.
165. Dignan FL, Amrolia P, Clark A, Cornish J, Jackson G, Mahendra P, et al. Diagnosis and management of chronic graft-versus-host disease. Br J Haematol. 2012;158(1):46–61.
166. Hashmi K. Graft versus host disease. J Pak Med Assoc. 2005;55(11):467–8.
167. Przepiorka D, Weisdorf D, Martin P, Klingemann HG, Beatty P, Hows J, et al. 1994 consensus conference on acute GVHD grading. Bone Marrow Transplant. 1995;15(6):825–8.
168. Filipovich AH, Weisdorf D, Pavletic S, Socie G, Wingard JR, Lee SJ, et al. National Institutes of Health consensus development project on criteria for clinical trials in chronic graft-versus-host disease: I. Diagnosis and staging working group report. Biol Blood Marrow Transplant. 2005;11(12):945–56.
169. Greinix HT, Loddenkemper C, Pavletic SZ, Holler E, Socie G, Lawitschka A, et al. Diagnosis and staging of chronic graft-versus-host disease in the clinical practice. Biol Blood Marrow Transplant. 2011;17(2):167–75.
170. Cutler C, Li S, Ho VT, Koreth J, Alyea E, Soiffer RJ, et al. Extended follow-up of methotrexate-free immunosuppression using sirolimus and tacrolimus in related and unrelated donor peripheral blood stem cell transplantation. Blood. 2007;109(7):3108–14.
171. Tay J, Tinmouth A, Fergusson D, Huebsch L, Allan DS. Systematic review of controlled clinical trials on the use of ursodeoxycholic acid for the prevention of hepatic veno-occlusive disease in hematopoietic stem cell transplantation. Biol Blood Marrow Transplant. 2007;13(2):206–17.
172. Ruutu T, Eriksson B, Remes K, Juvonen E, Volin L, Remberger M, et al. Ursodeoxycholic acid for the prevention of hepatic complications in allogeneic stem cell transplantation. Blood. 2002;100(6):1977–83.
173. Marks C, Stadler M, Hausermann P, Wolff D, Buchholz S, Stary G, et al. German-Austrian-Swiss Consensus Conference on clinical practice in chronic graft-versus-host disease (GVHD): guidance for supportive therapy of chronic cutaneous and musculoskeletal GVHD. Br J Dermatol. 2011;165(1):18–29.
174. Landfried K, Wolff D, Holler E. Pathophysiology and management of graft-versus-host disease in the era of reduced-intensity conditioning. Curr Opin Oncol. 2009;21 Suppl 1:S39–41.
175. Deeg HJ. How I, treat refractory acute GVHD. Blood. 2007;109(10):4119–26.
176. Saliba RM, de Lima M, Giralt S, Andersson B, Khouri IF, Hosing C, et al. Hyperacute GVHD: risk factors, outcomes, and clinical implications. Blood. 2007;109(7):2751–8.
177. MacMillan ML, Weisdorf DJ, Wagner JE, DeFor TE, Burns LJ, Ramsay NK, et al. Response of 443 patients to steroids as primary therapy for acute graft-versus-host disease: comparison of grading systems. Biol Blood Marrow Transplant. 2002;8(7):387–94.
178. Pidala J. Graft-vs-host disease following allogeneic hematopoietic cell transplantation. Cancer Control. 2011;18(4):268–76.
179. Greinix HT, Knobler RM, Worel N, Schneider B, Schneeberger A, Hoecker P, et al. The effect of intensified extracorporeal photochemotherapy on long-term survival in patients with severe acute graft-versus-host disease. Haematologica. 2006;91(3):405–8.

180. Dall'Amico R, Messina C. Extracorporeal photochemotherapy for the treatment of graft-versus-host disease. Ther Apher. 2002;6(4):296–304.
181. Willmot F, Robertson G. Senecio disease, or cirrhosis of the liver due to senecio poisoning. Lancet. 1920;196(5069):848–9.
182. Jacobs P, Miller JL, Uys CJ, Dietrich BE. Fatal veno-occlusive disease of the liver after chemotherapy, whole-body irradiation and bone marrow transplantation for refractory acute leukaemia. S Afr Med J. 1979;55(1):5–10.
183. Berk PD, Popper H, Krueger GR, Decter J, Herzig G, Graw Jr RG. Veno-occlusive disease of the liver after allogeneic bone marrow transplantation: possible association with graft-versus-host disease. Ann Intern Med. 1979;90(2):158–64.
184. Kumar S, DeLeve LD, Kamath PS, Tefferi A. Hepatic veno-occlusive disease (sinusoidal obstruction syndrome) after hematopoietic stem cell transplantation. Mayo Clin Proc. 2003;78(5):589–98.
185. DeLeve LD, Shulman HM, McDonald GB. Toxic injury to hepatic sinusoids: sinusoidal obstruction syndrome (veno-occlusive disease). Semin Liver Dis. 2002;22(1):27–42.
186. Coppell JA, Richardson PG, Soiffer R, Martin PL, Kernan NA, Chen A, et al. Hepatic veno-occlusive disease following stem cell transplantation: incidence, clinical course, and outcome. Biol Blood Marrow Transplant. 2010;16(2):157–68.
187. Hogan WJ, Maris M, Storer B, Sandmaier BM, Maloney DG, Schoch HG, et al. Hepatic injury after nonmyeloablative conditioning followed by allogeneic hematopoietic cell transplantation: a study of 193 patients. Blood. 2004;103(1):78–84.
188. Carreras E, Bertz H, Arcese W, Vernant JP, Tomas JF, Hagglund H, et al. Incidence and outcome of hepatic veno-occlusive disease after blood or marrow transplantation: a prospective cohort study of the European Group for Blood and Marrow Transplantation. European Group for Blood and Marrow Transplantation Chronic Leukemia Working Party. Blood. 1998;92(10):3599–604.
189. Shulman HM, Hinterberger W. Hepatic veno-occlusive disease–liver toxicity syndrome after bone marrow transplantation. Bone Marrow Transplant. 1992;10(3):197–214.
190. Jones RJ, Lee KS, Beschorner WE, Vogel VG, Grochow LB, Braine HG, et al. Venoocclusive disease of the liver following bone marrow transplantation. Transplantation. 1987;44(6):778–83.
191. McDonald GB, Sharma P, Matthews DE, Shulman HM, Thomas ED. Venocclusive disease of the liver after bone marrow transplantation: diagnosis, incidence, and predisposing factors. Hepatology. 1984;4(1):116–22.
192. Levitsky J, Sorrell MF. Hepatic complications of hematopoietic cell transplantation. Curr Gastroenterol Rep. 2007;9(1):60–5.
193. Bearman SI. The syndrome of hepatic veno-occlusive disease after marrow transplantation. Blood. 1995;85(11):3005–20.
194. Shulman HM, Fisher LB, Schoch HG, Henne KW, McDonald GB. Veno-occlusive disease of the liver after marrow transplantation: histological correlates of clinical signs and symptoms. Hepatology. 1994;19(5):1171–81.
195. Shulman HM, Gown AM, Nugent DJ. Hepatic veno-occlusive disease after bone marrow transplantation. Immunohistochemical identification of the material within occluded central venules. Am J Pathol. 1987;127(3):549–58.
196. Shulman HM, McDonald GB, Matthews D, Doney KC, Kopecky KJ, Gauvreau JM, et al. An analysis of hepatic venocclusive disease and centrilobular hepatic degeneration following bone marrow transplantation. Gastroenterology. 1980;79(6):1178–91.
197. Rubbia-Brandt L, Audard V, Sartoretti P, Roth AD, Brezault C, Le CM, et al. Severe hepatic sinusoidal obstruction associated with oxaliplatin-based chemotherapy in patients with metastatic colorectal cancer. Ann Oncol. 2004;15(3):460–6.
198. Rubbia-Brandt L, Lauwers GY, Wang H, Majno PE, Tanabe K, Zhu AX, et al. Sinusoidal obstruction syndrome and nodular regenerative hyperplasia are frequent oxaliplatin-associated liver lesions and partially prevented by bevacizumab in patients with hepatic colorectal metastasis. Histopathology. 2010;56(4):430–9.
199. DeLeve LD, Valla DC, Garcia-Tsao G. Vascular disorders of the liver. Hepatology. 2009;49(5):1729–64.

200. DeLeve LD. Hepatic microvasculature in liver injury. Semin Liver Dis. 2007;27(4): 390–400.
201. McCuskey RS. Morphological mechanisms for regulating blood flow through hepatic sinusoids. Liver. 2000;20(1):3–7.
202. McCuskey RS, Reilly FD. Hepatic microvasculature: dynamic structure and its regulation. Semin Liver Dis. 1993;13(1):1–12.
203. Cutler C, Kim HT, Ayanian S, Bradwin G, Revta C, Aldridge J, et al. Prediction of veno-occlusive disease using biomarkers of endothelial injury. Biol Blood Marrow Transplant. 2010;16(8):1180–5.
204. Rubbia-Brandt L. Sinusoidal obstruction syndrome. Clin Liver Dis. 2010;14(4):651–68.
205. Hubert C, Sempoux C, Horsmans Y, Rahier J, Humblet Y, Machiels JP, et al. Nodular regenerative hyperplasia: a deleterious consequence of chemotherapy for colorectal liver metastases? Liver Int. 2007;27(7):938–43.
206. Aloia T, Sebagh M, Plasse M, Karam V, Levi F, Giacchetti S, et al. Liver histology and surgical outcomes after preoperative chemotherapy with fluorouracil plus oxaliplatin in colorectal cancer liver metastases. J Clin Oncol. 2006;24(31):4983–90.
207. Faioni EM, Mannucci PM. Venocclusive disease of the liver after bone marrow transplantation: the role of hemostasis. Leuk Lymphoma. 1997;25(3–4):233–45.
208. Faioni EM, Krachmalnicoff A, Bearman SI, Federici AB, Decarli A, Gianni AM, et al. Naturally occurring anticoagulants and bone marrow transplantation: plasma protein C predicts the development of venocclusive disease of the liver. Blood. 1993;81(12):3458–62.
209. Scrobohaci ML, Drouet L, Monem-Mansi A, Devergie A, Baudin B, D'Agay MF, et al. Liver veno-occlusive disease after bone marrow transplantation changes in coagulation parameters and endothelial markers. Thromb Res. 1991;63(5):509–19.
210. Harper PL, Jarvis J, Jennings I, Luddington R, Marcus RE. Changes in the natural anticoagulants following bone marrow transplantation. Bone Marrow Transplant. 1990;5(1):39–42.
211. Vannucchi AM, Rafanelli D, Longo G, Bosi A, Guidi S, Saccardi R, et al. Early hemostatic alterations following bone marrow transplantation: a prospective study. Haematologica. 1994;79(6):519–25.
212. Catani L, Gugliotta L, Mattioli BM, Vianelli N, Gherlinzoni F, Miggiano MC, et al. Hypercoagulability in patients undergoing autologous or allogeneic BMT for hematological malignancies. Bone Marrow Transplant. 1993;12(3):253–9.
213. Collins PW, Gutteridge CN, O'Driscoll A, Blair S, Jones L, Aitchison R, et al. von Willebrand factor as a marker of endothelial cell activation following BMT. Bone Marrow Transplant. 1992;10(6):499–506.
214. Vollmar B, Menger MD. The hepatic microcirculation: mechanistic contributions and therapeutic targets in liver injury and repair. Physiol Rev. 2009;89(4):1269–339.
215. McCuskey RS. Sinusoidal endothelial cells as an early target for hepatic toxicants. Clin Hemorheol Microcirc. 2006;34(1–2):5–10.
216. Ho VT, Cutler C. Current and novel therapies in acute GVHD. Best Pract Res Clin Haematol. 2008;21(2):223–37.
217. McCune JS, Batchelder A, Deeg HJ, Gooley T, Cole S, Phillips B, et al. Cyclophosphamide following targeted oral busulfan as conditioning for hematopoietic cell transplantation: pharmacokinetics, liver toxicity, and mortality. Biol Blood Marrow Transplant. 2007;13(7): 853–62.
218. McDonald GB, Slattery JT, Bouvier ME, Ren S, Batchelder AL, Kalhorn TF, et al. Cyclophosphamide metabolism, liver toxicity, and mortality following hematopoietic stem cell transplantation. Blood. 2003;101(5):2043–8.
219. Giles FJ, Kantarjian HM, Kornblau SM, Thomas DA, Garcia-Manero G, Waddelow TA, et al. Mylotarg (gemtuzumab ozogamicin) therapy is associated with hepatic venoocclusive disease in patients who have not received stem cell transplantation. Cancer. 2001;92(2):406–13.
220. Hagglund H, Remberger M, Klaesson S, Lonnqvist B, Ljungman P, Ringden O. Norethisterone treatment, a major risk-factor for veno-occlusive disease in the liver after allogeneic bone marrow transplantation. Blood. 1998;92(12):4568–72.

221. Rozman C, Carreras E, Qian C, Gale RP, Bortin MM, Rowlings PA, et al. Risk factors for hepatic veno-occlusive disease following HLA-identical sibling bone marrow transplants for leukemia. Bone Marrow Transplant. 1996;17(1):75–80.
222. Frickhofen N, Wiesneth M, Jainta C, Hertenstein B, Heymer B, Bianchi L, et al. Hepatitis C virus infection is a risk factor for liver failure from veno-occlusive disease after bone marrow transplantation. Blood. 1994;83(7):1998–2004.
223. McDonald GB, Hinds MS, Fisher LD, Schoch HG, Wolford JL, Banaji M, et al. Veno-occlusive disease of the liver and multiorgan failure after bone marrow transplantation: a cohort study of 355 patients. Ann Intern Med. 1993;118(4):255–67.
224. Ayash LJ, Hunt M, Antman K, Nadler L, Wheeler C, Takvorian T, et al. Hepatic venoocclusive disease in autologous bone marrow transplantation of solid tumors and lymphomas. J Clin Oncol. 1990;8(10):1699–706.
225. DeLeve LD, Wang X. Role of oxidative stress and glutathione in busulfan toxicity in cultured murine hepatocytes. Pharmacology. 2000;60(3):143–54.
226. DeLeve LD. Glutathione defense in non-parenchymal cells. Semin Liver Dis. 1998;18(4):403–13.
227. DeLeve LD, Kaplowitz N. Importance and regulation of hepatic glutathione. Semin Liver Dis. 1990;10(4):251–66.
228. Teicher BA, Crawford JM, Holden SA, Lin Y, Cathcart KN, Luchette CA, et al. Glutathione monoethyl ester can selectively protect liver from high dose BCNU or cyclophosphamide. Cancer. 1988;62(7):1275–81.
229. DeLeve LD. Cellular target of cyclophosphamide toxicity in the murine liver: role of glutathione and site of metabolic activation. Hepatology. 1996;24(4):830–7.
230. Deeg HJ, Sullivan KM, Buckner CD, Storb R, Appelbaum FR, Clift RA, et al. Marrow transplantation for acute nonlymphoblastic leukemia in first remission: toxicity and long-term follow-up of patients conditioned with single dose or fractionated total body irradiation. Bone Marrow Transplant. 1986;1(2):151–7.
231. Carreras E. Veno-occlusive disease of the liver after hemopoietic cell transplantation. Eur J Haematol. 2000;64(5):281–91.
232. Ringden O, Ruutu T, Remberger M, Nikoskelainen J, Volin L, Vindelov L, et al. A randomized trial comparing busulfan with total body irradiation as conditioning in allogeneic marrow transplant recipients with leukemia: a report from the Nordic Bone Marrow Transplantation Group. Blood. 1994;83(9):2723–30.
233. Meresse V, Hartmann O, Vassal G, Benhamou E, Valteau-Couanet D, Brugieres L, et al. Risk factors for hepatic veno-occlusive disease after high-dose busulfan-containing regimens followed by autologous bone marrow transplantation: a study in 136 children. Bone Marrow Transplant. 1992;10(2):135–41.
234. Grochow LB. Busulfan disposition: the role of therapeutic monitoring in bone marrow transplantation induction regimens. Semin Oncol. 1993;20(4 Suppl 4):18–25.
235. Grochow LB, Jones RJ, Brundrett RB, Braine HG, Chen TL, Saral R, et al. Pharmacokinetics of busulfan: correlation with veno-occlusive disease in patients undergoing bone marrow transplantation. Cancer Chemother Pharmacol. 1989;25(1):55–61.
236. McKoy JM, Angelotta C, Bennett CL, Tallman MS, Wadleigh M, Evens AM, et al. Gemtuzumab ozogamicin-associated sinusoidal obstructive syndrome (SOS): an overview from the research on adverse drug events and reports (RADAR) project. Leuk Res. 2007;31(5):599–604.
237. Rio B, Andreu G, Nicod A, Arrago JP, Dutrillaux F, Samama M, et al. Thrombocytopenia in venocclusive disease after bone marrow transplantation or chemotherapy. Blood. 1986;67(6):1773–6.
238. Lassau N, Leclere J, Auperin A, Bourhis JH, Hartmann O, Valteau-Couanet D, et al. Hepatic veno-occlusive disease after myeloablative treatment and bone marrow transplantation: value of gray-scale and Doppler US in 100 patients. Radiology. 1997;204(2):545–52.
239. Shulman HM, Gooley T, Dudley MD, Kofler T, Feldman R, Dwyer D, et al. Utility of transvenous liver biopsies and wedged hepatic venous pressure measurements in sixty marrow transplant recipients. Transplantation. 1995;59(7):1015–22.

240. Carreras E, Granena A, Navasa M, Bruguera M, Marco V, Sierra J, et al. Transjugular liver biopsy in BMT. Bone Marrow Transplant. 1993;11(1):21–6.
241. Richardson PG, Ho VT, Giralt S, Arai S, Mineishi S, Cutler C, et al. Safety and efficacy of defibrotide for the treatment of severe hepatic veno-occlusive disease. Ther Adv Hematol. 2012;3(4):253–65.
242. Zhang L, Wang Y, Huang H. Defibrotide for the prevention of hepatic veno-occlusive disease after hematopoietic stem cell transplantation: a systematic review. Clin Transplant. 2012;26(4):511–9.
243. Haussmann U, Fischer J, Eber S, Scherer F, Seger R, Gungor T. Hepatic veno-occlusive disease in pediatric stem cell transplantation: impact of pre-emptive antithrombin III replacement and combined antithrombin III/defibrotide therapy. Haematologica. 2006;91(6):795–800.
244. Bearman SI, Lee JL, Baron AE, McDonald GB. Treatment of hepatic venocclusive disease with recombinant human tissue plasminogen activator and heparin in 42 marrow transplant patients. Blood. 1997;89(5):1501–6.
245. Richardson PG, Elias AD, Krishnan A, Wheeler C, Nath R, Hoppensteadt D, et al. Treatment of severe veno-occlusive disease with defibrotide: compassionate use results in response without significant toxicity in a high-risk population. Blood. 1998;92(3):737–44.

Chapter 12
Endoscopic Management of Biliary Obstruction

James H. Tabibian and Todd H. Baron

Introduction

Endoscopic retrograde cholangiography (ERC) was introduced approximately 10 years after the first description of fiber-optic gastrointestinal (GI) endoscopy and has since increasingly changed the management of biliary tract disorders [1]. ERC is generally performed under moderate sedation or with anesthesia support [2] using a side-viewing duodenoscope, which facilitates superior identification of the major papilla. The bile duct is cannulated under endoscopic and fluoroscopic guidance. A variety of catheters, guidewires, and stents are available to allow diagnostic and therapeutic maneuvers to be performed.

Over the past few decades, ERC has evolved from a purely diagnostic to an almost exclusively therapeutic procedure. Similarly, and in more recent years, endoscopic ultrasonography (i.e., endoscopic ultrasound [EUS]), a less invasive modality, has experienced noteworthy growth in facilitating diagnosis and treatment of biliary tract disorders. In this chapter, we discuss the therapeutic applications of GI endoscopy, including both ERC and EUS, for patients with benign and malignant biliary obstruction.

J.H. Tabibian, M.D.
Division of Gastroenterology & Hepatology, Department of Medicine, Mayo Clinic, Rochester, MN, USA

T.H. Baron, M.D. (✉)
Division of Gastroenterology & Hepatology, Advanced Therapeutic Endoscopy, Department of Medicine, University of North Carolina, 41041 Bioinformatics Blvd, CB 7080, Chapel Hill, NC, 27599-0001, USA
e-mail: todd_baron@med.unc.edu

E.J. Carey and K.D. Lindor (eds.), *Cholestatic Liver Disease*, Clinical Gastroenterology,
DOI 10.1007/978-1-4939-1013-7_12, © Springer Science+Business Media New York 2014

Diagnostic ERC: A Technique Now Largely Supplanted by Noninvasive Imaging

Owing to advancements in several noninvasive imaging modalities, use of ERC as a diagnostic tool in biliary disease is becoming less frequent. Magnetic resonance cholangiopancreatography (MRCP), facilitated by the high T2-signal intensity of bile as well as recent improvements in imaging and post-processing methodologies [3], has become the preferred modality for performing cholangiography. There remain, however, several indications for diagnostic ERC (Table 12.1).

It is herein worthwhile to comment on two of these indications, namely (1) primary sclerosing cholangitis (PSC) and (2) indeterminate biliary strictures, which can occur within or independent of PSC.

Primary Sclerosing Cholangitis (PSC)

PSC is an idiopathic, chronic cholangiopathy characterized by biliary fibroinflammation [4, 5], a median liver transplantation-free (LT) survival of 12–15 years [6, 7], and a predisposition to hepatobiliary malignancy, particularly cholangiocarcinoma (CCA) [6, 8, 9]. Despite clinical trials of numerous pharmacologic agents, medical therapy for PSC has yet to be established [4, 5, 10]. Although operative therapy with LT is effective for PSC, it is only performed in specialty centers and in select patients; furthermore, even in appropriate LT candidates, PSC and CCA can recur post-LT [11–13]. The diagnosis of PSC is based on cholangiography demonstrating biliary strictures or characteristic irregularity, liver histology demonstrating sclerosing cholangitis, and clinical features, particularly elevated serum alkaline phosphatase (ALK) [4, 14, 15].

ERC is indicated in the setting of presumed or known PSC when (1) the diagnosis is highly suspected but MRCP is negative or nondiagnostic, (2) cytologic sampling

Table 12.1 Applications of endoscopic retrograde cholangiography in biliary disease

Diagnostic
Primary sclerosing cholangitis
Indeterminate biliary strictures
Sphincter of Oddi manometry
Patient with contraindications to noninvasive imaging
Therapeutic
Common bile duct stones
Benign biliary strictures
Malignant biliary strictures
Primary sclerosing cholangitis
Transpapillary gallbladder drainage
Ampullary adenoma

is needed to rule out CCA, or (3) lesions requiring therapeutic intervention are anticipated (e.g., dominant biliary stricture with or without acute hepatobiliary decompensation). Regarding the first of these, it is important that proper techniques be followed to allow acquisition of optimal cholangiographic images, particularly in patients with possible early-stage PSC [16]; for example, complete filling of the intrahepatic ducts is essential to establish the diagnosis and is best achieved when the occlusion balloon catheter is positioned above the cystic duct takeoff. A negative ERC, of note, does not preclude the diagnosis of PSC, as a small fraction of patients will have small duct PSC only [17, 18]. The latter two points, i.e., cytologic sampling and management of dominant strictures, are discussed later in this chapter.

Indeterminate Biliary Strictures

Some biliary strictures cannot be readily classified as benign or malignant on the basis of noninvasive imaging studies, ERC, and/or conventional tissue sampling methods (i.e., wire-guided biliary brushing, intraductal forceps biopsy) [19]. Additional techniques that can be used to evaluate indeterminate strictures include (1) EUS, (2) intraductal ultrasonography [20], (3) probe-based confocal laser endomicroscopy [21–23], and (4) cholangioscopy with or without site-directed biopsy [24, 25]. There are two main methods of cholangioscopy: (1) passage of a cholangioscope through the working channel of the ERC scope and (2) passage of a small caliber, forward-viewing endoscope (4.9 mm) directly into the bilc duct. The latter is referred to as direct peroral cholangioscopy and can be technically challenging as the inherent mechanics and angulation do not readily permit a forward-viewing endoscope to be passed directly into the bile duct [26, 27]. However, these forward-viewing endoscopes achieve relatively superior optics (video rather than fiber optic) and have a larger working channel compared to cholangioscopes passed through the working channel of the ERC scope [28].

In a small proportion of patients, the etiology and nature of the stricture may remain unclear despite the aforementioned techniques, in which case the final diagnosis is established during long-term follow-up or by means of surgical or (repeated) nonsurgical tissue sampling.

Therapeutic ERC

The most common therapeutic application of ERC is for management of common bile duct (CBD) stones and palliation of malignant biliary obstruction. However, the range of options for endoscopic therapy of obstructive biliary disease (Table 12.2) has expanded substantially since its initial applications.

Table 12.2 Applications of endoscopic ultrasound in biliary disease

Diagnostic
Gallbladder
Stones
Sludge
Microlithiasis
Choledocholithiasis
Indeterminate biliary strictures
Ampullary lesions
Therapeutic
Transmural gallbladder drainage
Transgastric drainage of bilomas
Transgastric drainage of hepatic abscesses
Biliary drainage
Rendezvous
Hepaticogastrostomy
Choledochoduodenostomy

Benign Biliary Disease

Bile Duct Stones

ERC is frequently performed in patients with known choledocholithiasis or in those with at least a moderate clinical suspicion of choledocholithiasis [29]. In patients with cholelithiasis and low clinical suspicion of choledocholithiasis, noninvasive imaging studies (MRCP, transabdominal ultrasound) or less invasive EUS may be preferable as an initial step to avoid unnecessary ERC-related complications [30]. In patients with low clinical suspicion of choledocholithiasis in whom cholecystectomy is already planned, intraoperative cholangiography can be performed instead of preoperative ERC; if bile duct stones are identified, stone removal can be undertaken intraoperatively, thus reserving ERC for patients in whom stones are not extracted intraoperatively [30].

The standard method for stone removal is endoscopic sphincterotomy (ES) to enlarge the caliber of the papilla followed by stone extraction with an occlusion balloon or basket (Fig. 12.1). With this method >95 % of stones <1.5 cm can be removed successfully when performed by experienced endoscopists (and in the absence of underlying strictures or altered bilio-enteric anatomy) [31]. Larger stones may require more advanced techniques, which are discussed later.

An alternative to biliary sphincterotomy is balloon dilation of the papilla (i.e., balloon sphincteroplasty) using small-diameter balloons (4–8 mm) [32]. This technique was introduced to preserve sphincter of Oddi anatomy and function, particularly in young patients. The majority of published literature on balloon sphincteroplasty originates from outside the USA. Two meta-analyses of randomized trials of balloon sphincteroplasty versus ES have shown that the incidence of pancreatitis and need for mechanical lithotripsy are significantly higher while the

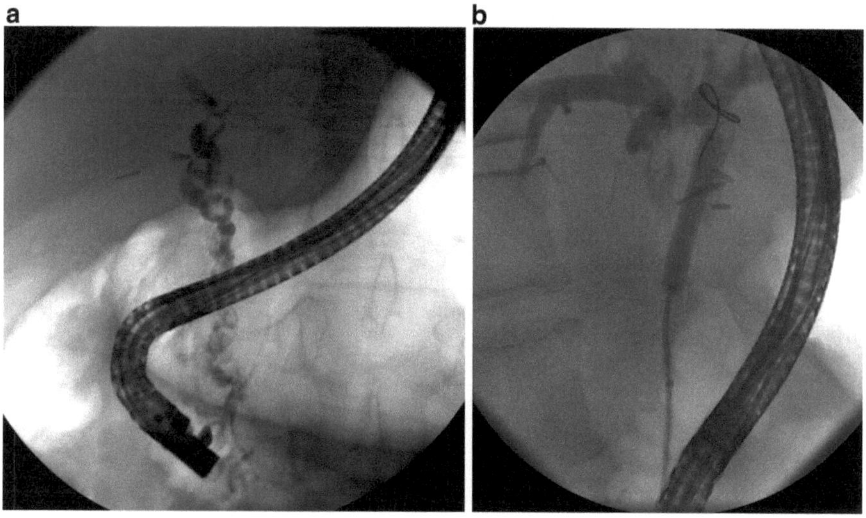

Fig. 12.1 Endoscopic management of choledocholithiasis. (**a**) Extensive choledocholithiasis seen throughout the extrahepatic biliary tree, particularly the common bile duct (gallbladder is surgically absent). (**b**) Removal of stones by endoscopic sphincterotomy followed by stone extraction with an occlusion balloon (as shown)

incidence of bleeding is significantly lower with balloon sphincteroplasty compared to standard ES [33, 34]. The only randomized clinical trial in the USA comparing balloon sphincteroplasty to ES was terminated early because of two deaths in young patients from post-ERC pancreatitis (PEP) after balloon sphincteroplasty, and thus the use of endoscopic balloon sphincteroplasty alone to extract stones as an alternative to ES has fallen out of favor in the USA [35, 36]. Nevertheless, sphincteroplasty still remains a viable option in patients with coagulopathy, persons with underlying portal hypertension (particularly Child's class C[33]), and those with altered anatomy (e.g., Billroth II gastrojejunostomy), wherein ES is technically difficult [33]. The use of prophylactic pancreatic duct stents and/or nonsteroidal anti-inflammatory drugs (NSAIDs) in these patients should be considered to prevent PEP when sphincteroplasty alone is used to remove stones.

Removal of large bile duct stones (generally defined as ≥1.5 cm in diameter) may require additional techniques such as lithotripsy in order to be removed successfully. One form of lithotripsy is *mechanical* lithotripsy, in which the stone is captured in a specialized large basket and crushed [37]; the fragments are then removed using standard extraction techniques. Another form of lithotripsy is *intraductal* lithotripsy, which is performed by passing laser or electrohydraulic catheters into the bile duct and fragmenting stones under direct endoscopic visualization via transpapillary choledochoscope [38]. Direct visualization is essential during intraductal lithotripsy to ensure that the lithotripsy device is directed at the stone and not the bile duct wall so as to prevent biliary epithelial or transmural injury.

Table 12.3 Principal causes of benign biliary strictures

Operative injury
Cholecystectomy
Resection of choledochal cyst or other hepatobiliary lesion
Liver transplantation (i.e., anastomotic biliary stricture)
Antrectomy
Pancreatitis
Ischemia (e.g., post-liver transplantation non-anastomotic strictures)
Portal biliopathy
Immunoglobulin G4-related cholangiopathy
Acquired immune deficiency syndrome (AIDS) cholangiopathy
Eosinophilic cholangitis
Idiopathic

Recently, the combination of biliary sphincterotomy and large-diameter (>12 mm and up to 20 mm) balloon dilation has been used to remove large stones and avoid the need for mechanical lithotripsy. This combination enlarges the lumen of the distal common bile duct and sphincterotomy opening, which represent the major limitations to successful extraction of large bile duct stones, and appears to be safe and is not associated with an increased risk of PEP.

When large stones cannot be removed, a biliary stent is placed to relieve biliary obstruction [39]; additional procedures can then be undertaken to remove residual stone burden.

Benign Biliary Strictures

Benign biliary strictures (BBSs) can occur due to a variety of causes (Table 12.3), although regardless of cause, endoscopic therapy generally consists of balloon dilation and placement of plastic biliary stents (Fig. 12.2) [40]. There is now substantial evidence that placement of multiple plastic stents side by side for a total of 6–12 months optimizes stricture resolution rates (>90 %) (Fig. 12.3) and minimizes recurrence as compared to placement of only one or two stents [41–44].

More recently, the use of 8–10 mm diameter fully covered self-expandable metal stents (SEMS), which are several times the diameter of individual plastic biliary stents, has emerged as a promising alternative in the treatment of non-hilar BBS (i.e., those involving the ductal confluence); however, these stents are costly and not yet approved in the USA for BBSs [45]. Chronic pancreatitis can result in formation of distal common bile duct strictures that are commonly refractory to endoscopic therapy with plastic stents, particularly in patients with calcific chronic pancreatitis [46]. In these cases, maximal multiple plastic stent therapy, or alternatively fully covered SEMS, can be attempted [47].

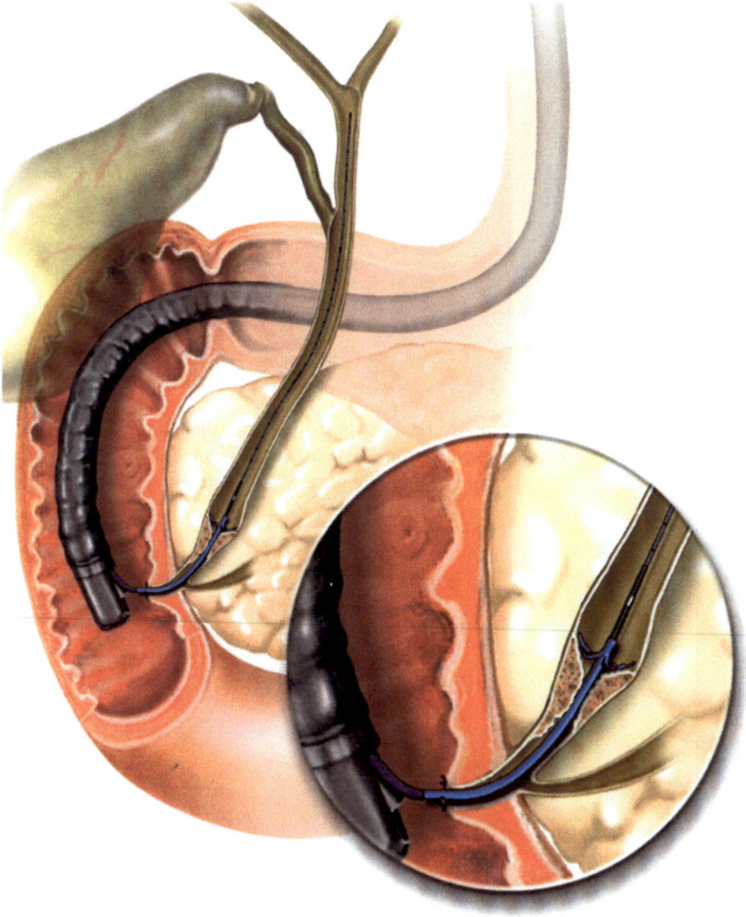

Fig. 12.2 Representative illustration of endoscopic stenting of (malignant) distal common bile duct stricture

Biliary Strictures in LT Patients

As with other benign biliary strictures, ERC is indicated for treatment of post-LT biliary strictures [44, 48]. Placement of multiple (up to 9 [44]) plastic biliary stents for a total of at least 12 months has been shown to optimize stricture resolution rates (Fig. 12.3) [44, 46, 48]. While the response to this multiple or "maximal" endoscopic stenting protocol is favorable for most BBSs (Fig. 12.4) [44, 49], therapeutic outcomes depend at least in part on the underlying etiology (e.g., non-anastomotic post-LT strictures are generally more challenging to treat) [43, 44, 50], time since LT [51], immunosuppressive regimen (sirolimus being a risk factor for adverse ERC outcomes) [52, 53], and endoscopist experience [54].

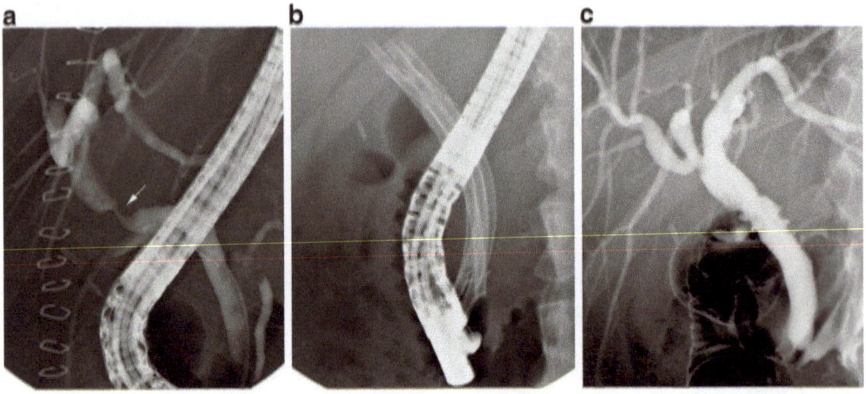

Fig. 12.3 Endoscopic management of benign, post-liver transplantation anastomotic biliary stricture (ABS). (**a**) Post-liver transplantation ABS (*arrow*) evident on ERC. (**b**) Endoscopic balloon dilation followed by placement of multiple plastic biliary stents. (**c**) ABS resolution

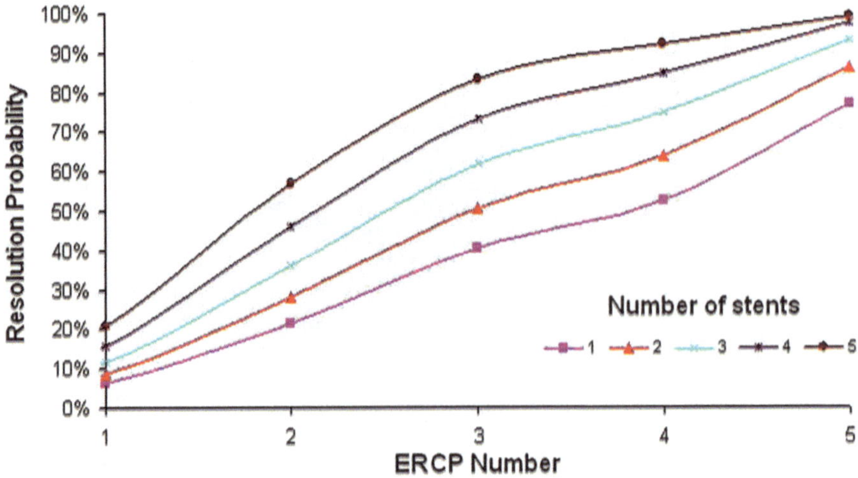

Fig. 12.4 Cox proportional hazard model demonstrating ABS resolution probability as a function of number of stents at each ERCP. Adapted from Tabibian JH, Asham EH, Han S, et al. Endoscopic treatment of postorthotopic liver transplantation anastomotic biliary strictures with maximal stent therapy (with video). Gastrointest Endosc 2010;71:505–12. With permission from Elsevier Limited

Malignant Biliary Obstruction

Endoscopic relief of malignant biliary obstruction is achieved by placement of one (distal) or more (hilar) large-bore (10 Fr) plastic stents or SEMS across the malignant stricture(s). The endoscopic approach depends on whether the obstructive is distal to the bifurcation of the common hepatic duct or involving the bifurcation (i.e., hilar obstruction).

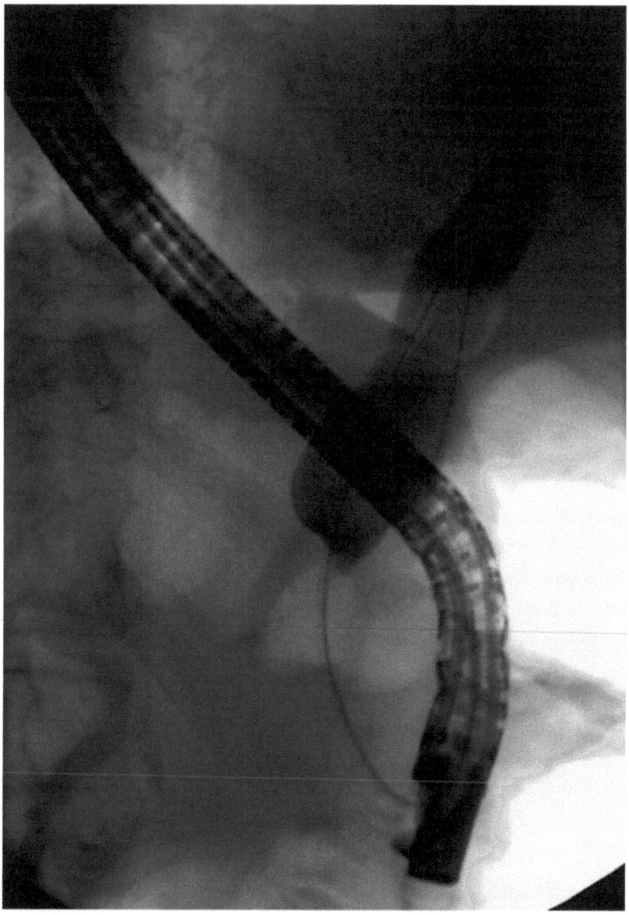

Fig. 12.5 Long distal common bile duct stricture with bird's beak appearance, highly suggestive of underlying malignancy

Malignant Distal (Non-hilar) Biliary Obstruction

Distal biliary obstruction due to malignancy (Fig. 12.5), regardless of etiology (e.g., CCA, pancreatic adenocarcinoma), can be effectively treated using a single biliary stent. ERC with biliary stent placement is now accepted as a viable alternative to palliative surgical bypass and can be performed safely in an outpatient setting [55]. Relief of obstruction is as effective as with surgical biliary bypass, but with lower morbidity and mortality, albeit with an increased re-obstruction rate [56].

The most common cause of distal bile duct obstruction is adenocarcinoma of the pancreatic head. The role of endoscopic biliary decompression in patients with distal bile duct obstruction due to pancreatic adenocarcinoma depends heavily on the clinical scenario, and in fact routine preoperative ERC for biliary decompression is discouraged in patients with surgically resectable disease. Several studies have shown

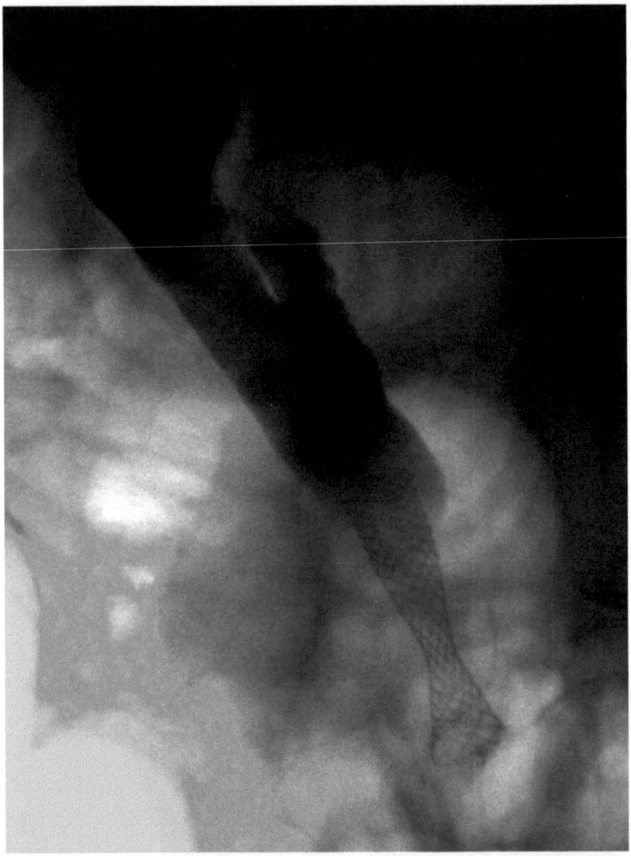

Fig. 12.6 Biliary self-expanding metal stent (SEMS) placed for palliation of a malignant distal biliary stricture

that preoperative endoscopic stent placement does not improve surgical outcome and in fact increases overall morbidity and adverse events from ERC that may result in delay of or even prohibit surgical resection [57, 58]. ERC is indicated, however, in cases complicated by acute cholangitis and severe pruritus [59]. ERC is also indicated when neoadjuvant chemoradiation is planned considering the prolonged period of time to surgical resection. In such cases, the use of a short-length (≤6 cm) SEMS (covered or uncovered) (Fig. 12.6) appears to be the best option based on data showing a higher rate of stent occlusion in patients receiving plastic biliary stents as compared to a SEMS [60, 61].

The main limitation to plastic stent placement is stent occlusion as a result of bacterial biofilm formation or reflux of food matter and as a function of time since stent placement [44, 62]; therefore, in the comparative trials of endoscopy versus surgery, the shorter length of initial hospital stay in the endoscopy group was offset by the need for subsequent hospitalizations and repeat ERC to manage plastic stent

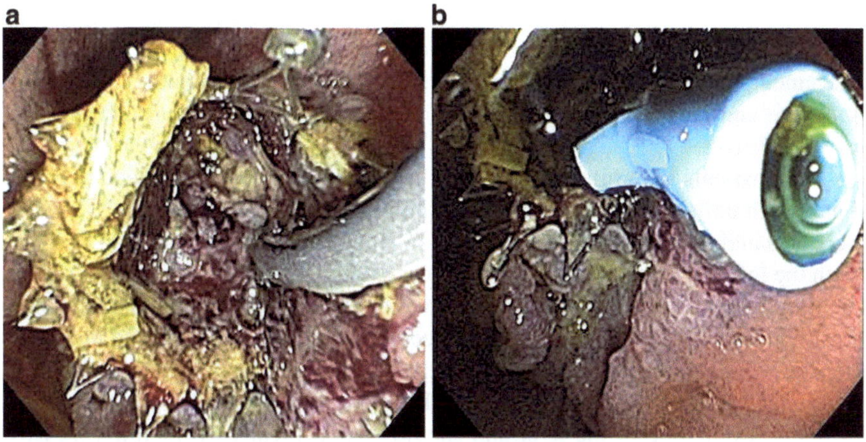

Fig. 12.7 Tumor ingrowth. (**a**) Ingrowth of tumor and debris is seen obstructing the lumen of a SEMS. (**b**) Palliation is provided by placement of a plastic biliary stent through the SEMS

occlusion. The use of SEMS has largely overcome the issue of bacterial biofilm formation, and randomized controlled trials have shown superior patency rates for uncovered biliary SEMS when compared to plastic stents [42, 63]. It is notable to recognize that the cost of a SEMS is substantially greater than that of a plastic stent; however, placement of a SEMS can be cost effective as long as projected life expectancy is longer than 3–6 months; thus, this should be taken into account when deciding between plastic and metal biliary stents [64].

Other factors to be considered in deciding between a plastic stent and a SEMS include a patient's adherence and ability to return for care, including management of stent occlusion. Uncovered SEMS occlusion is generally managed with placement of a plastic stent or a new SEMS within the existing one. Covered SEMS have been introduced more recently in an attempt to reduce tumor ingrowth (Fig. 12.7) and tissue hyperplasia through stent interstices and thereby potentially extending patency; although there may be less stent occlusion with covered SEMS, this appears to come with a greater cost, higher migration rates [65], and possibly an increased risk of acute cholecystitis [66, 67]. Advantages of covered SEMS are ease of removability and revision compared to uncovered SEMS, which can become imbedded into the surrounding bile duct. Removability may be particularly important in patients who are later found to have benign disease (e.g., autoimmune pancreatitis) or curable malignancy (e.g., lymphoma [68]).

Malignant Hilar Biliary Obstruction

Hilar biliary strictures may be caused by CCA (i.e., Klatskin tumor) or metastatic disease. The approach to biliary obstruction involving the hepatic hilum is endoscopically more challenging than that of distal biliary obstruction [69], with procedural and clinical success rates depending on biliary tract anatomy and endoscopist experience. Success rates also depend on the need for unilateral versus bilateral biliary stent placement, which is a function of potential for resectability, Bismuth classification, presence and location of liver atrophy, intrahepatic tumor burden, and presence of PSC [70].

Most patients with hilar malignant biliary obstruction will be adequately palliated with unilateral biliary stenting and drainage, i.e., with only one side being accessed and therefore endoscopically contaminated [71]; patients who have had both the left and right biliary systems accessed and injected with contrast require stenting of both to reduce the risk of acute cholangitis [72]. To avoid such contrast injection in cases where it is not necessary, guidewires are passed into intrahepatic ducts without injecting contrast using an imaging-guided (MRI, computed tomography [CT]) approach. Pre-ERC abdominal imaging may reveal atrophy of one lobe of the liver and should be specifically avoided during ERC since contamination will require drainage to prevent cholangitis but will likely not facilitate palliation.

Unlike patients with malignant *distal* biliary obstruction, the advantages of SEMS placement are not as clear-cut in patients with *hilar* disease, and re-intervention for management of stent occlusion can be particularly difficult when bilateral biliary stents have been placed [73]. In a prospective single-arm pilot study of SEMS in 17 patients with Bismuth type II and III hilar CCA, median stent patency was 12 months [74]. Similarly, in a non-comparative single-arm study, insertion of a Wallstent (a type of SEMS) was found to be safe and feasible and resulted in successful palliation without the need for further biliary intervention in 69 % of patients with nonresectable hilar CCA [75]. In a more recent prospective observational cohort study of patients with hilar tumors treated with plastic or metal stents, patients receiving metal stents had significantly lower rates of post-procedural complications and need for percutaneous drainage [76]. These encouraging results suggest that SEMS may offer similar benefits for malignant hilar biliary obstruction as they do for distal biliary obstruction.

To summarize regarding the role of endoscopic stenting in malignant hilar biliary obstruction, patients with unresectable hilar CCA who undergo ERC for palliation should receive unilateral stenting with unilateral contrast injection. One biliary stent, be it plastic or metal, is generally adequate to achieve palliation, although treatment may need to be individualized (e.g., extensive, bilateral stenting in some cases) [77]. SEMS appear to offer more durable palliation than plastic stents but are only cost effective when expected survival is at least 3 months, as mentioned above [78, 79]. Lastly, from an endoscopic perspective, achieving successful drainage is more difficult technically for hilar as compared to distal biliary obstruction.

For patients in whom jaundice does not resolve after endoscopic placement of plastic stents, several other endoscopically administered modalities can be used for palliation of unresectable hilar CCA [80]. Photodynamic therapy (PDT) is associated with significant improvements in cholestasis, quality of life, and survival (as compared with historical controls) and can be maintained for an extended period [81, 82]. However, the initial studies on PDT for hilar CCA were performed outside the USA, in countries where smaller, more flexible laser fibers are available. In the USA, biliary PDT is currently performed utilizing rigid laser fibers which are used for the treatment of neoplastic esophageal diseases. Nevertheless, PDT trials in the USA have shown promising results [83, 84] among select centers with expertise in this procedure.

More recently, intraductal radiofrequency ablation has been used to treat CCA [85]. The radiofrequency ablation probe is 10 Fr in diameter and flexible and can be used with standard electrosurgical generators. Preliminary data are promising, and indeed this technology may ultimately replace biliary PDT. Endoscopically delivered brachytherapy, either low dose or high dose, is also available, but this therapy is generally reserved for patients who are part of an LT protocol [86].

Primary Sclerosing Cholangitis with Indeterminate Dominant Strictures

In addition to the indications for diagnostic ERC in patients with PSC described above, patients with PSC may benefit from therapeutic ERC for several indications, including treatment of a dominant stricture or biliary lithiasis [87]. Patients with a dominant stricture usually present with progressive biliary obstruction and associated signs (e.g., rising serum alkaline phosphatase and/or bilirubin, acute cholangitis) and symptoms (e.g., pruritus, choluria). Endoscopic treatment of a dominant stricture involves balloon dilation, often in combination with short-term (<8 weeks) placement of a large-bore (10 Fr) stent. Success rates, with clinical, biochemical, and radiologic improvement as endpoints, have ranged from 65 to 100 % with this approach, although currently available endoscopic interventions are not thought to impact the long-term outcomes (i.e., CCA, need for LT, or death) of PSC [4, 88].

In addition to relieving biliary obstruction during ERC, attempts to exclude CCA should also be undertaken. Routine brush cytology has a low sensitivity in the patients with PSC, but the diagnostic yield can be augmented by also performing fluorescence in situ hybridization (FISH) on biliary brush specimens [8, 89]. Cholangioscopy may further improve detection of malignancy in these patients (Fig. 12.8), but published studies are limited, and reliability appears to be less in patients with PSC than in those with de novo strictures due to difficulty in distinguishing benign from malignant strictures [90]. More recently, probe-based confocal laser endomicroscopy has been used [23]. This technique requires pre-procedural injection of fluorescein contrast and use of a specialized probe that allows real-time visualization of cellularity [91]. More data are needed before this technique can be recommended routinely.

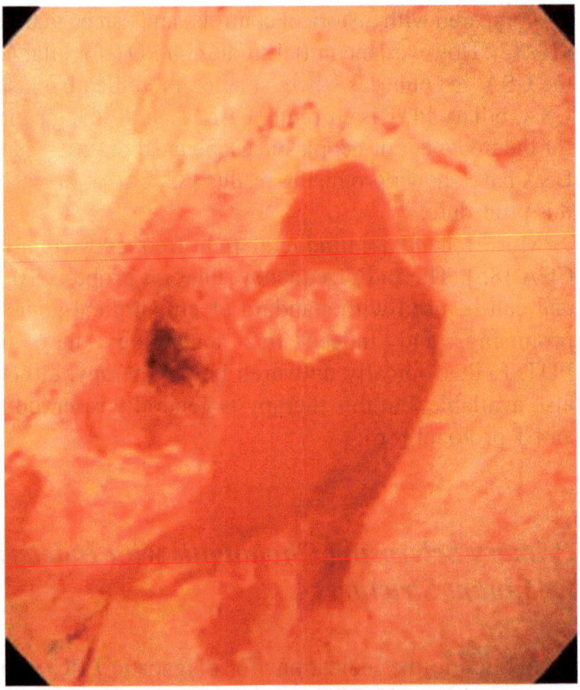

Fig. 12.8 Cholangioscopic image demonstrating tortuous blood vessels and biliary mucosal friability. A diagnosis of cholangiocarcinoma was ultimately made by a combination of diagnostic techniques

Diagnostic and Therapeutic Biliary Endoscopy in Patients with Altered Bilio-Enteric Anatomy

ERC was once considered impossible in patients with surgically altered anatomy, and instead percutaneous or surgical approaches were historically used. With increasing experience, however, initially using colonoscopies [92], and in the advent of balloon enteroscopy [54, 93], biliary endotherapy can now be achieved in patients with surgically altered anatomy, including patients with Roux-en-Y anastomoses and post-Whipple anatomy (Fig. 12.9). The most difficult anatomy is that following Roux-en-Y gastric bypass, in these patients, options include unique endoscopic approaches [94] or a combined endoscopic and laparoscopic assisted approach whereby access to the excluded stomach and antegrade passage of a standard side-viewing duodenoscope into the duodenum are possible [95]. Furthermore, percutaneous-endoscopic hybrid access approaches have been recently described to treat biliary diseases; "percutaneous assisted transluminal endoscopic therapy" (PATENT) [96] has been used to treat gallbladder disease and to access the excluded stomach in order to pass antegrade duodenoscopes in patients with RYGB anatomy. Using this approach, management of CBD stones and other obstructive biliary processes can be achieved entirely endoscopically [97].

Unfortunately, biliary cannulation with solely endoscopic (i.e., non-hybrid or percutaneously assisted) approaches remains technically difficult in patients with a

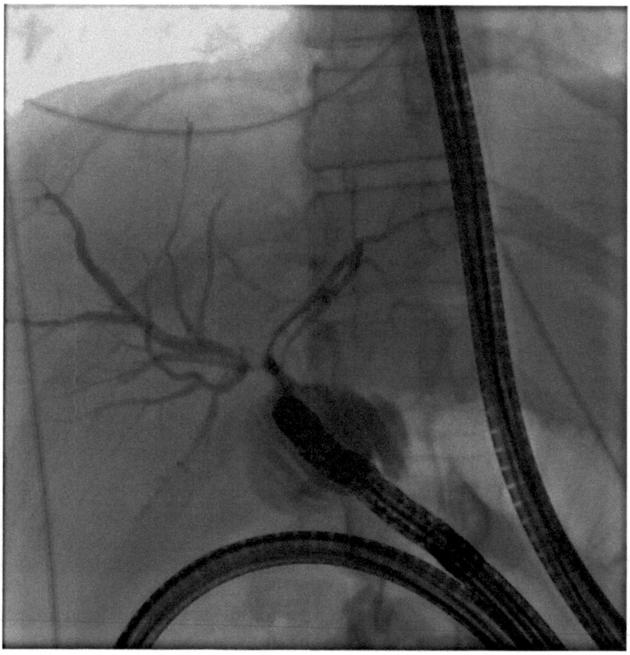

Fig. 12.9 ERC in a patient with Roux-en-Y bilio-enteric anatomy

native papilla since colonoscopes and balloon enteroscopes are forward viewing rather than side viewing. Nevertheless, in centers with extensive experience in biliary endoscopy (where such procedures should be performed given the technical demand and labor intensiveness), high procedural success rates can be achieved [54].

Endoscopic Ultrasonography

EUS combines endoscopy and ultrasound to less invasively provide high-resolution images of the biliary system without radiation or contrast exposure. Over the last decade, the role of EUS in facilitating diagnosis and treatment of biliary tract disorders has seen considerable expansion.

Diagnostic EUS

EUS is highly reliable in determining the cause of extrahepatic biliary obstruction, with an overall sensitivity of 97 % and specificity of 88 % [98]. For the diagnosis of bile duct stones, the sensitivity, specificity, and accuracy rates of EUS are 95 %,

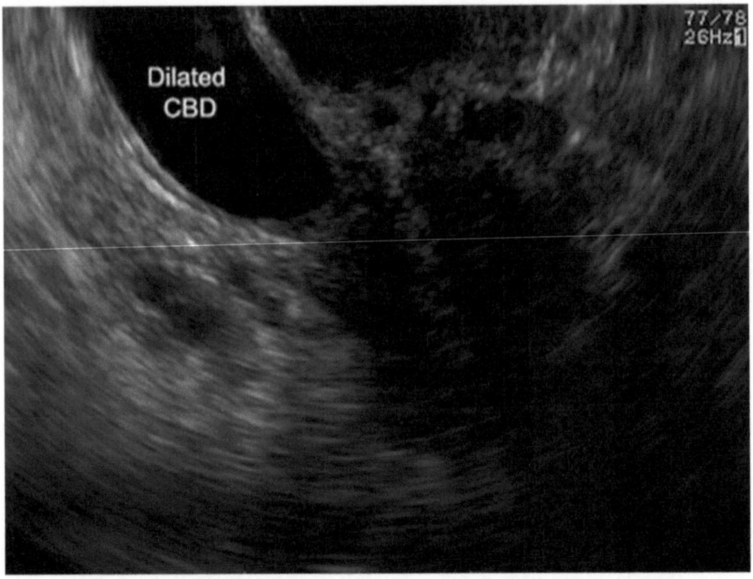

Fig. 12.10 Endoscopic ultrasound image demonstrating pancreatic head mass (*arrows*) and consequent upstream dilatation of the common bile duct

98 %, and 96 %, respectively [98]. Given that EUS is exquisitely sensitive for the diagnosis of choledocholithiasis as well as gallbladder sludge, cholelithiasis, and microlithiasis, it can be particularly useful among patients in whom there is a high suspicion of such pathology yet noninvasive imaging studies (e.g., transabdominal ultrasound, MRCP) have been unrevealing.

For detection of pancreatic tumors, EUS is more sensitive (range 93–100 %) than CT (53–77 %), transabdominal ultrasound (50–67 %), MRI (50–67 %), and ERC (≈90 %) [98]. Linear-array EUS (Fig. 12.10) allows directed tissue acquisition using fine-needle aspiration (FNA) techniques and is helpful in (1) establishing a tissue diagnosis of malignant biliary strictures when other modalities are negative [99], (2) staging CCA [100] and other biliary malignancies, and (3) evaluating for the presence of lymph node involvement in patients with malignant biliary strictures.

Therapeutic EUS

Applications of therapeutic EUS for biliary disease are now becoming widely recognized [101, 102]. In addition to the use of EUS to provide biliary access for ERC using a rendezvous approach, direct biliary drainage is now becoming an increasingly used approach [103].

Biliary Drainage

EUS-guided biliary access and drainage are performed by needle puncture followed by passage of FNA wire- and/or catheter-guided entry into the biliary system. This technique, which continues to gain favor in the emergence of new accessories specifically for this purpose, allows reliable and safe drainage of intrahepatics ducts via approaches (a) through the stomach into the left lobe (hepaticogastrostomy) [104–107] or (b) through the duodenum into the bile duct (choledochoduodenostomy) [108, 109]. Thereafter, drainage can be internalized through the papilla without requiring a rendezvous approach (although combination approaches can be useful as well) [110, 111]. This EUS-guided technique is especially helpful when cannulation of the bile duct fails or access to the papilla is not possible due to duodenal obstruction or other causes [112].

EUS can also facilitate other hepatobiliary drainage procedures, including (1) transgastric and transduodenal drainage of the gallbladder (as an alternative to percutaneous cholecystostomy in patients with acute cholecystitis [113] who are poor operative candidates for cholecystectomy) [114]; (2) transgastric drainage of hepatic abscesses [115]; and (3) transgastric drainage of bilomas [116].

Adverse Events

Adverse events (AEs) of ERC and EUS are well known and are categorized into five major types: sedation related, GI bleeding, perforation, PEP, and infection [117–119]. Risk factors for AEs generally depend on operator characteristics, patient characteristics, and degree of procedural invasiveness, and preventive measures can be optimized at each of these levels to minimize the frequency and severity of AEs.

ERC is increasingly being performed with anesthesia support, especially in more severely ill patients and in cases anticipated to be more complex, and thus endoscopists are faced with less frequent sedation-related cardiopulmonary complications. GI bleeding most often occurs after ES. Risk factors for post-ES bleeding include coagulopathy and institution of anticoagulation within 72 h of the sphincterotomy [120]. Perforation of the duodenum occurs in less than 1 % of patients and may require surgical management, especially when the lateral duodenal wall is injured [35, 121]. Infection occurs primarily in patients in whom drainage of the biliary tree after ERC is inadequate. Such patients include those with extensive intrahepatic PSC or advanced hilar tumors and those who have undergone failed stent placement for biliary obstruction. Accumulating data suggest that a lower ERC volume by an endoscopist is associated with a lower success rate and higher AE rate [122].

Rates of PEP vary depending on differences in patient selection and operator technique and experience. Patients at highest risk for PEP are young, otherwise healthy women, especially those with known or suspected SOD [123]; elderly patients and those with chronic pancreatitis or pancreatic cancer (or other causes of non-SOD biliary dilatation) have lower rates of pancreatitis. Prophylactic placement of a main pancreatic duct stent reduces the risk of pancreatitis in high-risk patients and nearly eliminates the risk of severe pancreatitis [124]. More recently, the use of rectally administered NSAIDs (indomethacin) immediately after the ERC has been shown to significantly decrease the risk of PEP in patients at high risk for this AE [123–125].

Management of most AEs is nonoperative and can include pharmacotherapy, repeat endoscopy, or interventional radiological approaches. Even most perforations can now be managed nonoperatively [121]; this is facilitated by early recognition of perforation and improved closure devices. Nevertheless, it is important to have all relevant disciplines (hospitalists, critical care specialists, interventional radiologists, and surgeons) available to manage patients with perforation and other AEs.

Other AEs associated with management of biliary obstruction include stent migration (proximally or distally) and leakage between EUS-guided puncture site and biliary tree.

Conclusions

Endoscopic management of biliary obstruction has progressed impressively over the last 30 years. A wide array of biliary diseases can now be treated endoscopically using ERC, with high success rates and low adverse event rates in experienced centers. Furthermore, EUS is now emerging as an additional therapeutic tool for biliary diseases. Continued advancements in both ERC and EUS are anticipated.

Funding Sources JHT is supported by NIH T32 DK007198.

References

1. McCune WS. ERCP at thirty years: an interview with Dr. William S. McCune (1909–1998). Gastrointest Endosc. 1998;48:643–4.
2. Papachristou G, Gleeson F, Papachristou D, et al. Endoscopist administered sedation during ERCP: impact of chronic narcotic/benzodiazepine use and predictive risk of reversal agent utilization. Am J Gastroenterol. 2007;102:738–43.
3. Tabibian JH, Macura SI, O'Hara SP, et al. Micro-computed tomography and nuclear magnetic resonance imaging for noninvasive, live-mouse cholangiography. Lab Invest. 2013;93: 733–43.
4. Tabibian JH, Lindor KD. Primary sclerosing cholangitis: a review and update on therapeutic developments. Expert Rev Gastroenterol Hepatol. 2013;7:103–14.
5. O'Hara SP, Tabibian JH, Splinter PL, et al. The dynamic biliary epithelia: molecules, pathways, and disease. J Hepatol. 2013;58:575–82.
6. Wiesner RH, Grambsch PM, Dickson ER, et al. Primary sclerosing cholangitis: natural history, prognostic factors and survival analysis. Hepatology. 1989;10:430–6.
7. Farrant JM, Hayllar KM, Wilkinson ML, et al. Natural history and prognostic variables in primary sclerosing cholangitis. Gastroenterology. 1991;100:1710–7.

8. Tabibian JH, Lindor KD. Challenges of cholangiocarcinoma detection in patients with primary sclerosing cholangitis. J Anal Oncol. 2012;1:50–5.
9. Kaplan GG, Laupland KB, Butzner D, et al. The burden of large and small duct primary sclerosing cholangitis in adults and children: a population-based analysis. Am J Gastroenterol. 2007;102:1042–9.
10. Tabibian JH, Weeding E, Jorgensen RA, et al. Randomised clinical trial: vancomycin or metronidazole in patients with primary sclerosing cholangitis – a pilot study. Aliment Pharmacol Ther. 2013;37:604–12.
11. Alabraba E, Nightingale P, Gunson B, et al. A re-evaluation of the risk factors for the recurrence of primary sclerosing cholangitis in liver allografts. Liver Transpl. 2009;15:330–40.
12. Graziadei IW. Live donor liver transplantation for primary sclerosing cholangitis: is disease recurrence increased? Curr Opin Gastroenterol. 2011;27:301–5.
13. Landaverde C, Ng V, Sato A, et al. De-novo cholangiocarcinoma in native common bile duct remnant following OLT for primary sclerosing cholangitis. Ann Hepatol. 2009;8:379–83.
14. Chapman R, Fevery J, Kalloo A, et al. Diagnosis and management of primary sclerosing cholangitis. Hepatology. 2010;51:660–78.
15. Beuers U, Boberg KM, Chapman RW, et al. EASL clinical practice guidelines: management of cholestatic liver diseases. J Hepatol. 2009;51:237–67.
16. Gardner TB, Baron TH. Optimizing cholangiography when performing endoscopic retrograde cholangiopancreatography. Clin Gastroenterol Hepatol. 2008;6:734–40.
17. Angulo P, Maor-Kendler Y, Lindor KD. Small-duct primary sclerosing cholangitis: a long-term follow-up study. Hepatology. 2002;35:1494–500.
18. Tabibian JH, Masyuk AL, Masyuk TV, LaRusso NF. Cholangiocyte physiology. Compr Physiol. 2013;3:541–65.
19. Papachristou G, Smyrk T, Baron T. Endoscopic retrograde cholangiopancreatography tissue sampling: when and how? Clin Gastroenterol Hepatol. 2007;5:783–90.
20. Varadarajulu S, Eloubeidi M, Wilcox C. Prospective evaluation of indeterminate ERCP findings by intraductal ultrasound. J Gastroenterol Hepatol. 2007;22:2086–92.
21. Shah R, Langer D, Antillon M, et al. Cholangioscopy and cholangioscopic forceps biopsy in patients with indeterminate pancreaticobiliary pathology. Clin Gastroenterol Hepatol. 2006;4:219–25.
22. Victor DW, Sherman S, Karakan T, et al. Current endoscopic approach to indeterminate biliary strictures. World J Gastroenterol. 2012;18:6197–205.
23. Heif M, Yen RD, Shah RJ. ERCP with probe-based confocal laser endomicroscopy for the evaluation of dominant biliary stenoses in primary sclerosing cholangitis patients. Dig Dis Sci. 2013;58:2068–74.
24. Draganov PV, Chauhan S, Wagh MS, et al. Diagnostic accuracy of conventional and cholangioscopy-guided sampling of indeterminate biliary lesions at the time of ERCP: a prospective, long-term follow-up study. Gastrointest Endosc. 2012;75:347–53.
25. Petersen BT. Cholangioscopy for special applications: primary sclerosing cholangitis, liver transplant, and selective duct access. Gastrointest Endosc Clin N Am. 2009;19:579–86.
26. Moon JH, Terheggen G, Choi HJ, et al. Peroral cholangioscopy: diagnostic and therapeutic applications. Gastroenterology. 2013;144:276–82.
27. Osanai M, Itoi T, Igarashi Y, et al. Peroral video cholangioscopy to evaluate indeterminate bile duct lesions and preoperative mucosal cancerous extension: a prospective multicenter study. Endoscopy. 2013;45:635–42.
28. Nishikawa T, Tsuyuguchi T, Sakai Y, et al. Comparison of the diagnostic accuracy of peroral video-cholangioscopic visual findings and cholangioscopy-guided forceps biopsy findings for indeterminate biliary lesions: a prospective study. Gastrointest Endosc. 2013;77:219–26.
29. Frossard JL, Morel PM. Detection and management of bile duct stones. Gastrointest Endosc. 2010;72:808–16.
30. Williams E, Green J, Beckingham I, et al. British Society of Gastroenterology. Guidelines on the management of common bile duct stones (CBDS). Gut. 2008;57:1004–21.

31. Carr-Locke D. Therapeutic role of ERCP in the management of suspected common bile duct stones. Gastrointest Endosc. 2002;56:S170–4.
32. Maple JT, Ikenberry SO, Anderson MA, et al. The role of endoscopy in the management of choledocholithiasis. Gastrointest Endosc. 2011;74:731–44.
33. Baron T, Harewood G. Endoscopic balloon dilation of the biliary sphincter compared to endoscopic biliary sphincterotomy for removal of common bile duct stones during ERCP: a meta-analysis of randomized, controlled trials. Am J Gastroenterol. 2004;99:1455–60.
34. Weinberg B, Shindy W, Lo S. Endoscopic balloon sphincter dilation (sphincteroplasty) versus sphincterotomy for common bile duct stones. Cochrane Database Syst Rev. 2006;4, CD004890.
35. Fatima J, Baron T, Topazian M, et al. Pancreaticobiliary and duodenal perforations after periampullary endoscopic procedures: diagnosis and management. Arch Surg. 2007;142:448–54.
36. Disario J, Freeman M, Bjorkman D, et al. Endoscopic balloon dilation compared with sphincterotomy for extraction of bile duct stones. Gastroenterology. 2004;127:1291–9.
37. Baron T. Endoscopy for bile duct stones. Minerva Gastroenterol Dietol. 2005;51:289–301.
38. Piraka C, Shah R, Awadallah N, et al. Transpapillary cholangioscopy-directed lithotripsy in patients with difficult bile duct stones. Clin Gastroenterol Hepatol. 2007;5:1333–8.
39. Katsinelos P, Kountouras J, Paroutoglou G, et al. Combination of endoprostheses and oral ursodeoxycholic acid or placebo in the treatment of difficult to extract common bile duct stones. Dig Liver Dis. 2008;40:453–9.
40. Baron Sr TH, Davee T. Endoscopic management of benign bile duct strictures. Gastrointest Endosc Clin N Am. 2013;23:295–311.
41. Zepeda-Gomez S, Baron TH. Benign biliary strictures: current endoscopic management. Nat Rev Gastroenterol Hepatol. 2011;8:573–81.
42. Dumonceau JM, Tringali A, Blero D, et al. Biliary stenting: indications, choice of stents and results: European Society of Gastrointestinal Endoscopy (ESGE) clinical guideline. Endoscopy. 2012;44:277–98.
43. Tabibian JH, Asham EH, Goldstein L, et al. Endoscopic treatment with multiple stents for post-liver-transplantation nonanastomotic biliary strictures. Gastrointest Endosc. 2009;69: 1236–43.
44. Tabibian JH, Asham EH, Han S, et al. Endoscopic treatment of postorthotopic liver transplantation anastomotic biliary strictures with maximal stent therapy (with video). Gastrointest Endosc. 2010;71:505–12.
45. Baron TH. Covered self-expandable metal stents for benign biliary tract diseases. Curr Opin Gastroenterol. 2011;27:262–7.
46. Costamagna G, Bulajic M, Tringali A, et al. Multiple stenting of refractory pancreatic duct strictures in severe chronic pancreatitis: long-term results. Endoscopy. 2006;38:254–9.
47. Perri V, Boskoski I, Tringali A, et al. Fully covered self-expandable metal stents in biliary strictures caused by chronic pancreatitis not responding to plastic stenting: a prospective study with 2 years of follow-up. Gastrointest Endosc. 2012;75:1271–7.
48. Adler DG, Baron TH, Davila RE, et al. ASGE guideline: the role of ERCP in diseases of the biliary tract and the pancreas. Gastrointest Endosc. 2005;62:1–8.
49. Pasha SF, Harrison ME, Das A, et al. Endoscopic treatment of anastomotic biliary strictures after deceased donor liver transplantation: outcomes after maximal stent therapy. Gastrointest Endosc. 2007;66:44–51.
50. Graziadei IW, Schwaighofer H, Koch R, et al. Long-term outcome of endoscopic treatment of biliary strictures after liver transplantation. Liver Transpl. 2006;12:718–25.
51. Thethy S, Thomson B, Pleass H, et al. Management of biliary tract complications after orthotopic liver transplantation. Clin Transplant. 2004;18:647–53.
52. Tabibian JH, Yeh HC, Singh VK, et al. Sirolimus may be associated with early recurrence of biliary obstruction in liver transplant patients undergoing endoscopic stenting of biliary strictures. Ann Hepatol. 2011;10:270–6.
53. Tabibian JH, Girotra M, Yeh HC, et al. Sirolimus based immunosuppression is associated with need for early repeat therapeutic ERCP in liver transplant patients with anastomotic biliary stricture. Ann Hepatol. 2013;12:563–9.

54. Azeem N, Tabibian JH, Baron TH, et al. Use of a single-balloon enteroscope compared with variable-stiffness colonoscopes for endoscopic retrograde cholangiography in liver transplant patients with Roux-en-Y biliary anastomosis. Gastrointest Endosc. 2013;77:568–77.
55. Taylor M, McLeod R, Langer B. Biliary stenting versus bypass surgery for the palliation of malignant distal bile duct obstruction: a meta-analysis. Liver Transpl. 2000;6:302–8.
56. Ferreira LE, Baron TH. Endoscopic stenting for palliation of malignant biliary obstruction. Expert Rev Med Devices. 2010;7:681–91.
57. Sewnath M, Karsten T, Prins M, et al. A meta-analysis on the efficacy of preoperative biliary drainage for tumors causing obstructive jaundice. Ann Surg. 2002;236:17–27.
58. van der Gaag NA, Rauws EA, van Eijck CH, et al. Preoperative biliary drainage for cancer of the head of the pancreas. N Engl J Med. 2010;362:129–37.
59. Bonin EA, Baron TH. Preoperative biliary stents in pancreatic cancer. J Hepatobiliary Pancreat Sci. 2011;18:621–9.
60. Wasan S, Ross W, Staerkel G, et al. Use of expandable metallic biliary stents in resectable pancreatic cancer. Am J Gastroenterol. 2005;100:2056–61.
61. Singh A, Lee JH. Self-expanding metal stents for preoperative biliary drainage in patients receiving neoadjuvant therapy for pancreatic cancer. J Gastrointest Oncol. 2012;3:304–5.
62. Weickert U, Venzke T, König J, et al. Why do bilioduodenal plastic stents become occluded? A clinical and pathological investigation on 100 consecutive patients. Endoscopy. 2001;33:786–90.
63. Moss AC, Morris E, Leyden J, et al. Malignant distal biliary obstruction: a systematic review and meta-analysis of endoscopic and surgical bypass results. Cancer Treat Rev. 2007;33: 213–21.
64. Pop GH, Richter JA, Sauer B, et al. Bridge to surgery using partially covered self-expandable metal stents (PCMS) in malignant biliary stricture: an acceptable paradigm? Surg Endosc. 2011;25:613–8.
65. Nakai Y, Isayama H, Komatsu Y, et al. Efficacy and safety of the covered Wallstent in patients with distal malignant biliary obstruction. Gastrointest Endosc. 2005;62:742–8.
66. Saleem A, Leggett CL, Murad MH, et al. Meta-analysis of randomized trials comparing the patency of covered and uncovered self-expandable metal stents for palliation of distal malignant bile duct obstruction. Gastrointest Endosc. 2011;74:321–7. e1–3.
67. Almadi MA, Barkun AN, Martel M. No benefit of covered vs uncovered self-expandable metal stents in patients with malignant distal biliary obstruction: a meta-analysis. Clin Gastroenterol Hepatol. 2013;11:27–37. e1.
68. Bakken JC, Baron TH. Metal stents and biliary obstruction secondary to lymphoma: a tale of caution. Dig Dis Sci. 2010;55:3636.
69. Rerknimitr R, Angsuwatcharakon P, Ratanachu-ek T, et al. Asia-Pacific consensus recommendations for endoscopic and interventional management of hilar cholangiocarcinoma. J Gastroenterol Hepatol. 2013;28:593–607.
70. Kozarek RA. Malignant hilar strictures: one stent or two? Plastic versus self-expanding metal stents? The role of liver atrophy and volume assessment as a predictor of survival in patients undergoing endoscopic stent placement. Gastrointest Endosc. 2010;72:736–8.
71. De Palma G, Galloro G, Siciliano S, et al. Unilateral versus bilateral endoscopic hepatic duct drainage in patients with malignant hilar biliary obstruction: results of a prospective, randomized, and controlled study. Gastrointest Endosc. 2001;53:547–53.
72. Chang W, Kortan P, Haber G. Outcome in patients with bifurcation tumors who undergo unilateral versus bilateral hepatic duct drainage. Gastrointest Endosc. 1998;47:354–62.
73. Siddiqui A, Shahid H, Sarkar A, et al. Stage of hilar cholangiocarcinoma predicts recurrence of biliary obstruction in patients with metal stents. Clin Gastroenterol Hepatol. 2013;11: 1169–73.
74. Peters R, Williams S, Lombard M, et al. The management of high-grade hilar strictures by endoscopic insertion of self-expanding metal endoprostheses. Endoscopy. 1997;29:10–6.
75. Cheng J, Bruno M, Bergman J, et al. Endoscopic palliation of patients with biliary obstruction caused by nonresectable hilar cholangiocarcinoma: efficacy of self-expandable metallic Wallstents. Gastrointest Endosc. 2002;56:33–9.

76. Perdue D, Freeman M, Disario J, et al. The ERCP Outcome Study (ERCOST) group. Plastic versus self-expanding metallic stents for malignant hilar biliary obstruction: a prospective multicenter observational cohort study. J Clin Gastroenterol. 2008;42:1040–6.
77. Costamagna G, Tringali A, Petruzziello L, et al. Hilar tumours. Can J Gastroenterol. 2004; 18:451–4.
78. Gerges C, Schumacher B, Terheggen G, et al. Expandable metal stents for malignant hilar biliary obstruction. Gastrointest Endosc Clin N Am. 2011;21:481–97. ix.
79. Mukai T, Yasuda I, Nakashima M, et al. Metallic stents are more efficacious than plastic stents in unresectable malignant hilar biliary strictures: a randomized controlled trial. J Hepatobiliary Pancreat Sci. 2013;20:214–22.
80. Ortner M, Liebetruth J, Schreiber S, et al. Photodynamic therapy of nonresectable cholangiocarcinoma. Gastroenterology. 1998;114:536–42.
81. Wiedmann M, Berr F, Schiefke I, et al. Photodynamic therapy in patients with non-resectable hilar cholangiocarcinoma: 5-year follow-up of a prospective phase II study. Gastrointest Endosc. 2004;60:68–75.
82. Ortner M. Photodynamic therapy for cholangiocarcinoma. J Hepatobiliary Pancreat Surg. 2001;8:137–9.
83. Kahaleh M, Mishra R, Shami V, et al. Unresectable cholangiocarcinoma: comparison of survival in biliary stenting alone versus stenting with photodynamic therapy. Clin Gastroenterol Hepatol. 2008;6:290–7.
84. Baron T. Photodynamic therapy: standard of care for palliation of cholangiocarcinoma? Clin Gastroenterol Hepatol. 2008;6:266–7.
85. Wadsworth CA, Westaby D, Khan SA. Endoscopic radiofrequency ablation for cholangiocarcinoma. Curr Opin Gastroenterol. 2013;29:305–11.
86. Simmons DT, Baron TH, Petersen BT, et al. A novel endoscopic approach to brachytherapy in the management of Hilar cholangiocarcinoma. Am J Gastroenterol. 2006;101:1792–6.
87. Gluck M, Cantone N, Brandabur J, et al. A twenty-year experience with endoscopic therapy for symptomatic primary sclerosing cholangitis. J Clin Gastroenterol. 2008;42:1032–9.
88. McLoughlin M, Enns R. Endoscopy in the management of primary sclerosing cholangitis. Curr Gastroenterol Rep. 2008;10:177–85.
89. Charatcharoenwitthaya P, Enders F, Halling K, et al. Utility of serum tumor markers, imaging, and biliary cytology for detecting cholangiocarcinoma in primary sclerosing cholangitis. Hepatology. 2008;48:1106–17.
90. Tischendorf J, Krüger M, Trautwein C, et al. Cholangioscopic characterization of dominant bile duct stenoses in patients with primary sclerosing cholangitis. Endoscopy. 2006;38: 665–9.
91. Loeser CS, Robert ME, Mennone A, et al. Confocal endomicroscopic examination of malignant biliary strictures and histologic correlation with lymphatics. J Clin Gastroenterol. 2011;45:246–52.
92. Chahal P, Baron TH, Poterucha JJ, et al. Endoscopic retrograde cholangiography in post-orthotopic liver transplant population with Roux-en-Y biliary reconstruction. Liver Transpl. 2007;13:1168–73.
93. Saleem A, Baron TH, Gostout CJ, et al. Endoscopic retrograde cholangiopancreatography using a single-balloon enteroscope in patients with altered Roux-en-Y anatomy. Endoscopy. 2010;42:656–60.
94. Baron TH, Song LM, Ferreira LE, et al. Novel approach to therapeutic ERCP after long-limb Roux-en-Y gastric bypass surgery using transgastric self-expandable metal stents: experimental outcomes and first human case study (with videos). Gastrointest Endosc. 2012;75: 1258–63.
95. Saleem A, Levy MJ, Petersen BT, et al. Laparoscopic assisted ERCP in Roux-en-Y gastric bypass (RYGB) surgery patients. J Gastrointest Surg. 2012;16:203–8.
96. Abu Dayyeh BK, Baron TH. Development of a hybrid percutaneous-endoscopic approach for the complete clearance of gallstones. Clin Gastroenterol Hepatol. 2012;10:947–9.

97. Law R, Wong Kee Song LM, Petersen BT, et al. Single-session ERCP in patients with previous Roux-en-Y gastric bypass using percutaneous-assisted transprosthetic endoscopic therapy: a case series. Endoscopy. 2013;45:671–5.
98. Tse F, Barkun J, Romagnuolo J, et al. Nonoperative imaging techniques in suspected biliary tract obstruction. HPB (Oxford). 2006;8:409–25.
99. Ohshima Y, Yasuda I, Kawakami H, et al. EUS-FNA for suspected malignant biliary strictures after negative endoscopic transpapillary brush cytology and forceps biopsy. J Gastroenterol. 2011;46:921–8.
100. Levy MJ, Heimbach JK, Gores GJ. Endoscopic ultrasound staging of cholangiocarcinoma. Curr Opin Gastroenterol. 2012;28:244–52.
101. Gleeson F, Levy M. Endoscopic ultrasound (EUS) guided access and therapy of pancreatico-biliary disorders. Minerva Gastroenterol Dietol. 2008;54:151–60.
102. Khashab MA, Varadarajulu S. Endoscopic ultrasonography as a therapeutic modality. Curr Opin Gastroenterol. 2012;28:467–76.
103. Sarkaria S, Lee HS, Gaidhane M, et al. Advances in endoscopic ultrasound-guided biliary drainage: a comprehensive review. Gut Liver. 2013;7:129–36.
104. Shami V, Kahaleh M. Endoscopic ultrasonography (EUS)-guided access and therapy of pancreatico-biliary disorders: EUS-guided cholangio and pancreatic drainage. Gastrointest Endosc Clin N Am. 2007;17:581–93.
105. Ang T, Teo E, Fock K. EUS-guided transduodenal biliary drainage in unresectable pancreatic cancer with obstructive jaundice. JOP. 2007;8:438–43.
106. Kahaleh M, Hernandez A, Tokar J, et al. Interventional EUS-guided cholangiography: evaluation of a technique in evolution. Gastrointest Endosc. 2006;64:52–9.
107. Park do H. Endoscopic ultrasonography-guided hepaticogastrostomy. Gastrointest Endosc Clin N Am. 2012;22:271–80. ix.
108. Perez-Miranda M, Barclay RL, Kahaleh M. Endoscopic ultrasonography-guided endoscopic retrograde cholangiopancreatography: endosonographic cholangiopancreatography. Gastrointest Endosc Clin N Am. 2012;22:491–509.
109. Yamao K, Bhatia V, Mizuno N, et al. EUS-guided choledochoduodenostomy for palliative biliary drainage in patients with malignant biliary obstruction: results of long-term follow-up. Endoscopy. 2008;40:340–2.
110. Kahaleh M, Artifon EL, Perez-Miranda M, et al. Endoscopic ultrasonography guided biliary drainage: summary of consortium meeting, May 7th, 2011, Chicago. World J Gastroenterol. 2013;19:1372–9.
111. Gupta K, Perez-Miranda M, Kahaleh M, et al. Endoscopic ultrasound-assisted bile duct access and drainage: multicenter, long-term analysis of approach, outcomes, and complications of a technique in evolution. J Clin Gastroenterol. 2013;47(10):857–60.
112. Khashab MA, Fujii LL, Baron TH, et al. EUS-guided biliary drainage for patients with malignant biliary obstruction with an indwelling duodenal stent (with videos). Gastrointest Endosc. 2012;76:209–13.
113. Jang JW, Lee SS, Song TJ, et al. Endoscopic ultrasound-guided transmural and percutaneous transhepatic gallbladder drainage are comparable for acute cholecystitis. Gastroenterology. 2012;142:805–11.
114. Baron TH, Topazian MD. Endoscopic transduodenal drainage of the gallbladder: implications for endoluminal treatment of gallbladder disease. Gastrointest Endosc. 2007;65:735–7.
115. Noh SH, Park do H, Kim YR, et al. EUS-guided drainage of hepatic abscesses not accessible to percutaneous drainage (with videos). Gastrointest Endosc. 2010;71:1314–9.
116. Shami V, Talreja J, Mahajan A, et al. EUS-guided drainage of bilomas: a new alternative? Gastrointest Endosc. 2008;67:136–40.
117. Anderson MA, Fisher L, Jain R, et al. Complications of ERCP. Gastrointest Endosc. 2012;75:467–73.
118. Early DS, Acosta RD, Chandrasekhara V, et al. Adverse events associated with EUS and EUS with FNA. Gastrointest Endosc. 2013;77:839–43.

119. Balmadrid B, Kozarek R. Prevention and management of adverse events of endoscopic retrograde cholangiopancreatography. Gastrointest Endosc Clin N Am. 2013;23:385–403.
120. Ferreira L, Baron T. Post-sphincterotomy bleeding: who, what, when, and how. Am J Gastroenterol. 2007;102:2850–8.
121. Baron TH, Wong Kee Song LM, Zielinski MD, et al. A comprehensive approach to the management of acute endoscopic perforations (with videos). Gastrointest Endosc. 2012;76:838–59.
122. Kapral C, Duller C, Wewalka F, et al. Case volume and outcome of endoscopic retrograde cholangiopancreatography: results of a nationwide Austrian benchmarking project. Endoscopy. 2008;40:625–30.
123. Freeman M. Understanding risk factors and avoiding complications with endoscopic retrograde cholangiopancreatography. Curr Gastroenterol Rep. 2003;5:145–53.
124. Elta G. Temporary prophylactic pancreatic stents: which patients need them? Gastrointest Endosc. 2008;67:262–4.
125. Elmunzer BJ, Scheiman JM, Lehman GA, et al. A randomized trial of rectal indomethacin to prevent post-ERCP pancreatitis. N Engl J Med. 2012;366:1414–22.

Index

E.J. Carey and K.D. Lindor (eds.), *Cholestatic Liver Disease*, Clinical Gastroenterology,
DOI 10.1007/978-1-4939-1013-7, © Springer Science+Business Media New York 2014

D

MIX
Papier aus verantwortungsvollen Quellen
Paper from responsible sources
FSC® C105338

If you have any concerns about our products,
you can contact us on
ProductSafety@springernature.com

In case Publisher is established outside the EU,
the EU authorized representative is:
Springer Nature Customer Service Center GmbH
Europaplatz 3, 69115 Heidelberg, Germany

Printed by Libri Plureos GmbH
in Hamburg, Germany